Recent Results in Cancer Research 62

Fortschritte der Krebsforschung
Progrès dans les recherches sur le cancer

Edited by

V. G. Allfrey, New York · M. Allgöwer, Basel
K. H. Bauer, Heidelberg · I. Berenblum, Rehovoth
F. Bergel, Jersey · J. Bernard, Paris · W. Bernhard,
Villejuif · N. N. Blokhin, Moskva · H. E. Bocke,
Tübingen · W. Braun, New Brunswick · P. Bucalossi,
Milano · A. V. Chaklin, Moskva · M. Chorazy,
Gliwice · G. J. Cunningham, Richmond
G. Della Porta, Milano · P. Denoix, Villejuif
R. Dulbecco, La Jolla · H. Eagle, New York
R. Eker, Oslo · R. A. Good, New York
P. Grabar, Paris · R. J. C. Harris, Salisbury
E. Hecker, Heidelberg · R. Herbeuval, Vandocuvre
J. Higginson, Lyon · W. C. Hueper, Fort Myers
H. Isliker, Lausanne · J. Kieler, Kobenhavn
W. H. Kirsten, Chicago · G. Klein, Stockholm
H. Koprowski, Philadelphia · L. G. Koss, New York
G. Martz, Zürich · G. Mathé, Villejuif
O. Mühlbock, Amsterdam · W. Nakahara, Tokyo
L. J. Old, New York · V. R. Potter, Madison
A. B. Sabin, Charleston, S.C. · L. Sachs, Rehovoth
E. A. Saxén, Helsinki · C. G. Schmidt, Essen
S. Spiegelman, New York · W. Szybalski, Madison
H. Tagnon, Bruxelles · R. M. Taylor, Toronto
A. Tissières, Genève · E. Uehlinger, Zürich
R. W. Wissler, Chicago

Editor in Chief: P. Rentchnick, Genève

Tactics and Strategy in Cancer Treatment

Edited by Georges Mathé

With 75 Figures

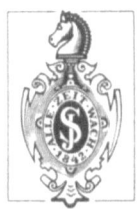

Springer-Verlag
Berlin Heidelberg New York 1977

EORTC-Symposium. Held in Paris on June 24/25, 1976

Professor GEORGES MATHÉ
Institut de Cancérologie et d'Immunogénétique
(INSERM), Hôpital Paul-Brousse, 14 – 16 Ave.
Paul-Vaillant Couturier and Institut Gustave-Roussy,
16 bis Ave. Paul-Vaillant Couturier,
94800 Villejuif (France)

Sponsored by the Swiss League against Cancer

ISBN 978-3-642-81176-0   ISBN 978-3-642-81174-6 (eBook)
DOI 10.1007/978-3-642-81174-6

Library of Congress Cataloging in Publication Data. European Organization for
Research on Treatment of Cancer. Tactics and strategy in cancer treatment. (Recent
results in cancer research; 62). Proceedings of the annual general meeting of the
EORTC, which was held in Paris in June 1976, and sponsored by the Swiss League
against Cancer. Bibliography: p. Includes index. 1. Cancer-Congresses. I. Mathé,
Georges, 1922–   . II. Schweizerische Nationalliga für Krebsbekämpfung und
Krebsforschung. III. Title. IV. Series.
RC261.R35 vol. 62 [RC270.8]   616.9′94′008s   [616.9′94′06]   77-21315

© by Springer-Verlag Berlin · Heidelberg 1977
Softcover reprint of the hardcover 1st edition 1977

Typesetting: William Clowes & Sons Limited, London, Beccles and Colchester/
England.

2125/3140-543210

Preface

Tactics is the art of combining the action of troops or the proper means of different arms with the object of obtaining the maximum success at combat.

Strategy is the art of combining the action of all the military forces with a view to victory.

This work, which publishes the communications at the Annual General Meeting of the EORTC, which was held in Paris in June 1976, was devoted to tactics and to the therapeutic strategy with a view to the recovery of cancer patients.

Table of Contents

II. General Strategy

List of Contributors

M. Abbes, Centre Antoine Lacassagne, 36, avenue de la Voie Romaine, F-06000 Nice.

J. L. Amiel, Service d'Hématologie de l'Institut Gustave-Roussy, 16 bis, avenue Paul-Vaillant-Couturier, F-94800 Villejuif.

K. D. Bagshawe, Department of Medical Oncology, Charing Cross Hospital (Fulham), Fulham Palace Road, London W6 8RF/U.K.

A. Baron, Centre Médico-Chirurgical de Bligny, F-91640 Briis-sous-Forges.

J. G. Bekesi, Department of Neoplastic Diseases, Mount Sinai School of Medicine, and Hospital of the City University of New York, New York, N.Y. 10029/USA.

D. Belpomme, Institut de Cancérologie et d'Immunogénétique, Hôpital Paul-Brousse, et Service d'Hématologie de l'Institut Gustave-Roussy, 14–16, avenue Paul-Vaillant-Couturier, F-94800 Villejuif.

M. Benoit, Hôpital Bichat, 170, boulevard Ney, F-75018 Paris.

R. Berthier, Groupe Hospitalier des Affections Sanguines et Tumorales, Centre Hospitalier Régional et Universitaire de Grenoble, F-38700 La Tronche.

G. R. Blumenschein, Departments of Developmental Therapeutics and Medicine, The University of Texas System Cancer Center, M. D. Anderson Hospital and Tumor Institut, 6723 Bertner Avenue, Houston, Tex. 77030/USA.

G. Bonadonna, Istituto Nazionale Tumori, Via Venezian 1, I-Milan.

C. Bourut, Institut de Cancérologie et d'Immunogénétique, Hôpital Paul-Brousse, 14–16, avenue Paul-Vaillant-Couturier, F-94800 Villejuif.

G. Brule, Department of Cancer Therapy, Unité La Grange, Institut Gustave-Roussy, F-77176 Savigny-le-Temple.

M. Bruley-Rosset, Institut de Cancérologie et d'Immunogénétique, Hôpital Paul-Brousse, 14–16, avenue Paul-Vaillant-Couturier, F-94800 Villejuif.

M. A. Burgess, Departments of Developmental Therapeutics and Medicine, The University of Texas System Cancer Center, M. D. Anderson Hospital and Tumor Institute, 6723 Bertner Avenue, Houston, Tex. 77030/USA.

A. Buzdar, Departments of Developmental Therapeutics and Medicine, The University of Texas System Cancer Center, M. D. Anderson Hospital and Tumor Institute, 6723 Bertner Avenue, Houston, Tex. 77030/USA.

Y. Cachin, Département de Chirurgie Cervico-Faciale et O.R.L., Institut Gustave-Roussy, 16 bis, avenue Paul-Vaillant-Couturier, F-94800 Villejuif.

P. P. CARBONE, Division of Clinical Oncology, Department of Human Oncology and Department of Medicine, University of Wisconsin, Madison, Wis. 53706/USA.

S. K. CARTER, Northern California Cancer Program, 1801 Page Mill Road, Suite 200, Bldg. B, Palo Alto, Cal. 94304/USA.

A. CATTAN, Institut Jean Godinot, 45, rue Cognacq-Jay, F-51000 Reims.

J. CHAUVERGNE, Fondation Bergonié, 180, rue de Saint-Genès, F-33076 Bordeaux Cédex.

Y. COHEN, Department of Oncology, Rambam Medical Center, Aba Khoushi School of Medicine, The Technion, Haifa/Israel.

E. H. COOPER, The University of Leeds, Department of Experimental Pathology and Cancer Research, School of Medicine, Leeds LS2 9NL/U.K.

M. DANA, Hôpital Américain de Neuilly, 63, boulevard Victor-Hugo, F-92202 Neuilly-sur-Seine.

A. J. S. DAVIES, Chester Beatty Research Institute, Institute of Cancer Research, Royal Cancer Hospital, Fulham Road, London SW3 6JB/U.K.

G. DECROIX, Service de Pneumologie, Université Pierre et Marie Curie, Centre Hospitalier Universitaire Saint-Antoine, 184, rue de Faubourg Saint-Antoine, F-75571 Paris Cédex 12.

M. DELGADO, Institut de Cancérologie et d'Immunogénétique, Unité Fred-Siguier de l'Hôpital Paul-Brousse et Service d'Hématologie de l'Institut Gustave-Roussy, 14–16, avenue Paul-Vaillant-Couturier, F-94800 Villejuif.

F. DE VASSAL, Institut de Cancérologie et d'Immunogénétique, Unité Fred-Siguier de l'Hôpital Paul-Brousse et Service d'Hématologie de l'Institut Gustave-Roussy, 14–16, avenue Paul-Vaillant-Couturier, F-94800 Villejuif.

V. DJUROVIC, Laboratoire d'Immunothérapie du Cancer, Service de Pneumologie, Hôpital Saint-Antoine, 184, rue du Faubourg Saint-Antoine, F-75571 Paris Cédex 12.

G. DUTRANOY, Hôpital de la Pitié, 47, boulevard de l'Hôpital, F-75013 Paris.

F. ECONOMIDES, Institut de Cancérologie et d'Immunogénétique, Hôpital Paul-Brousse, 14–16, avenue Paul-Vaillant-Couturier, F-94800 Villejuif.

K. FELLOWS, Children's Hospital Medical Center, Sidney Farber Cancer Institute and Harvard Medical School, Boston, Mass/USA.

E. FREI, III, Children's Hospital Medical Center, Sidney Farber Cancer Institute and Harvard Medical School, Boston, Mass/USA.

H. GAUTIER, Centre Médico-Chirurgical de Bligny, F-91640 Briis-sous-Forges.

R. GENSER, Centre Hospitalier de Sarreguemines, F-57200 Sarreguemines.

M. A. GIL, Service d'Hématologie de l'Institut Gustave-Roussy, 16, avenue Paul-Vaillant-Couturier, F-94800 Villejuif.

J. U. GUTTERMAN, Department of Developmental Therapeutics, The University of Texas System Cancer Center, M. D. Anderson Hospital and Tumor Institute, 6723 Bertner Avenue, Houston, Tex. 77030/USA.

O. HALLE-PANNENKO, Institut de Cancérologie et d'Immunogénétique, Hôpital Paul-Brousse, 16, avenue Paul-Vaillant-Couturier, F-94800 Villejuif.

M. HAYAT, Institut de Cancérologie et d'Immunogénétique, Hôpital Paul-Brousse et Service d'Hématologie de l'Institut Gustave-Roussy, 16, avenue Paul-Vaillant-Couturier, F-94800 Villejuif.

E. M. HERSH, Department of Developmental Therapeutics. The University of Texas System Cancer Center, M. D. Anderson Hospital and Tumor Institute, 6723 Bertner Avenue, Houston, Tex. 77030/USA.

B. HOERNI, Fondation Bergonié, 180, rue Saint-Genès, F-33076 Bordeaux Cédex.

J. F. HOLLAND, Department of Neoplastic Diseases, Mount Sinai School of Medicine and Hospital of the City University of New York, New York, N.Y. 10029/USA.

D. HOLLARD, Groupe Hospitalier des Affections Sanguines et Tumorales, Centre Hospitalier Régional et Universitaire de Grenoble, F-38700 La Tronche.

G. N. HORTOBAGYI, Department of Developmental Therapeutics and Medicine, The University of Texas System Cancer Center, M. D. Anderson Hospital and Tumor Institute, 6723 Bertner Avenue, Houston, Tex. 77030/USA.

P. HUGUENIN, Centre Médico-Chirurgical de Bligny, F-91640 Briis-sous-Forges.

N. JAFFE, Children's Hospital Medical Center, Sidney Farber Cancer Institute, and Harvard Medical School, 44 Binney Street, Boston, Mass. 02115/USA.

B. JAMAIN, Hôpital Bichat, 170, boulevard Ney, F-75018 Paris.

C. JASMIN, Institut de Cancérologie et d'Immunogénétique, Hôpital Paul-Brousse, et Service d'Hématologie de l'Institut Gustave-Roussy, 16, avenue Paul-Vaillant-Couturier, F-94800 Villejuif.

B. KELLER, Hôpital de Strasbourg, 1, place de l'Hôpital, F-67000 Strasbourg.

H. O. KLEIN, Medical Clinic, University of Cologne, Josef-Stelzmann-Strasse 9, D-5000 Cologne 41.

C. LAGARDE, Fondation Bergonié, 180, rue Saint-Genès, F-33076 Bordeaux Cédex.

I. LANSAC, Centre Hospitalier Régional et Universitaire Bretonneau, F-37033 Tours Cédex.

H. LE BRIGAND, Centre Chirurgical Marie-Lannelongue, 133 Avenue de la Resistance, F-92350 Le Plessis Robinson.

J. LEMERLE, Pediatric Oncology Department, Institut Gustave-Roussy, 16 bis, avenue Paul-Vaillant-Couturier, F-94800 Villejuif.

G. LE LORIER, Hôpital Rothschild, 43, boulevard de Picpus, F-75012 Paris.

A. LETESSIER, Hôpital Bichat, 170, boulevard Ney, F-75018 Paris.

P. LEVASSEUR, Centre Chirurgical Marie-Lannelongue, 133 Avenue de la Resistance, F-92350 Le Plessis Robinson.

J. LHERITIER, Institut de Cancérologie et d'Immunogénétique, Hôpital Paul-Brousse, 16, avenue Paul-Vaillant-Couturier, F-94800 Villejuif.

D. MACHOVER, Institut de Cancérologie et d'Immunogénétique, Unité Fred-Siguier de l'Hôpital Paul-Brousse, et Service d'Hématologie de l'Institut Gustave-Roussy, 16, avenue Paul-Vaillant-Couturier, F-94800 Villejuif.

J. S. MALPAS, Imperial Cancer Research Fund, St Bartholomew's Hospital, West Smithfield, London EC1A 7BE/U.K.

G. MATHÉ, Institut de Cancérologie et d'Immunogénétique, Hôpital Paul-Brousse, et Service d'Hématologie de l'Institut Gustave-Roussy, 14–16, avenue Paul-Vaillant-Couturier, F-94800 Villejuif.

R. MAURUS, Service de Pédiatrie, Hôpital Universitaire Saint-Pierre, 320, rue Haute, B-1000 Brussels.

M. MERLIER, Centre Chirurgical Marie-Lannelongue, 133 Avenue de la Resistance, F-92350 Le Plessis Robinson.

J. L. MISSET, Institut de Cancérologie et d'Immunogénétique, Unité Fred-Siguier de l'Hôpital Paul-Brousse, et Service d'Hématologie de l'Institut Gustave-Roussy, 16, avenue Paul-Vaillant-Couturier, F-94800 Villejuif.

P. MORIN, Centre Médico-Chirurgical de Bligny, F-91640 Briis-sous-Forges.

M. MUSSET, Unité Fred-Siguier de l'Hôpital Paul-Brousse, et Service d'hématologie de l'Institut Gustave-Roussy, 16, avenue Paul-Vaillant-Couturier, F-94800 Villejuif.

L. OLSSON, Department of Tumor Virology, Institute of Medical Microbiology, University of Copenhagen, 30, Juliane Mariesvej, DK-2100 Copenhagen.

T. PALANGIE, Institut de Cancérologie et d'Immunogénétique, Hôpital Paul-Brousse, 16, avenue Paul-Vaillant-Couturier, F-94800 Villejuif.

R. PARROT, Centre Médico-Chirurgical de Bligny, F-91640 Briis-sous-Forges.

J. PENA-ANGULO, Institut de Cancérologie et d'Immunogénétique, et Service d'Hémato-logie de l'Institut Gustave-Roussy, 16, avenue Paul-Vaillant-Couturier, F-94800 Villejuif.

L. PIANA, Clinique Obstétrique et Gynécologique de Marseille, Hôpital de la Conception, 144, rue Saint-Pierre, F-13005 Marseille.

J. L. PICO, Institut de Cancérologie et d'Immunogénétique, Unité Fred-Siguier de l'Hôpital Paul-Brousse, et Service d'Hématologie de l'Institut Gustave-Roussy, 16, avenue Paul-Vaillant-Couturier, F-94800 Villejuif.

J. M. PIQUET, Hôpital Rothschild, 43, boulevard de Picpus, F-75012 Paris.

M. POISSON, Centre Médico-Chirurgical de Bligny, F-91640 Briis-sous-Forges.

P. POUILLART, Institut de Cancérologie et d'Immunogénétique, Hôpital Paul-Brousse, 16, avenue Paul-Vaillant Couturier, F-94800 Villejuif.

L. H. REES, Department of Chemical Pathology, St. Bartholomew's Hospital, London EC1A 8BE/U.K.

S. P. RICHMAN, Department of Developmental Therapeutics, The University of Texas System Cancer Center, M. D. Anderson Hospital and Tumor Institute, 6723 Bertner Avenue, Houston, Tex. 77030/USA.

H. G. ROBERT, Hôpital de la Pitié, 47, boulevard de l'Hôpital, F-75013 Paris.

E. ROBINSON, Department of Oncology, Rambam Medical Center, Aba Khoushi School of Medicine, The Technion, Haifa/Israel.

A. ROJAS-MIRANDA, Centre Chirurgical Marie-Lannelongue, 133 Avenue de la Resistance, F-92350 Le Plessis Robinson.

C. ROSENFELD, Institut de Cancérologie et d'Immunogénétique, Hôpital Paul-Brousse, 14–16, avenue Paul-Vaillant-Couturier, F-94800 Villejuif.

A. Rossi, Istituto Nazionale Tumori, Via Venezian 1, I-20133 Milan.

J. Salat-Baroux, Hôpital Rothschild, 43, boulevard de Picpus, F-75012 Paris.

M. Schneider, Centre Antoine Lacassagne, 36, avenue de la Voie Romaine, F-06000 Nice.

M. Schwarz, Department of Developmental Therapeutics, The University of Texas System Cancer Center, M. D. Anderson Hospital and Tumor Institute, 6723 Bertner Avenue, Houston, Tex. 77030/USA.

L. Schwarzenberg, Institut de Cancérologie et d'Immunogénétique, Hôpital Paul-Brousse, 16, avenue Paul-Vaillant-Couturier, F-94800 Villejuif.

H. Serment, Clinique Obstétricale et Gynécologique de Marseille, Hôpital de la Conception, 144, rue Saint-Pierre, F-13005 Marseille.

P. H. Smith, Department of Urology, St James' University Hospital, Beckett Street, Leeds LS9 7TF/U.K.

J. J. Sotto, Groupe Hospitalier des Affections Sanguines et Tumorales, Centre Hospitalier Régional et Universitaire de Grenoble, F-38700 La Tronche.

J. H. Soutoul, Centre Hospitalier Régional et Universitaire Bretonneau, F-37033 Tours Cédex.

J. Stjernswärd, Ludwig Institute for Cancer Research, Lausanne Branch, CH-1066 Epalinges and Department of Radiotherapy, Cantonal University Hospital, Lausanne/Switzerland.

C. K. Tashima, Department Medicine, The University of Texas System Cancer Center, M. D. Anderson Hospital and Tumor Institute, 6723 Bertner Avenue, Houston, Tex. 77030/USA.

D. Traggis, Children's Hospital Medical Center, Sidney Farber Cancer Institute and Harvard Medical School, Boston, Mass/USA.

P. Valagussa, Istituto Nazionale Tumori, Via Venezian 1, I-20133 Milan.

G. Vawter, Children's Hospital Medical Center, Sidney Farber Cancer Institute and Harvard Medical School, Boston, Mass/USA.

U. Veronesi, Istituto Nazionale Tumori, Via Venezian 1, I-20133 Milan.

C. Wapler, Centre Chirurgical Marie-Lannelongue, 133 Avenue de la Resistance, F-92350 Le Plessis Robinson.

H. Watts, Children's Hospital Medical Center, Sidney Farber Cancer Institute, and Harvard Medical School, Boston, Mass/USA.

R. Weiner, Division of Medical Oncology, University of Florida, Gainesville, Fl./USA.

J. A. Whittaker, Department of Haematology, University Hospital of Wales and Welsh National School of Medicine, Heath Park, Cardiff, CF4 4XW/U.K.

G. Zographos, Service de Gynécologie, 124, Cours Lieutaud, F-13006 Marseille.

B. Zylberberg, Hôpital Bichat, 170, boulevard Ney, F-75018, Paris and Hôpital Rothschild, 43, boulevard de Picpus, F-75012 Paris.

I. Tactics

Tactics in Cancer Treatment: Introduction

G. MATHÉ

Four weapons are now available for the treatment of the various cancers: surgery, radiotherapy, chemotherapy, and immunotherapy. However competent the oncologist is, he can never be sure of using these weapons to their best advantage for each patient.
Immunotherapy [1] is still in its infancy; clinical data are very few, but experimental results, on the other hand, are so numerous that the clinical immunotherapist should check that he is aware of them all before establishing a protocol.
Chemotherapy [2] is older, and the progress of the last 10 years has been in improving the operational use of each drug and drug combinations rather than in multiplying the number of agents. But progress in chemotherapy is far from finished, and all serious chemo-therapists are conscious that their patients have much to gain from a more scientific application of oncostatics.
Radiotherapy [3] has also seen considerable progress with the acquisition of high-energy radiations and their improved usage, but side effects are still considerable even though this is a local therapy.
Surgery [4], the oldest form of cancer therapy, is the one which is least based on scientific data, hence the numerous contradictory surgical practices; some surgeons systematically remove the regional lymph nodes in stage I melanoma, and others no less systematically do not. Hence the need for research in this field in order to develop a methodology as scientific as that in the fields of the other cancer weapons.
It is the object of the first part of this meeting to consider some of the tactical problems of cancer treatment.

References

1. MATHÉ, G.: Cancer active immunotherapy: immunoprophylaxis and immunorestoration. An introduction. Heidelberg-New York: Springer-Verlag, 1976.
2. CLARYSSE, A., KENIS, Y., MATHÉ, G.: Cancer chemotherapy: its role in the treatment strategy of hematologic malignancies and solid tumors. Heidelberg-New York: Springer Verlag, 1976.
3. TUBIANA, M., DUTREIX, J., DUTREIX, A., JOCQUEY, P.: Bases physiques de la radiothérapie et de la radiobiologie. Paris: Masson et Cie, 1963.
4. SAEGESSER, F., PETTAVEL, J.: Oncologie chirurgicale. Paris: Masson et Cie, 1971.

1. Surgery

Effects of the Removal of the Regional Lymph Nodes on the Survival of Mice Bearing B16 Melanoma or EAkR Lymphosarcoma

F. ECONOMIDES and M. BRULEY-ROSSET

Summary

This work presents data concerning the effect of tumor excision accompanied or not by the removal of the regional lymph node (RLN) on the survival time of mice bearing the EAkR lymphosarcoma or the B16 melanoma. The operations were performed at various times to study this effect in relation to tumor size.

Early tumorectomy, on day 6 for the EAkR lymphosarcoma, on day 10 for the B16 melanoma, significantly prolonged the survival time. The additional removal of the RLN abolished this beneficial effect. In the case of the EAkR lymphosarcoma, a beneficial effect on the survival time was, in contrast, observed after total excision of the tumor accompanied by RLN removal performed on day 8. The two surgical procedures were ineffective in increasing the survival time when they were applied after the 8th day for the EAkR lymphosarcoma and after the 10th day for the B16 melanoma.

These results suggest that the preservation of the RLN may be favorable for the host, at least at an early stage of the tumor growth.

Introduction

An important dilemma facing the clinical oncologist is whether or not the regional lymph node (RLN) should be routinely removed in cancer patients. The RLN in neoplastic disease has been considered to play an important role, both mechanic and immunologic, in the tumor-bearing host. It has been shown [5, 3, 4], however, that the node is much less effective as a filter or a trap for tumor cells than as the site of the initial recognition of tumor antigens. Concerning the effect of the ablation of the RLN on tumor development, CRILE [2] claims the immunologic disadvantage of the procedure, particularly if performed at an early stage of the disease when the host still bears a tumor of limited volume.

This study was undertaken to show the effect of the removal of the RLN together with the major tumor mass on the survival of tumor-bearing mice; surgery was performed at various times so that this effect could be studied in relation to tumor volume.

Materials and Methods

Inbred female C57Bl/6 and (C57Bl/6 × DBA/2)F1 mice of 8–10 weeks of age were purchased from Iffa Credo Laboratories and were grafted with either EAkR lymphosarcoma or B16 melanoma. The EAkR lymphosarcoma was induced in C57Bl/6 mice by injecting leukemic cells obtained from AkR mice in which leukemia grew spontaneously. The tumor was kept in ascitic form by weekly intraperitoneal inoculations of 5×10^6 cells. For our study, the (C57Bl/6 $\times$ DBA/2)F1 mice were used in which subcutaneous injections of the leukemic cells into the right inguinal area resulted in solid tumor growth.

B16 melanoma which arose spontaneously in C57Bl/6 mice was maintained by subcutaneous injections of 10^6 tumor cells into the same site as above.

Tumor Challenge

Preliminary studies were done to determine the minimal dose of tumor cells required to kill 100% of the animals. This was found to be 5×10^6 cells/mouse for the EAkR lymphosarcoma injected s.c. and 10^6 cells/mouse for the B16 melanoma (Figs. 1 and 3). A single cell suspension was obtained from the latter by removing a part of the main mass taking care to avoid every necrotic or hemorrhagic area. The viable part was minced and rinsed in Hank's balanced salt solution. Viability evaluated by trypan blue exclusion was about 40%. The median survival time was determined and results were expressed in mortality. The chi square (X^2) and the nonparametric Wilcoxon tests were used in the melanoma and lymphosarcoma cases respectively in order to evaluate significance of results yielded by the control and experimental groups.

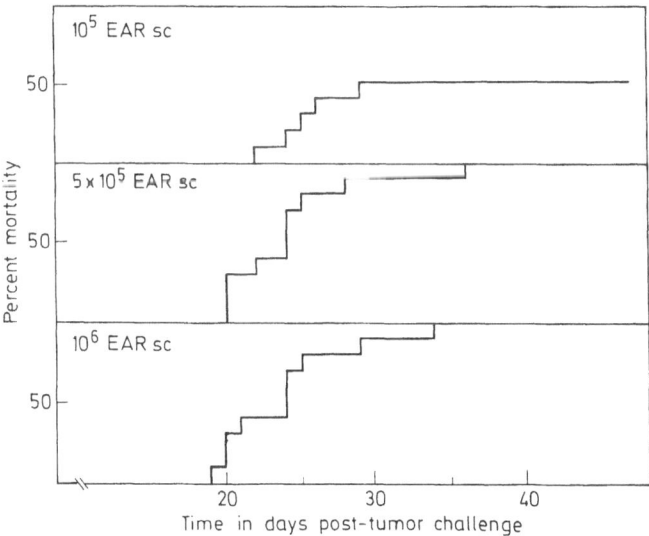

Fig. 1. Mortality of (C57Bl/6 $\times$ DBA/2)F1 mice in relation to the number of inoculated EAkR cells

Surgery

Two surgical procedures were performed (1) tumorectomy of the visible mass and (2) tumorectomy plus excision of the RLN.

Operations were done using both modalities at day 6, 8, and 10 after inoculation of the EAkR lymphosarcoma and at day 10, 14, and 18 on the melanoma-bearing mice. The nodes were sent soon after excision for histologic examination.

Results

EAkR Lymphosarcoma

Fig. 1 shows the mortality of mice in relation to the number of inoculated cells. When 10^5 cells were injected subcutaneously, 50% of the mice died of progressive tumor growth, the others remaining free of disease. When 5×10^5 and 10^6 cells were given subcutaneously, all mice died within 35 days. Since no difference was observed between the two last groups, a dose of 5×10^5 cells per mouse was chosen for the experiments to follow. All animals treated with surgery developed progressively growing tumor nodules at the same site and died. The operation failed to cure the animals because lymph node metastases were already present. Results presented in Fig. 2 show that surgery on day 6 significantly prolonged the survival of the group submitted to tumorectomy alone ($p < 0.02$), as compared with the control group, contrary to the group in which additional removal of the node was performed. No significant difference in the survival of those mice over the control was observed. The lymph nodes on day 6 were not palpable on examination before excision, but histologically, the first signs of infiltration could be seen.

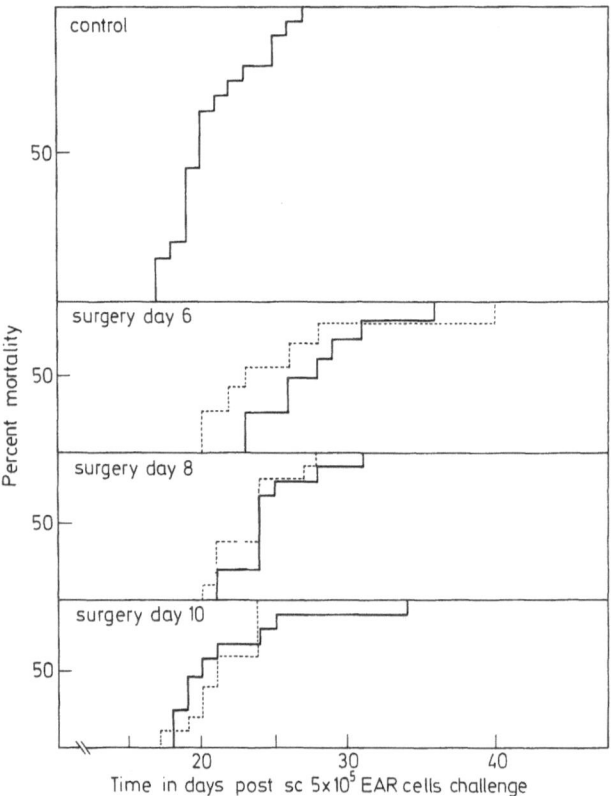

Fig. 2. Mortality of (C57Bl/6 × DBA/2)F1 mice bearing EAkR lymphosarcoma after surgery performed on days 6, 8, and 10, using two operational modalities: tumorectomy alone (————) and tumorectomy plus RLN excision (. . . .)

On the other hand, surgery on day 8 was beneficial no matter whether the lymph node was preserved or not ($p < 0.01$). When it was performed on the 10th day, however, no significant prolongation of survival was seen.

At histologic examination of the RLN, the cortical sinus was found to be infiltrated with tumor cells on day 8 and the germinal center full of macrophages. In the groups on which no surgery was performed, metastases in the contralateral inguinal nodes were detected; this was not found in the operated mice.

B16 Melanoma

Fig. 3 presents the survival of mice after inoculation of different doses of tumor cells. Since this tumor spread largely, the surgical intervention was only able to reduce the tumor mass whatever the time of the operation was: the 10th, 14th, or 18th day after inoculation. Simple tumor resection on day 10 yielded a significant result in survival ($p < 0.05$), but not the additional removal of the inguinal node. Surgery on days 14 and 18 made no difference in survival between the groups submitted to the two surgical modalities although the rate of death was slower for animals which underwent simple tumorectomy on day 18 (Fig. 4).

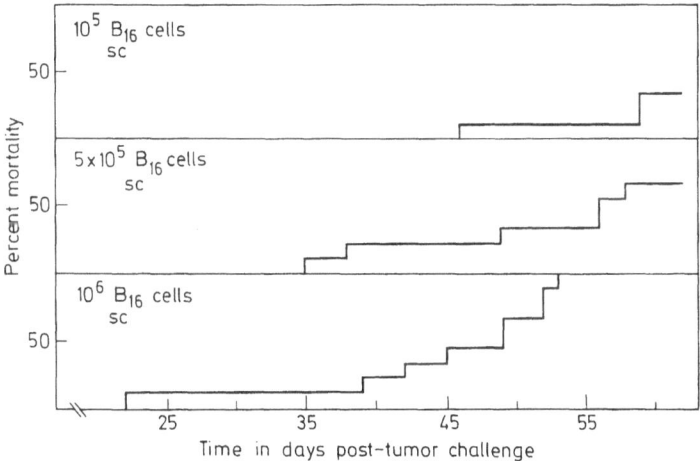

Fig. 3. Mortality of C57Bl/6 mice in relation to the number of inoculated B16 melanoma cells

Discussion

From the above-mentioned experiments, we could conclude that for both models removal of the regional lymph node together with the main tumor mass appeared to be disadvantageous for the animals when the primary tumor was small, that is, when surgery was performed on day 6 for EAkR lymphosarcoma and day 10 for B16 melanoma. This is in accordance with the findings of FIDLER et al. and CRILE who claim that the RLN may be important in the early stage of the disease whereas at a later stage, it could be removed without reducing the benefit of surgery.

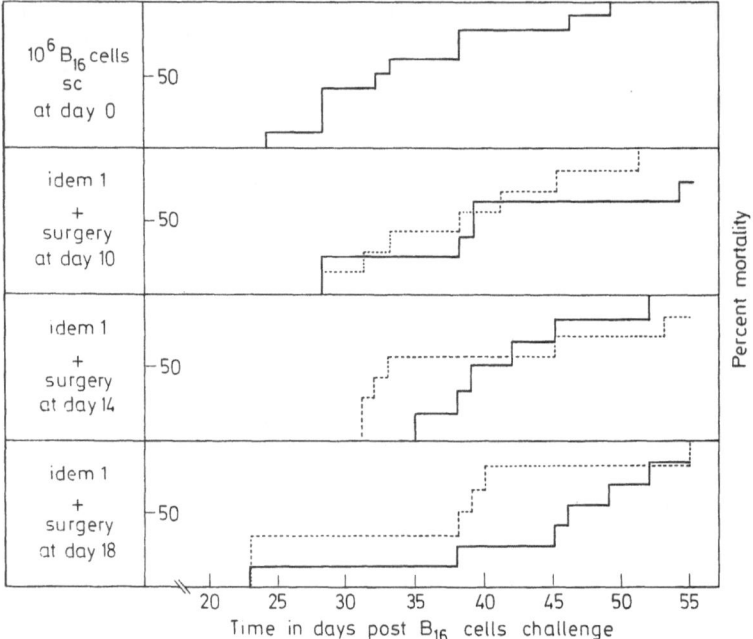

Fig. 4. Mortality of C57Bl/6 mice bearing the B16 melanoma following surgery performed on days 10, 14, and 18 after tumor inoculation.
(————) tumorectomy alone
(. . . .) tumorectomy plus RLN excision

The concept of the role of the RLN in the "defense" mechanism of the host as a relay for transfer of the information of the initial recognition of the tumor antigens to further immunologic centers has been postulated by GOLDFARB and HARDY [5] and MITCHISON [6]. The latter was able to transfer tumor immunity by transplanting the RLN to another animal whereas transplantation of the contralateral LN or spleen cells did not bring about the same effect.

According to GOLDFARB and HARDY [5], the initial response of the RLN occurred when tumor nodules were first palpable, the day of maximal response depending upon the inoculum dose of tumor cells. These authors have also shown that the immunologic activity of the RLN in a C3H mammary adenocarcinoma reached its maximum on day 7 and in other distant nodes on day 14.

In our experiments with the EAkR lymphosarcoma, the tumor on the 6th day after inoculation was either not palpable or had a diameter of up to 5 mm of length. On the 8th day, the length was 5–10 mm. This implies that the reaction of the node may already begin even before the tumor is palpated. The effect of tumorectomy was not modified by simultaneous excision of the RLN later in the course of the disease in our two models. This might be due to the fact that these infiltrated nodes are no longer important to systemic immunity and to the host's defensive mechanism [3], although in the case of B16 melanoma our preliminary results seemed to suggest that preservation of the lymph node retards the death rate of the animals.

Another experimental model [1] reports the increased incidence and extent of pulmonary metastases when the regional lymph nodes were removed in early surgical treatment whereas later they were no longer affected by this procedure.

More experiments on different models would be required before a definite conclusion is drawn and even extrapolated to man which is not to be decided at the moment.

References

1. CRILE, G.: The effect on metastasis of removing or irradiating regional lymph nodes of mice. Surg. Gynec. Obstet. *126*, 1272 (1968).
2. CRILE, G.: Possible role of uninvolved regional nodes in preventing metastasis from breast cancer. Cancer *24*, 1283 (1969).
3. FIDLER, I. J., McWILLIAMS, R. W., NIELSEN, S. B., BUDMEN, M. B.: Role of the regional lymph node in neoplasia: cellular mediated reactivity in vitro by autologous regional and distant lymph nodes or peripheral blood lymphocytes of dogs with spontaneous neoplasms. Immunol. Comm. *4*, 325 (1975).
4. FISHER, B., FISHER, E. R.: Barrier function of lymph node to tumor cells and erythrocytes. I and II. Cancer *20*, 1914 (1967).
5. GOLDFARB, P. M., HARDY, M. A.: The immunologic responsiveness of regional lymphocytes in experimental cancer. Cancer *35*, 778 (1975).
6. MITCHISON, N. A.: Passive transfer of transplantation immunity. Proc. Roy. Soc. (B) *142*, 72 (1954).

Regional Lymph Node Dissection in Melanoma of the Limbs Stage I — A Cooperative International Trial (WHO Collaborating Centers for diagnosis and treatment of melanoma)

U. VERONESI

From September 1967 to January 1974, a clinical trial was carried out by the W.H.O. Collaborating Centres for the Evaluation of Methods of Diagnosis and Treatment of Melanoma to evaluate the efficacy of elective node dissection in the treatment of malignant melanoma of the extremities with clinically uninvolved regional lymph nodes. Seventeen institutes from 12 countries participated in the trial; 553 cases were involved. Cases classified as $T_{1-2-3}N_0M_0$ only, not more than 5 cm in their largest dimension, and without fixation to the fascia were included. Only cases which had never been treated or in which the previous treatment consisted in excisional biopsy of the primary tumor less than 4 weeks before admission to the trial were included. Patients were randomized into two groups. 1) those to be submitted to excision of primary melanoma and simultaneous regional dissection, 2) those to be submitted to excision of primary melanoma and regional node dissection at the time of appearance of metastases. Only cases with adequate histologic diagnosis were included in the trial. In all cases, the original diagnosis made by the local pathologist was reviewed by a panel of five pathologists. Of the cases of malignant melanoma of the limbs classified as $T_{1-2-3}N_0M_0$, 490 were untreated and 63 had undergone limited excision of the primary melanoma less than 4 weeks before definitive treatment; 103 were males and 450 were females. Excision plus elective node dissection was performed in 267 patients, and excision of the primary melanoma was performed in 286. Regardless of how the data were analyzed (by sex, site of origin, maximum diameter of primary, Clark's level, or Breslow's thickness), no differences in survival were found in the two series. The incidence of regional node metastases was evaluated in 395 cases followed up for at least 5 years. Occult node metastases were observed in 38 (19.7%) out of 193 cases submitted to elective node dissection; out of 202 cases submitted to excision only of primary melanoma, 49 (24.2%) developed regional metastases during the follow-up period. The statistical analysis showed no difference in survival between these two subgroups of patients.

Data yielded by this clinical trial show that immediate node dissection does not improve the prognosis of malignant melanoma of the limbs. The survival curves of cases submitted to excision of primary melanoma followed by a regional lymph node dissection at the time of appearance of node metastases and of cases submitted to excision and elective regional node dissection, are identical. Elective node dissection failed to improve the prognosis no matter how the figures were analyzed. Moreover, the rate of local recurrences and "in transit" metastases was not different for the two groups.

It can be concluded that elective node dissection in malignant melanoma of the limbs is not warranted as long as the patient can be kept under strict clinical control.

2. Chemotherapy

Effectiveness of Murine Leukemia Chemotherapy According to the Immune State: Reconsideration of Correlations Between Chemotherapy, Tumour Cell Killing, and Survival Time

G. Mathé, O. Halle-Pannenko, and C. Bourut

Summary

Cyclophosphamide (CPM) chemotherapy (134 mg/kg) of L1210 leukemia is less efficient in mice previously immunodepressed by antithymocyte serum (ATS) than in non-ATS pretreated mice. On the other hand, administration of a higher dose of CPM (403 mg/kg), which kills a greater number of leukemic cells but induces an immunodepression, according to the skin graft test, results in a shorter survival time than does the administration of a lower dose of CPM (134 mg/kg), capable of killing fewer leukemic cells but not inducing such an immunodepression. Thus, it appears that: (1) the antileukemic effect of the same dose of a chemotherapeutic drug is less efficient in immunodepressed than in nonimmuno-depressed hosts, and (2) calculation of the number of neoplastic cells killed by a given chemotherapy by extrapolation from the survival time may lead to erroneous conclusions.

Introduction

Skipper et al. [1] showed in mice a correlation between the number of L1210 leukemia cells grafted and the survival time of the host. From this observation they deduced that, after grafting a known number of leukemic cells, the effectiveness of a chemotherapy could be expressed by the number of cells killed, as estimated from the survival time. Later, some investigators were tempted to express the results of an L1210 leukemia chemotherapy by the number of killed cells instead of by the survival time. In the following experiments we have studied whether, in view of the immunosuppressive effects of the majority of chemotherapeutic agents, this modality of expression can lead to erroneous conclusions. In the first experiment, we compared the effects of the same doses (134 mg/kg) of cyclo-phosphamide (CPM) administered either alone or in combination with antithymocyte serum (ATS). In the second experiment, the effects of two different doses of CPM, one which is *not* immunosuppressive (134.5 mg/kg) and one which *is* immunosuppressive (403.4 mg/kg), were compared. In both experiments, the survival time of the mice after grafting of L1210 leukemia cells was estimated. In a third experiment, the immunosuppressive action of doses of 134.5 mg/kg and 403.4 mg/kg of CPM were compared by estimating their effect on the rejection time of an allogeneic skin graft.

Materials and Methods

First Experiment

In all experimental groups, 10^3 L1210 leukemia cells were grafted i.v. to 10-week-old (C57B1/6 × DBA/2)F1 mice on day 0. The control mice (group 1) received no further treatment. Group 2 mice received 0.25 ml ATS injected i.p. on days -8, -6, -3, and -1. In group 3, CPM was administered at a dose of 134 mg/kg on day $+1$, and in group 4, ATS was administered as in group 2 and CPM as in group 3. Each experimental group contained 16–20 mice. The immunosuppressive activity of the ATS was previously verified in skin graft experiments: ATS was injected i.p. at a dose of 0.25 ml on day -1 before and days $+3$ and $+5$ after skin grafting; it prolonged the survival of C₃H skin grafts on 10-week-old (C57B1/6 × DBA/2)F1 recipients for 16 days, as compared with untreated controls.

Second Experiment

In all experimental groups, 10^4 L1210 leukemia cells were grafted s.c. on day 0 to mice of the same age and same genetic constitution as those in the first experiment.
Eighteen mice received no further treatment and served as controls (group 1), 9 mice received 134.5 mg/kg of CPM on day $+6$ (group 2), and 19 mice received 403.4 mg/kg on day $+6$ (group 3).

Third Experiment

The rejection time of C57B1/6 tail skin, grafted at day 0 onto adult Swiss mice, was studied in all experimental groups. Eight untreated recipients were used as controls (group 1). Seven recipients were treated with 134.5 mg/kg of CPM on day -1 (group 2), and 7 recipients with the same dose of CPM on day $+1$ (group 3); 9 recipients were treated with 403.4 mg/kg of CPM on day -1 (group 4), and 9 recipients with the same dose of CPM at day $+1$ (group 5). The skin graft technique was performed and the rejection time estimated as previously described by our colleagues [2].

Results

The results of the first experiment (Fig. 1) show that ATS administered alone does not significantly affect the survival time of L1210 leukemia-bearing mice (100% of the animals had died by day 11 after grafting) as compared with the untreated control group (50% of the animals had died by day 10 and 100% by day 11 after grafting). However, the association of the ATS treatment with CPM chemotherapy decreases the antileukemic effect of CPM chemotherapy administered alone ($P < 0.03$) (50% of the animals were dead by day 32 and only 30% alive on day 100, compared with 84% of the animals treated with CPM alone being still alive on day 100 after grafting).
The results of the second experiment (Fig. 2a) show that compared with the untreated control group (100% of the animals had died by day 17), CPM administered at a dose of 403.4 mg/kg is less efficient in curing mice with L1210 leukemia (50% of the animals had

died by day 16 and only 5% survived to day 40 after grafting) (P < 0.05) than is CPM
administered at a dose of 134.5 mg/kg (50% of the animals had died by day 22 and 44%
were still surviving on day 40 after grafting) (P < 0.001).
The results of the third experiment (Fig. 2b) show that treatment of skin graft recipients
with a dose of 134.5 mg/kg of CPM (either before or after the graft) does not significantly
modify the rejection time of an allogeneic skin graft as compared with the untreated control

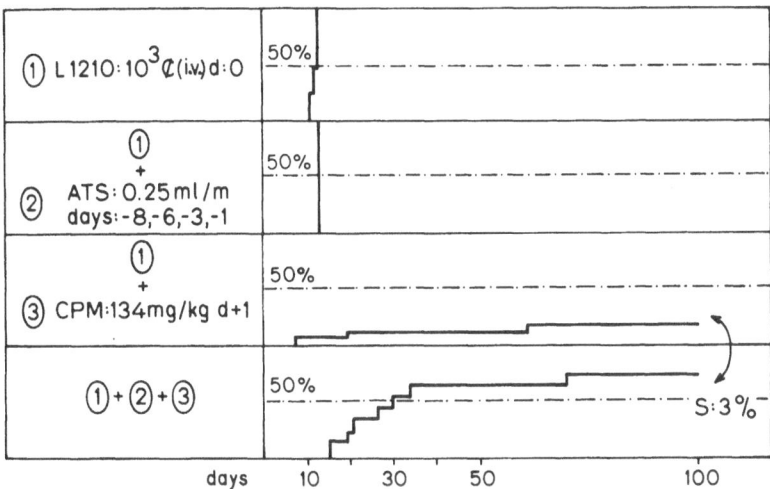

Fig. 1. Effect of ATS-induced immunodepression on the oncostatic power of CPM chemotherapy.
Results are expressed in percentage of cumulative mortality of leukemia-bearing mice. Statistical
significance is calculated by Wilcoxon's nonparametric test

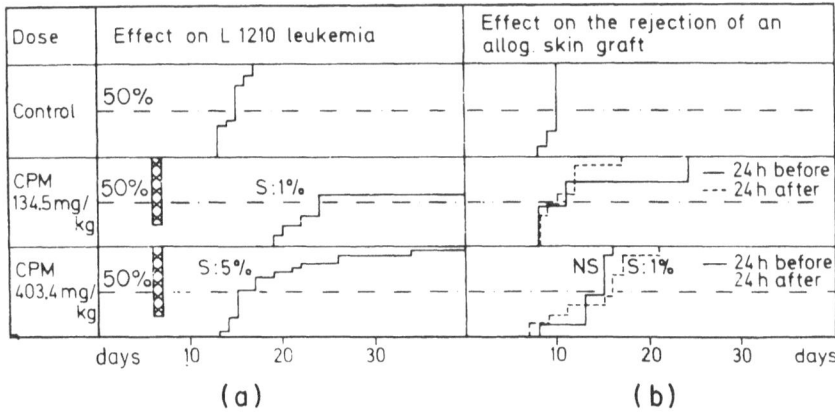

Fig. 2a and b. Correlation between the inferior oncostatic power of a high dose of CPM, 403.4 mg/kg, as
compared with 134.5 mg/kg (a) and its immunosuppressive effect demonstrated by skin graft tests (b).
Results are expressed in percentage of cumulative mortality for L1210 leukemia-bearing mice and in
percentage of cumulative rejection time for allogeneic skin grafts. Statistical significance is calculated by
Wilcoxon's nonparametric test

group (50% of the grafts were rejected in all cases by days 10/11 after grafting), whereas, treatment with a dose of 403.4 mg/kg of CPM administered 1 day after grafting significantly (P < 0.01) delayed the time of skin graft rejection (50% of the grafts were rejected by day 16 after grafting).

Discussion

Results obtained in the present experiments suggest that chemotherapy applied to immunodepressed hosts is less efficient than that applied to nonimmunodepressed hosts. In the first experiment, the immunodepression induced by ATS significantly reduced the antileukemic effect of CPM chemotherapy (134 mg/kg) in L1210 leukemia-bearing mice. In the second experiment, the higher dose of CPM (403.4 mg/kg presumed to be capable of killing a greater number of leukemic cells) was less efficient in curing mice with L1210 leukemia than the lower dose of CPM (134.5 mg/kg presumed to be capable of killing fewer leukemic cells). In the third experiment, skin graft survival time was significantly prolonged after the administration of 403.4 mg/kg of CPM but was unaffected by the administration of 134.5 mg/kg of CPM. These last results reflect the immunosuppressive effect of the higher dose and nonimmunosuppressive effect of the lower dose of CPM, and they provide a rational explanation for the apparently paradoxical phenomenon observed in the experiments on chemotherapy of L1210 leukemia: the fact that higher, rather than lower, doses of CPM induce an immunosuppression may explain why chemotherapy with the same high doses is less effective against L1210 leukemia.

From these observations, it can be deduced that: (1) chemotherapy may be less efficient in immunodepressed patients than in immunologically normal subjects, a phenomenon which we have observed in patients submitted to chemotherapy for bronchus cancer, and (2) calculation of the number of neoplastic cells killed by a given chemotherapy by extrapolation from the survival time may lead to erroneous conclusions.

References

1. Skipper, H. E., Schobel, F. H., Wilcox, W. S.: Experimental evaluation of potential anticancer agents. XIII. On the criteria and kinetics associated with "curability" of experimental leukaemia. Cancer Chemoth. Rep. 35, 1–111 (1964).
2. Tenenbaum, R., Mery, A. M., Amiel, J. L.: Nouvelle technique de greffe de peau chez la souris. Rev. Franç. Et. Clin. Biol. 10, 1106–1108 (1961).

Chemotherapy of Tumours in Immuno-deprived Mice

A. J. S. DAVIES*

In most spheres of biomedical research there are two discernible influences. The clinician for his part is a pragmatist whose rationale for acting is tempered by the necessity to act. The nonclinical worker with less pressure upon him is less inclined to make a virtue out of necessity. From the existence of these two viewpoints has arisen the broad notion that the clinician is less scientific than his non-clinical colleagues. He is, but not much. Both often have to practise a brand of empiricism which is scandalously bare of scientific principles when operating at the level of the whole organism or the organ or the tissue or the cell or even such macromolecular aggregates as cell membranes. But, despite this, the possibility of doing something rather than maintaining a state of lordly, intellectually-inspired, inactivity is seductive.

Cancer chemotherapy for example has, on the one hand, the practising clinicians who meet to discuss individual cases and who arrive at a course of action based, it appears, on the information contained in a few battered pocket books. On the other hand, the back-room chemist plots how the removal or addition of this or that radical from a particular compound may influence its use in the hands of the clinicians. Nowadays, we must also consider the often faceless breed of organisation men who conspire to ensure that the right kind of information is generated and moved in the right direction. Out of this melting pot of confusion there arises the miasma which at any one point in time can be regarded as the state of the art. I want to deal with a particular aspect of this.

The watchword of those in both clinical and experimental chemotherapy is selectivity; how can a tumour be damaged in such a way as to minimise damage to the tumour-bearing patient? In such a situation and often with uncritical disregard of the evidence, the requisite specificity has been assumed. The tumour has been seen as some kind of greyhound among somatic cells with an abnormally high speed of division and a vast capacity for regeneration. In contrast, the normal cell populations have been seen as pedestrian with restricted possibilities for recovery after damage. Thus, in designing drugs for treatment of cancer, much emphasis has been put on poisons likely to interfere with highly metabolically active cells. It must be allowed that compounds have been produced, successfully in the sense that the tumour of the patient to whom they have been administered has regressed without irreparable damage to bone marrow, skin or gut. This success has served as the somewhat shaky foundation for an enormous superstructure of cancer chemotherapy drug screening and synthesis. The specificity which is apparent from the clinical results could, however, be spurious. It could equally well be argued that tumours regress under the influence of chemotherapeutic drugs because they consist in the main of feeble, genetically unbalanced cell populations, whose principle advantage, in a powerfully selective environment, is their heterogeneity which is not characteristic of normal somatic cells. Whatever the truth of this conundrum, it cannot be denied that most cancer chemotherapeutic compounds are noxious in the extreme and that they can rarely be administered except in malignant conditions.

---

* 'I wish to thank my colleagues at the Chester Beatty Research Institute and Dr. H. J. G. BLOOM and Mr. N. BRADLEY of the Royal Marsden Hospital for sharing their results with me and allowing me to include them in this paper. Work at the Chester Beatty Research Institute (Institute of Cancer Research: Royal Cancer Hospital) is supported by grants from the Medical Research Council and the Cancer Research Campaign.'

Against such a background, it seems that much effort is put into combinations and permutations of known drugs; the contemporary literature is depressingly short of information about 'new' compounds. There is a search for new drugs based either on vast screening programmes which deal with previously untested compounds or variants of agents of known efficacy in the anticancer field. There are also efforts to chase molecules into the labyrinthine biochemical pathways of living cells in order to elucidate so-called structure-activity relationships. (The adoption of such a catch phrase tends to pre-empt discussion by assuming the relationships rather than setting out to discover them). The endocrinologists play a role in that some tumours show a residual, or perhaps even new, sensitivity to hormones which can facilitate tumour growth regulation. This last approach has an appeal to the biologist and in recent years it has been joined by immunotherapy, a set of procedures designed to influence tumour growth on the assumption that tumours elicit an immune response from their hosts. This is a rather esoteric form of chemotherapy which perhaps works and perhaps it works for the reasons its protagonists think it works. To an outsider, however, the practises of immunotherapists do seem to be buttressed by enthusiasm.

We have chosen in our own work to do three things in relation to chemotherapy. Firstly, to determine whether antibodies can be used as carriers of chemotherapeutic agents to tumours in relation to which the antibodies are specifically reactive. Secondly, to explore the possibility that the outcome of chemotherapy can be influenced by the immune response. And thirdly, to determine whether human tumours growing in immunologically inactive mice can usefully be considered as targets for chemotherapeutic agents.

I do not wish to consider the first of these activities in any detail except to state the principles. It is an assumption that in some if not all tumour situations there are produced in the host organism antibodies which have some specificity for the tumour. Or that, even if such auto-antibodies never exist, antibodies of the requisite specificity can be induced by an appropriate sequence of immunisation and absorption using another organism as the antibody producer. Or that, in the event of both autochthonous and homologous or heterologous antibody proving inadequately specific, it is possible artificially to approach the problem by using a tumour as a target for a drugged antibody (to use the phrase coined by one of my namesakes). For example, drugged mouse-antihuman antibody could be used in mice against a human tumour which would be the only target for the antibody and its burden. From this last approach could derive a technology for specific attack on cells which even if it fails as an antitumour device might be useful for attacking protozoan extracellular parasites or even viruses.

Can the outcome of cancer chemotherapy be influenced by the immune status of the host organism? The answer briefly is yes—in a number of experimental systems. The principle is that if the rate of transplanted tumour growth can be influenced by the immune status of the host, then the outcome of chemotherapy against that tumour can be similarly affected. For example, the Gardner lymphosarcoma is a tumour which originated in C3H mice. If a few hundred thousand cells are transplanted, it will usually grow up the immunological gradient to kill CBA mice. In a normal animal, it is possible to cure the tumour by an injection of asparaginase. In an animal which has been immunologically reduced by adult thymectomy and irradiation, the tumour regresses under the influence of asparaginase but always grows again [1]. It should be noted about this system that the growth rate and lethality of this tumour are only slightly higher in immunologically incompetent mice. Thus, a slight difference in growth control exercised by a slight immune mechanism can lead to a totally different outcome to chemotherapeutic treatment.

This particular system lends itself to a different kind of model building. If T cell-deprived mice never survive tumours plus chemotherapy and normal mice always do, it is possible to pose the question as to how many T cells a mouse has to have to give it a 50% chance of survival. The answer is surprisingly between $1-2 \times 10^6$ nonimmune cells and tenfold fewer immune cells. Veritably a few lymphocytes can have a powerful effect.

Such experiments can be used to test putative immunopotentiating agents such as levamisole, BCG and *Corynebacterium parvum*. It should be remembered that the method involves a deliberate homograft of malignant cells and that the immunological relationship between tumour and host thus generated may be quite unlike any such relationship in the autochthonous situation.

Let me now consider a slightly different example. The Walker tumour grows rapidly and lethally in most strains of rats. Its growth rate is, subterminally, slower in normal than in immunologically reduced rats, but the lethal outcome is the same. To initiate growth of the Walker in rats requires a trochar implant of 10–20×10^6 cells. The ascites form of the Walker will not grow subcutaneously in normal rats. In immunologically normal mice, of course, the Walker tumour will not grow at all but in T cell-deprived mice it grows very well. Its growth rate is slow—it is always fast in rats. In mice it is encapsulated whereas in rats it is extensively invasive. In mice it sometimes regresses, in rats if it grows then it kills. In mice single ascites cells will often initiate a tumour in a subcutaneous situation. It is tempting to suppose that the alteration in pattern of growth of the Walker in mice as compared with rats is related to the relaxation of immunological pressure against the tumour. The evidence such as it is implies that this is not the case but that there exists some other reason connected perhaps with the xenografting procedure. It is tempting to suppose that here is operating some nonimmunological defence mechanism which might be operative under normal circumstances in controlling tumour growth. It is revealed in the present experiments by exaggerating the foreignness of the tumour artificially. It is possible that such a mechanism would operate against human tumours growing in rodents (*vide infra*). If it did, then the subsequent alteration of growth pattern might reduce the use of the system for the testing of chemotherapeutic agents.

What is the outcome of chemotherapy of the Walker tumour in rats and in mice? Using 5 aziridino-2,4-dinitrobenzamide (CB 1954), a well-loved chemotherapeutic agent, it emerged that despite the big differences in growth characteristics in the two species, the outcome of chemotherapy is comparable and largely biased by the lower toxicity of CB 1954 in mice.

It must be noted in these experiments that, in any mouse in which the Walker tumour grew and regressed, whether spontaneously or under the influence of drugs, the animal was subsequently resistant to challenge with the Walker. Thus, a minimally effective immunological system can generate effective immunity under conditions of chronic antigenic stimulation, but it may take some time to do so. I am not sure whether these experiments teach us more about cancer chemotherapy or about immunity. They bring us on to the next topic which is that of the human xenograft growing in variously immunologically incompetent mice.

We have chosen to concentrate our efforts on three systems. Firstly, the testing of a variety of known chemotherapeutic agents against a battery of human tumours. Secondly, the testing of a few selected agents against human gliomas growing in mice. Thirdly, we have attempted a limited study of low grade chemotherapy against a human breast carcinoma. Our initial attempts with a battery of human tumours growing in adult thymectomized irradiated and bone marrow reconstituted mice revealed that hexamethylmelamine (HMM) was active against three of the seven human carcinomas involved (publication pending). 4-hydroxy-4-methylcyclophosphamide was active against a carcinoma of the colon but not of one of the bronchus. BCNU had some activity against the two carcinomas of the colon we had on trial. So far 80 dose-response curves have been performed on some 17 compounds without any particularly surprising results except with HMM, which is not markedly active against mouse tumours. There are undeniably problems. The host mice might not be sufficiently immunologically suppressed to grow tumours. This has been circumvented by selecting for treatment those animals in which tumours have attained a certain size. Not all tumours grow progressively in the controls which could of course be due to some residual immunological potential. The tumours are slow growing which is aggravating to those used to dealing with rapidly growing rodent tumours. Two good points are that the rate of growth and pattern of differentiation in mice are usually similar to those in the human of origin. So far, no kinetic studies have been performed to determine whether the mitotic rate and cell loss fractions are similar.

At the moment, the adoption of a human tumour screen in mice is an intelligent departure from previous screening procedures. It could be that certain agents are effective against human tumours but not those of mice because of different intermediary metabolism of the drug in the two species.

Our second project, with gliomas, has a slightly different intent. We have grown and transplanted 13 of 46 human gliomas in T cell-deprived mice. One of these, a grade IV astrocytoma, has been used as a target for either BCNU or CCNU. The results are quite straightforward—the tumours can be cured but usually at the expense of the life of the mouse. Either of the two compounds given once a week for 5 weeks at a dose level per injection of 10 mg/kg has this effect.

Dianhydrogalactitol—one of the new wonder drugs—only caused cessation of growth of the tumour at dose levels (8 mg/kg/injection) at which some animals died during treatment. HMM could cause nearly complete regression of the tumour at dose levels nearly those causing bone marrow failure. Tumours recovered from those treated animals and retransplanted were insensitive to further treatment with HMM. In an anomalous experiment, treatment of a human breast carcinosarcoma was attempted with melphalan before the tumours were palpable. In the controls, no tumours grew, but in the low dose treated groups tumours appeared. At higher doses no tumours were apparent. The most obvious explanation for such an apparent paradox is that the chemotherapeutic agent was immunosuppressive and facilitated tumour growth in the otherwise inadequately suppressed mouse hosts. At higher doses the antitumour effect was apparent.

Gliomas are singularly intractable tumours and these attempts to determine how to treat them might succeed. The major difficulty is to maintain a low grade state of cautious optimism when the pressure from granting authorities tends to elicit exaggerated claims of importance.

Lastly, I wish to discuss our attempts to grow breast tumours in congenitally athymic nude mice (nu/nu). About 10% of all the 100 or so tumours we have implanted (each one 16 times) have shown some form of progressive growth in nude mice. When growth has occurred, the similarities between the tumour in the original condition and when transplanted have been more impressive than the differences. Parts of those tumours which failed to grow have in most instances survived for long periods of time. The early postimplantation events have been studied and it is not obvious that failure to grow is due to an immunological rejection. The issue could in part be related to the capacity of the graft adequately to survive postimplantation isochaemic necrosis. It remains to be seen whether implantation of smaller or even larger pieces in better vascularized places is successful.

One of the tumours which did grow was treated with repeated low doses of melphalan over a period of many weeks. The tumour growth rate was slightly reduced without notable effects on the host.

These studies represent the attempts of a nonclinical immunologist to work in the more clinically orientated field of chemotherapy. The findings are preliminary and give presently little indication of their eventual value.

Reference

1. CARTER, R. L., CONNORS, T. A., WESTON, B. J., DAVIES, A. J. S.: Treatment of a mouse lymphoma by L-asparaginase: success depends on the host's immune response. Int. J. Cancer *11*, 345–357 (1973).

Treatment of Malignant Gliomas and Brain Metastases in Adults Using a Combination of Adriamycine, VM 26, and CCNU Results of a Type II Trial

P. Pouillart, G. Mathé, T. Palangie, J. Lheritier, M. Poisson, P. Huguenin, H. Gautier, P. Morin, and R. Parrot

The conventional treatment currently applied in malignant brain tumors in adults consists of surgery, often followed by irradiation of the brain. The prognosis is not encouraging, as the survival median does not exceed 11 months [8, 17]. Studies by Frankel and German [5] showed that where surgery alone is used, the survival median is about 6 months after extensive *exeresis* and two, 5 months after partial exeresis. After simple biopsy, the spontaneous survival median is 10 months. Comparable results were reported in the retrospective work of Roth and Elwidge. Radiotherapy increases the survival median established after surgical treatment alone by about 4 months (Frankel and German [5]). Experimental results in animals [16], which were later confirmed in man [7, 10, 19, 20, 21, 23, 24, 4, 6], have shown the potential value of chemotherapy and led to the development of new therapeutic methods, despite the limited number of drugs available and the fact that their combined effect has not been studied [11].

The introduction of nitrosourea derivatives—BCNU, ie., 1-3 A (2 chloroethyl) 1 nitro-sourea and CCNU, i.e., (1.2 chloroethyl)-3 cyclohexyl-1-nitrosourea, which are *liposoluble* and easily penetrate the blood-brain barrier—has made direct access possible to the tumor site. BCNU is active in inoperable glioblastoma [20]. Systematically administered after surgery, alone, or in combination with radiotherapy, it significantly prolongs the survival of patients treated [21, 2].

Vincristine was also shown to be effective [10], but the results were disappointing when it was combined with BCNU [4].

In animals, VM 26 proved effective in treating intracerebrally grafted tumors; this fact, as well as the drug's *liposolubility* and its action on glioblastomas (which differs from that of nitrosoureas) [18] and also the potentializing effect of sequential VM 26 and CCNU administration [12], led us to conduct an experiment combining both these drugs. The clinical results observed in patients with nonresectable glioblastomas are comparable to those obtained by other authors who used CCNU alone [13]. By introducing adriamycine into this therapeutic sequence, we were recently able to increase the effectiveness of the previous combination in animals.

In the present work, we have analyzed the therapeutic results obtained by cyclic and sequential administration of adriamycine, VM 26, and CCNU in 43 patients with nonresectable glioblastoma and 30 patients with cerebral metastases.

Patients and Methods

Seventy-seven patients, presented in Table 1, were included in this study, beginning in October, 1973.

Table 1. Classification of patients included in the trial

Malignant gliomas		43
Chordomas		2
Medulloblastomas		2
Metastases	Bronchial tumors	13
	Breast tumors	8
	Others	9
Total		77

All patients suffered from an inoperable or recurring tumor and had undergone surgery, with or without radiotherapy.

1. Glioblastomas

The average age of the 43 patients in this trial (12 women and 31 men) was 52.8 years, the youngest being 20 and the oldest 71.

Age	No of patients
< 40	5
40–50	9
50–60	17
60–71	12

In 22 patients, the tumors were surgically nonresectable, either because of their size or their site. Seventeen patients had residual tumors following surgery, and six patients a recurring tumor after a first operation.

2. Brain Metastasis

These patients were classified according to the origin of their tumor, as shown in Table 1. All the patients in this study, at the time of diagnosis, presented at least one other visceral metastatic localization which justified their inclusion in a chemotherapy protocol.

Treatment

Patients were submitted to intermittent cyclic sequential chemotherapy. Each 5-day cycle of treatment included direct i.v. administration on day 1 of 45 mg/m 2 adriamycine; on days 2 and 3, VM 26 (60 mg/m 2 per day) in 250 ml of isotonic glucose solution, in rapid 1½-hour infusions, and on days 4 and 5, CCNU *p.o.*, at a dose of 60 mg/m 2 per day.

Each cycle of treatment was only resumed once hematologic restoration was completed, that is, when the leukocyte count was four-fifths of the patient's initial treatment count and the platelet count half the initial count.

In the course of this therapeutic trial, treatment was stopped in cases of complete failure or in the case of intolerance to VM 26. In all other cases, chemotherapy cycles were repeated regularly whenever the patient's hematologic state permitted.

Adjuvant treatments, particularly symptomatic "antihypertension" treatments, were applied right at the beginning of the trial.

Before undergoing the first cycle of chemotherapy, all the patients were given an optimal dose of methylprednisolone which made it possible to reduce the intensity of *intracranium* hypertension syndrome manifestations. During this initial phase of treatment, before administration of the first chemotherapy cycle, patients were also given a daily 500 ml perfusion of 10% glucose hypertonic solution, a 500 ml infusion of hypertonic mannitol, and 100 mg furosemide, injected i.v.

These adjuvant treatments are administered after the conclusion of each chemotherapy cycle for at least 6 days. Doses of methylprednisolone were then gradually reduced to the minimum effective dose and replaced by 1 mg per day of late ACTH (synthetic corticostimulin). The reduction and discontinuance of the doses of corticoids were taken into account when assessing the therapeutic results.

Fifteen patients were submitted to additional treatment comprising a daily i.m. injection of 100 mg/m 2 chlorpromazine. The treatment began 24 hours before the beginning of the chemotherapy cycle and ceased 24 hours after the cycle ended. In all cases, we considered that corticoids and anticonvulsive drugs had no antitumoral effects in themselves and that the transitory clinical neurologic improvements often observed were only due to the reduction of the peritumoral edema.

Evaluating the Results

Intracranium tumors develop within a restricted space and their evolution depends on three factors: tumor growth, the development of the peritumoral edema, and the extension to vital neurologic centers. Results were evaluated taking into account the interaction of these factors. Each patient included in the trial underwent a general, neurologic, and biological checkup. The diagnosis was either based on a histologic study of the tumor to be operated on or on the correlation between the data provided by the patient's clinical development and by gammaencephalography and arteriography [8, 9].

In 25 cases, gammaencephalography was repeated every 3 months. All the patients were under steroid therapy at the beginning of chemotherapy protocol. Clinical development was judged by the modification of focal neurologic signs stabilized from corticoids, and the patient's general behaviour was studied every week, and later at longer intervals. These signs can be classified into four stages in decreasing order of gravity:

1. Stage IV: The patient is in a coma.
2. Stage III: The patient is conscious, but his neurologic condition requires constant assistance.
3. Stage II: The patient is conscious and can look after his basic needs.
4. Stage I: The patient can resume all his activities.

Improvement was defined as a regression of neurologic signs enabling the patient to progress by at least two stages within a minimum of 2 months.

The final overall assessment of the therapeutic effects was based on the evolution of the survival curve for the entire group of patients included in the trial.

Results

1. Tolerance

All patients underwent the trials considered in this study between 2 and 17 months ago.

a) Digestive Disorders
Digestive disorders such as nausea and vomiting, due to the administration of adriamycine and CCNU, varied from one patient to another. During chemotherapy, they were reported in 70% of the cases treated but were never acute enough to necessitate the treatment being stopped.
Such disorders subsided completely within 24 hours of the end of a chemotherapy treatment cycle and only responded sporadically to the administration of metoclopramide. However, the chloropromazine injections given to 15 patients seemed to us remarkably effective.

b) Hematologic Disorders
The intervals between chemotherapy cycles were solely determined on the basis of the time required for complete hematologic restoration. *Leukopenia* was moderate and recovery was on the average complete between the 15th and 20th day after the end of the cycle. There were no cases of infection, but *thrombopenia* increased from one cycle to another with increasingly slow restoration. During these trials, *combination chemotherapy* was only resumed once the platelet count had attained at least 50% of the pretreatment level. The results, shown in Table 2, indicate a steady increase in the average duration of the interval between chemotherapy cycles. From the first to sixth cycles, the duration of this interval increased from 31.6 to 42.2 days, the seventh interval lasting 65.5 days. In all, 170 cycles of treatment were administered to the 43 glioblastoma cases included in the trials, and the average interval between cycles lasted 36.6 days.

Table 2. Average increase in the intervals between chemotherapy cycles

Interval No.	No. of patients	Length of interval
1	40	31.6 days
2	33	35.5 days
3	25	36.1 days
4	20	37.8 days
5	16	42.2 days
6	13	38.8 days
7	9	65.5 days
Overall number of treatment cycles for 43 patients[a]		36.3 days

[a] In six cases, clinical relapse occurred in the course of a very long interval which lasted on an average 86.6 days.

Thrombopenia was never less than 75,000: mm 3 before the fifth chemotherapy cycle. After the sixth cycle, it dropped to 40,000 in seven patients, but there were no cases of hemorrhage. Platelet restoration took a long time in six patients—86.6 days on an average (ranging 65–125 days), during which clinical relapse occurred.

c) General Disorders
Alopecia was present in 43 patients studied in this trial. *Melanodermia* was also present but in variable intensity. Its origin is unclear but might possibly be due to adriamycine [14].

d) Neurologic Disorders
The only noticeable neurologic complication was intensification of the sign intracranium hypertension during or between treatment cycles. It was observed during the second chemotherapy cycle in 11 cases and during the third cycle in three cases. Such signs disappeared within 3 days and their intensity was always attenuated by absorption of corticoids. No deaths were imputable to the increase of HT/C.

Therapeutic Results

Objective clinical improvement as defined above occurred in 31 patients, that is, in 72% of the cases considered. The clinical condition of 12 others continued to worsen despite the treatment administered (Table 3). Whenever clinical improvement was observed, it occurred during the first 2 months following chemotherapy. Mere stabilization of a patient's initial clinical condition or continued progress after the 2nd month were some of the factors for a bad prognosis that occurred in 12 patients, i.e., in 28% of the cases treated.

Table 3. Malignant gliomas in adults: results observed (subjective neurologic improvements)

Improvement[a]	31	72%
Stabilization[a]	3	7%
Failures	9	21%
Total	43	

[a] Improvement is defined as a regression of the objective neurologic symptoms lasting at least 2 months.

Twenty-five out of the 31 patients whose condition improved as a result of the treatment were subjected to a regular trimonthly cinegammagraphic checkup (Prof. Ag. D. ANCRI). Objective regression of the pathologic image was noted in 16 cases; it was complete in five cases and partial in 11. In all, chemotherapy had an objective effect in 21 out of 25 patients studied, but in five cases the image was stabilized. The objective clinical effect noted did not completely correspond to the scintigraphic improvements recorded since scintigraphy showed a growth in the size of the infected site in four patients whose objective clinical condition had apparently improved, probably related to a delayed effect of steroid therapy (Table 6).
The effect of combined chemotherapy on survival is shown in Fig. 1. The survival median is 180 days. Thereafter, the number of deaths roughly equals the number of patients who survive, taken over the same lapse of time; and at the moment, out of 22 patients surviving for more than 6 months, 12 are in satisfactory condition and ten are in remission 180–510 days after treatment.

Table 4. Malignant gliomas in adults: scintigraphic results
observed after 3 months treatment

Spreading of infected site	4
Stabilization of infected site	5
< 50% regression	6
> 50% regression	5
Disappearance of site	5
	25

25 out of 31 cases that improved as a result of the treatment
were kept under regular cinegammagraphic observation.

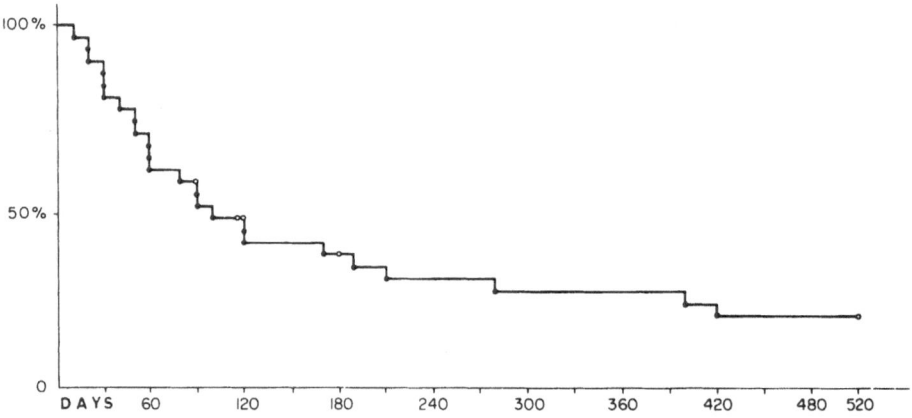

Fig. 1. Survival curve for cerebral metastasis patients

Factors That May Affect Chemotherapy Results

The results given in Table 5 show that the initial site of the tumor does not affect the results
of chemotherapy, neither does the tumor's extensive but unilateral character have any part
in determining its response to drugs.

Table 5. Malignant gliomas in adults: effects of chemotherapy, classified according to tumor site

	Frontal	Temporal	Parietal	Extensive tumor
Number of patients	12	14	8	9
Number of survivals on 15.4.1975	5	6	5	3
Survival median	189 days	181 days	188 days	190 days

When its initial site is frontal, the survival median is 189 days; when it is temporal, the median is 181 days; when it is parietal, 188 days; and for extensive but unilateral tumors, it is 190 days. It should, however, be noted that four patients had particularly serious tumors either located in the central grey nucleii or which had spread to the bilateral frontal or callous mass (*corps calleux*).

If one takes into account the treatments received by patients prior to this trial, the survival median for patients having undergone partial tumor *resectioning* is 185 days and may be compared to the 185-day median observed for patients considered inoperable (Table 6). So far, survival medians have proved identical, but 12 out of 21 patients have survived in the first group and eight out of 22 in the second.

Table 6. Effects of chemotherapy, according to tumor size

	Patients included in the trial after partial tumor *exeresis*	Inoperable tumor patients included in the trial
Number of patients	21	22
Survival median on 15.4.75	185 days (30–400)	188 days (40–506)
Number of survivals	12	8
Average survival periods for diseased patients	154 days	168 days

The initial site of the tumor conditions the early appearance of alarming symptoms leading to the investigations necessary for diagnosis. The first signs of what are originally left temporal tumors may be very striking and include speech difficulties and abnormal handwriting. These disorders worsen in a rapid and spectacular fashion, and the diagnosis is often established when the tumor is still small. On the other hand, tumors that start in the right temporal zone show no such outward signs for a long time. In such cases, the survival median is 190 days, and three patients out of the eight included in the trial are still alive. For those in the left temporal group, the survival median was 270 days, with three out of six patients surviving (Table 7). In all cases, the response to chemotherapy was achieved during the first 2 months*.

Table 7. Malignant gliomas in adults: effect of tumor site on chemotherapy results (effects of chemotherapy according to tumor site)

	Tumor site	
	Right Temporal	Left Temporal
Survival median	190 days (40–400)	280 days (134–446)
Number of patients	8	6
Number of survivals	3	3

Whatever the results, chemotherapy is regularly applied whenever the patient's hematologic state allows. In cases where such treatment continued uninterrupted, *regrowth* occurred mainly after the sixth cycle of treatment (Table 7). In this trial, scintigraphic relapses always preceded recurrence of clinical symptoms.

Table 8. Malignant gliomas in adults: date of clinical and/or scintigraphic relapse

After 3 cycles of treatment	2
After 4 cycles of treatment	3
After 5 cycles[a] of treatment	2
After 6 cycles[a] of treatment	9

[a] 22 patients survived for more than 6 months.
 10 died between the 180th and 300th day.
  2 are at present in a state of scintigraphic relapse.
 10 are in a satisfactory clinical and scintigraphic condition.

Two chordoma and two medulloblastoma patients were included in this study. The efficiency of the drug combinations used was satisfactory, but not enough time has elapsed in order to assess the effect of such improvement on their survival.

2. Brain Metastasis

Thirty patients with brain metastasis were included in this study. They all had peripheral tumor lesions.

Thirteen patients with epidermoid bronchial cancer brain metastases received from one to three cycles of treatment. The neurologic symptoms were in regression for 2 months in three patients. Only one patient is alive 120 days after treatment, and the mean survival time of these group A patients is 72 days.

Six out of eight cases of brain metastasis caused by breast cancer underwent subjective improvement, and their neurologic symptoms regressed for at least 2 months. One woman patient returned to a normal neurologic condition, and there has been no recurrence of her initial scintigraphic features for the past 14 months. The survival median of this group of patients is 240 days (range 20–510 days).

Neurologic improvements were observed in three of the nine other patients included in this trial, but no objective cinegammagraphic regression was noted. The survival median for these nine patients was 109 days, with only one patient now alive after 180 days (Tables 9 and 10; Fig. 1).

Discussion

Forty-three patients with glioblastoma and 30 patients with multiple brain metastasis were treated by sequential administration of adriamycine, VM 26, and CCNU. For the patients suffering from glioblastoma, the clinical response rate was 72% and the objective cinegammagraphic response 58%.

Taking into account the criteria applied to selection of patients for this noncomparative trial, the results are encouraging as far as the duration of survival is concerned. For a series of comparable patients treated by simple outside decompression, the survival median was 2 months [5]. In our series, 90% of the patients survived into the 2nd month, the overall survival median being 6 months with the extreme limit up to the 17th month. In the case of four patients who have now had over a year's treatment, there have so far been no neurologic or cinegammagraphic consequences due to their initial tumor.

High rates of objective response (50%) were obtained with the administration of BCNU alone [20]. CCNU has a comparable efficiency but seems easier to handle and less toxic

Table 9. Secondary cerebral tumors: results

Bronchial cancer metastases: 13 Patients

1. *Clinical development*
   Improvement   3
   Stabilization 1
   Failure   9

2. *Scintigraphic development:* after the 3rd cycle
   50% regression

Breast cancer metastases: 8 Patients

1. *Clinical development*
   Improvement   6
   Stabilization 1
   Failure   1

2. *Scintigraphic development:* after the 3rd cycle
   Complete remission: 1

Various cancer metastases: 9 Patients

1. *Clinical development*
   Improvement   3
   Stabilization 1
   Failure   5

Table 10. Results observed in 30 cerebral metastasis cases submitted to a chemotherapy combination

	Metastases bronchial epidermoid cancer	Metastases breast cancer	Metastases other types of cancer
Number of patients	13	8	9
Number of survivals	1/13	3/8	1/9
Average period of survival	72 days	246 days	109 days

[15, 3]. The results obtained by SKLANSKY et al. using VM 26 [18] indicate that the drug is especially effective in cases of resistance to nitrosoureas. Earlier trials using combinations of individually active drugs (VCR and BCNU) proved disappointing in the treatment of glioblastoma.

A comparison of the results obtained in this trial as regards survival, based on references to groups treated respectively by surgery only and by surgery combined with radiotherapy, shows that for those of our patients who did not respond to other forms of treatment, such combinations of drugs made it possible to achieve results similar to those obtained from a group for which the prognosis was apparently less grim. Using this combination, FEWER et al. [4] obtained less satisfactory results than those obtained by the use of BCNU alone*.

---

* J. HILDEBRAND [7], using a combination of CCNU, vincristine, and MTX, reported results comparable to those achieved by administrating CCNU alone.

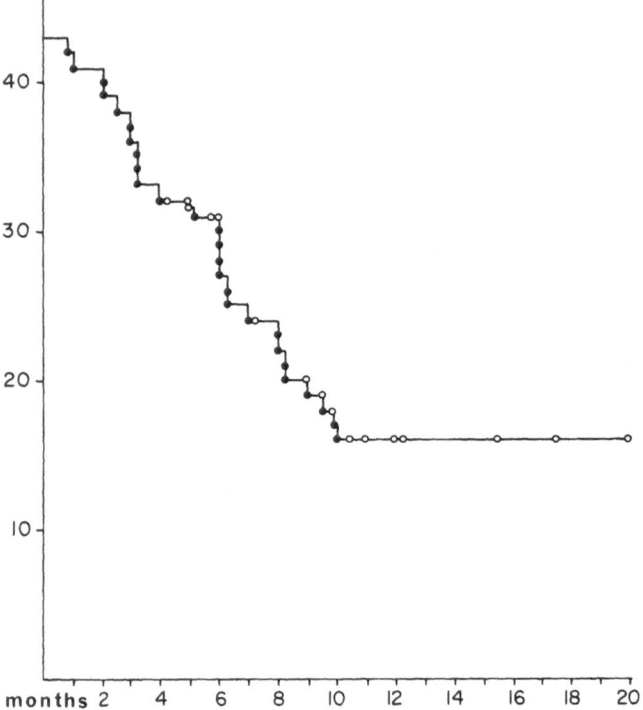

Fig. 2. Survival curve for 43 glioma patients

Using a combination of CCNU, vincristine, and methotrexate, HILDEBRAND et al. [7] reported results comparable to those achieved by administering CCNU alone. A non-comparative trial combining VM 26 and CCNU [13] led to a neurologic improvement in 60% of patients and a final 6-months survival median [13]. The small number of patients involved in this trial did not enable its results to be compared to those obtained by administration of CCNU alone.

However, our subsequent trial included 43 glioblastoma cases (Fig. 2), and evaluation of the results bring out the following five points for discussion:

1. Neurologic improvement always occurred during the first month of treatment and the absence of effect after the second cycle is the cause of a bad prognosis. Any rises in intracranium hypertension due to chemotherapy were easily kept under control by the treatment and did not cause any deaths.

2. There was no absolute correlation between the clinical effects and objective cinne-gammagraphic regression observed. Twenty percent of the patients who had improved neurologically showed a deterioration on scanning. This discrepancy between results had earlier been noted by FEWER et al. Apart from cases where chemotherapy did not modify the tumor's clinical development, all patients who showed an increase in or only stabiliza-tion of the initial tumor size died within the first 6 months. Consequently, there seems to be an exact correlation between prognosis during chemotherapy and the modifications observed in cinegammagraphy [1].

3. According to the results given in Tables 6 and 7, initial tumor size does not seem to alter the treatment's effect on survival. The different tumor sites appear to be sensitive to chemotherapy to an identical degree. A significant difference was, however, noted between the two groups of patients whose tumors originated in the left and right temporal zones respectively.

4. Even in cases where the clinical response was the most spectacular, it was imperative to continue the treatment. An earlier trial had shown that its discontinuance was quickly followed by resumption of tumor growth. The therapeutic technique used means that the interval between cycles increases, from the fifth cycle, and the possibilities of prolonged treatment are thus reduced. There is, moreover, a correlation between the length of the intervals between cycles and the frequency of clinical and scintigraphic relapses. Although it is still too early to formulate a final opinion, the survival median observed for the 43 glioblastoma patients who were given the triple drug combination specified above and were all initially inoperable may be compared to the median reported for earlier series of patients treated by radiotherapy after partial or no *resectioning* [5].

5. In conclusion, it seems that adriamycine is not useful in this type of combination for the treatment of patients with glioblastomas.

6. The low sensitivity of cerebral metastases to the effects of these treatments was remarkable in this trial. Except for one woman patient suffering initially from multiple breast cancer metastases that completely disappeared 14 months ago, the condition of all the other patients in the trial improved little or did not improve at all as a result of the treatment. The slight effects of chemotherapy under these conditions had already been noted [7]. In patients with metastasis of breast cancer, the efficiency of chemotherapy on peripheral localizations was generally *greater* in all the cases than the efficiency on brain metastasis.

Summary

Forty-three patients with inoperable and/or recurring malignant gliomas and 30 patients with multiple recurring brain metastases were treated with a combination of adriamycine (45 mg/m 2 and 4-dimethyl-epipodophyllotoxin D-thenylidene (VM 26) (60 mg/m 2 for 2 days) with 1-(2-chloroethyl)-3-cyclohexyl-1-nitroso-urea (CCNU) (60 mg/m 2 for 2 days). These cycles of treatment were repeated as soon as the hematologic restoration was complete. The treatment was well-tolerated and the clinical condition of 31 out of 43 glioblastoma patients improved during the 2 months after the beginning of the treatment.

Six out of eight patients with breast cancer metastases, one out of 13 with bronchial cancer metastases, and three out of nine with other types of cancer metastases also benefitted from the treatment. Examination of the results obtained reveals the following characteristics:

1. A low degree of efficiency of this combination in the treatment of brain metastases, except for breast cancer metastases.

2. Absence of complete correlation between the clinical results observed and the cine-gammagraphic developments

3. Similarity of the results independent of the initial localization

4. Establishment of a 6-month median survival period, with ten patients at present in a state of apparently complete remission, 180–506 days after beginning of the treatment

References

1. ANCRI, D.: La cinégammagraphie cérébrale. Rev. Neurol. *125*, 131–154 (1971).
2. ARMENTROUT, S. A., FOLTZ, E., VERMUND, H., OTIS, P. T.: Comparison of post-operative irradiation alone and in combinations with BCNU (NSC 409.962) in the management of malignant gliomas. Cancer Chemoth., Rep. *58*, 841–844 (1974).
3. FEWER, D., WILSON, C. B., BOLDREY, E. B., ENOT, K. J.: Phase II study of 1(2-chloroethyl.)3 cyclohexyl-1 nitrosourea (CCNU-NSC 79037) in treatment of brain tumours. Cancer Chemoth. Rep. *56*, 421–427 (1972).
4. FEWER, D., WILSON, C. B., BOLDREY, E. B., ENOT, K. J., POWELL, M. R.: The chemotherapy of brain tumours clinical experience with carmustine (BCNU) and vincristine. J.A.M.A. *222*, 549–552 (1972).
5. FRANKEL, S. A., GERMAN, W. J.: Glioblastoma multiforme (review of 219 cases with regard to natural history, pathology, diagnostic methods and treatment). J. Neuro Surg. *15*, 489 (1958).
6. GOLDSMITH, M. A., CARTER, S. K.: Glioblastoma multiforme, a review of therapy. Cancer Treat. Review *1*, 153–165 (1974).
7. HILDEBRAND, J. H., BRIHAYE, J., WAGENKNECHT, L., MITCHEL, J., KENIS, Y.: Combination chemotherapy with 1(2-chloroethyl) 3 cyclohexyl-1 nitrosourea (CCNU), vincristine, and methotrexate in primary and metastasis brain tumours. A preliminary report. Europ. J. Cancer *9*, 627–634 (1973).
8. JELSMA, R., BUCY, C.: Glioblastoma multiforme. Arch. Neurol. *20*, 161–171 (1969).
9. KRAYENBUHL, H. A., YASARGIL, M. G.: Cerebral angiography. London: Butterworths and Co., 1968, pp. 272–273.
10. LASSMAN, L., PEARCE, G. W., GANG, J.: Sensitivity of intracranial gliomata vincristine sulfate. Lancet (1965) I, 296–297.
11. LEVIN, V. A., WILSON, CH.B.: Chemotherapy: the agents in current use. Sem. in Oncology *2*, 63–67 (1975).
12. POUILLART, P., HOANG THY HUONG, T., BRUGERIE, E., LHERITIER, J.: Sequential administration of two oncostatic drugs: study of modalities for pharmacodynamic potentiations. Biomedicine *21*, 471–479 (1974).
13. POUILLART, P., SCHWARZANBERG, L., AMIEL, J. L., MATHE, G., HUGUENIN, P., MORIN, P., BARON, A., LAPARRE CH., PARROT, R.: Combinaisons chimiothérapiques de drogues se potentialisant. III. Application aux tumeurs du système nerveux central. Nouv. Press Med. *4*, 721–724 (1975).
14. PRATT, C. B., SHANKS, E. C.: Hyperpigmentation of nails from doxorubicin. J.A.M.A. *228*, 460 (1974).
15. ROSENBLUM, M. L., REYNOLDS, A. F., SMITH, K. A., RUMACK, B. H., WALCKER: Chloroethyl-cyclo-hexyl-nitrosourea (CCNU) in the treatment of malignant brain tumours. J. Neurol. Surg. *39*, 306–324 (1973).
16. SCHABEL, F. M., Jr., JOHNSTON, F. P., CALEB, G. S.: Experimental evaluation of potential anticancer agents. VIII. Effects of certain nitrosoureas on intra cerebral L1210 leukaemias. Cancer Research *23*, 725–733 (1963).
17. SHAPIRO, W. R., POSNER, J. B.: The chemotherapy of brain tumours. A clinical and experimental review. In: Recent Advances in Neurology. Plum, F. (ed.).   :   , 1969, pp. 149–235.
18. SKLANSKY, B. D., MANN-KAPLAN, R. S., REYNOLDS, A. F., ROSENBLUM, M. L., WALKER, M. D.: 4' Demethyl-epipodophylotoxin . D. Thenylidene glucoside (PT6) in the treatment of malignant intracranial neoplasms. Cancer *33*, 460–467 (1974).
19. TRIARTE, P. V., HANANIAN, J., CORTNER, J. A.: Central nervous system leukaemia with 1-3 bis (2 chloroethyl)-1 nitrosourea (BCNU). Cancer *19*, 1187–1194 (1966).
20. WALKER, M. D., HURWITZ, B. S.: BCNU (1,3 bis (2-chloroethyl)-1 nitrosourea: NSC—409.962) in the treatment of malignant brain tumours. Cancer Chemoth. Rep. *4*, 263–273 (1970).
21. WALKER, M. D., GEHAM, E. A.: An evaluation of 1,3 bis (2 chloroethyl)-1 nitrosourea (BCNU) and irradiation alone and in combination for the treatment of malignant glioma. Ann. Meet. Am. Ass. Cancer Res. *13* (Abstract No. 63) (1972).
22. WALKER, M. D.: Chemotherapy: adjuvant to surgery and radiation therapy. Seminars in Oncology *2*, 69–72 (1975).
23. WILSON, C. B., BOLDREY, E. B., ENOT, K. J.: 1,3 bis (2 chloroethyl)-1 nitrosourea (NSC 409962) in the treatment of malignant brain tumours. Cancer Chemoth. Rep. *54*, 273–281 (1970).
24. WILSON, C. B., HOSHINO, T.: Current trials in the chemotherapy brain tumours with special references to glioblastoma. J. Neurol. Surg. *31*, 589–603 (1969).

3. Immunotherapy

Immunologic and Cytokinetic Parameters of BCG-Induced Growth Control of a Murine Leukemia

L. OLSSON

Introduction

Administration of immune adjuvants such as BCG may lead to tumor-growth control in some tumor-host relationships [8]. It is assumed that this tumor-growth control is induced by immunologic mechanisms, and this assumption has been given some support by in vitro studies on the cytotoxic effects on tumor cells of various humoral and cellular functions of the immune system. However, the importance of immunologic mechanisms remains to be demonstrated directly in vivo, and in addition, the cytokinetic pertubations in the tumor cell population due to immune adjuvant have not been studied.

Both the immunologic and cytokinetic aspects of BCG-induced tumor growth control are indispensable for a rational protocol combining chemotherapy and BCG, and we have, therefore, performed some studies to elucidate these aspects [10, 11]. The present paper thus partly describes the relationship between various tumor-cell cytotoxic immune mechanisms of the host and tumor growth and partly some cytokinetic perturbations in the tumor cell population induced by BCG. The consequences of these studies for future protocols combining chemotherapy and immunestimulation with BCG are also discussed.

Materials and Methods

A detailed description of materials and methods is given elsewhere [10, 11]. Briefly, female mice of an inbred C57Bl/6 strain (Orléans La Source, France) were used at 9–10 weeks of age and were inoculated i.p. on day 0 with 10^5 isogeneic tumor cells from a transplantable, lymphoid leukemia (EAkR) [1]. The tumor cells (TC) had a physiologic age of 6 days at inoculation for the experiments. The mice were randomized into a control group and a BCG-treated group. The latter received weekly injections i.v. of 1.0 mg BCG (7×10^6 viable u/mg) (Pasteur Institute, France), starting on day +1 after tumor inoculation and given a maximum of eight times. Both the control group and the BCG group were further randomized into subgroups: one group of 30 mice for the survival curve, and groups of varying size for determination of the tumor growth curve and the detailed immunologic and cytokinetic analyses. The dates of use of the latter groups were decided a priori, and serum and lymphoid cells from spleen and lymph nodes collected from each mouse.

The tumor growth curve was determined by counting every 2nd day, from the time of inoculation, the number of tumor cells in the ascites using the method of KLEIN and RÉVÉSZ [7].

Cytotoxicity Assays Tumor cells with a physiologic age of 6 days and aspirated under sterile conditions were used as target cells in all the following tests:

1. Complement-dependent cytotoxic antibodies (CDCA). The source of complement was fresh rabbit serum [2] of 10^6 cells/ml in RPMI-1640 medium. Tumor cells were incubated with antibody in various dilutions in wells of microplates (Falcon Plastics, No. 3040) at 37°C for 30 min. The cells were washed twice after incubation in a dilution of 1:24 and incubated for 45 min at 37°C. The cytotoxic index was estimated by trypan blue.

2. Direct lymphocyte-mediated cytotoxicity (DLC). All tests were performed in microplate. TC were incubated with the lymphoid cells on a rocking platform for 18 hours at 37°C in a humified atmosphere of 95% O_2 and 5% CO_2. TC:lymphocyte ratio was 1:100.

3. Antibody-dependent lymphocyte-mediated cytotoxicity (ADLMC). The same microplate technique as for the DLC assay was employed. Serum and lymphoid cells were from the same mouse. The TC:lymphocyte ratio was in all experiments 1:100, while serum was added in dilution 1:225. Incubation condition and length were as for the DLC assay.

The cytotoxic index was computed as (CW-EW)/CW. 100%, where CW is the number of TC in control wells and EW the TC number in experimental wells.

The cell kinetic analysis was performed on days 4, 10, and 18 after tumor-cell inoculation. The stathmokinetic method [5] was used to evaluate the percentage of tumor cells entering mitoses per hour (mitotic rate, MR). On the day of the kinetic analysis, eight control and eight BCG-treated mice were injected with Colcemid ^{R} (CIBA) at 11 a.m., and at the same time, the ascitic tumor cell number in eight other mice from each group was determined and smears prepared for evaluation of the mitotic index, autoradiography, and cytophotometry (see below). The Colcemid-treated mice were killed 3 hours later (i.e., at 2 p.m.), and again smears were prepared of the ascitic cell population and the percentage of mitoses in the tumor cell population (mitotic index, MI), for each mouse at least 1000 tumor cells, and the mitotic rate then computed. To estimate the percentage of DNA-synthesizing tumor cells in the ascites, the mice used for MI-determination at 11 a.m. received an injection i.v. of $10 \mu Ci[^3H]$-TdR (sp.a. 25 Ci/mM; CEA, France) at 10 a.m. Slides for autoradiography were dipped in Kodak K-2 emulsion, exposed for 10 days, developed, fixed, and stained with May-Grünwald-Giemsa and the percentage of labeled tumor cells (labelling index, LI) was determined for each mouse among at least 1000 cells.

Cytophotometry was used to determine the percentage of distribution of the ascitic tumor cell population within the mitotic cell cycle. The slides were Feulgen-stained [10] and a Zeiss UMSP-I was used for the measurements.

Statistics

Wilcoxons nonparametric test was used in all significant tests.

Results

Table 1 shows that the median survival time of control mice was significantly below the median survival time of BCG-treated mice that died. It is furthermore seen that BCG treatment cured about 24% of the mice.

The tumor growth curve (Fig. 1) of control mice followed the classic gompertizian form. The mice in the BCG-treated group are seen to be subdivided into two groups: one group

Table 1. Survival of mice inoculated i.p. on day 0 with 10^5 EAkR-leukemic, not treated or treated with weekly injections i.v. of 1.0 mg BCG

	Controls	BCG-treated 1 mg i.v./week
Median survival time of mice that died of leukemia	15.6 ± 2.2 (SE) days	17.3 ± 3.7 (SE) [a]days
Percent of mice cured	0	24

[a] Significantly ($p < 0.05$) different from controls.

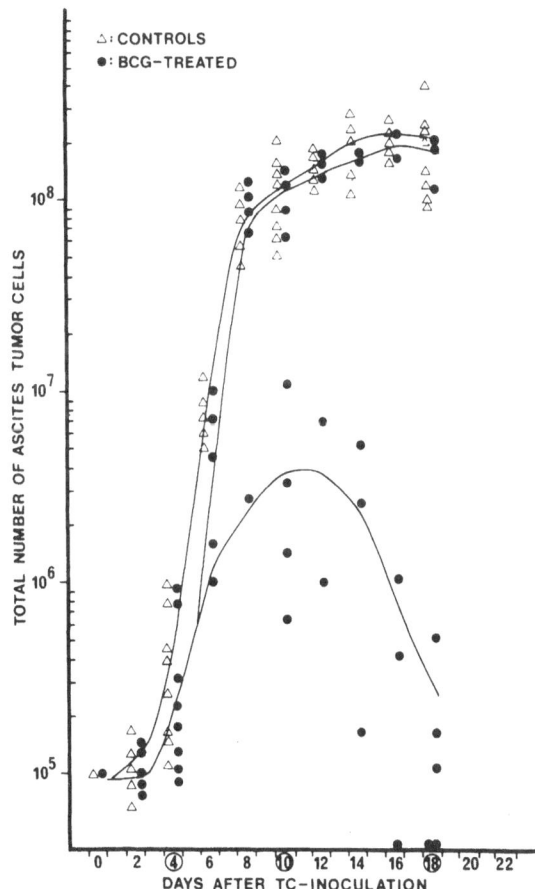

Fig. 1. Total number of tumor cells in the ascites at various times after inoculation i.p. of 10^5 tumor cells on day 0. The growth curve of control mice was drawn by hand through the control mean of each test day. BCG-treated mice were from day 6 on and for the rest of the experimental period clearly divided into one group with values at the control level and another group with values below the controls. Two growth curves for the BCG group were therefore drawn, one through the means of values at the control level and one through the means of values below the controls. Each point was obtained from a different mouse. Note that the ordinate scale is logarithmic

with a tumor mass equal to that of the controls and another group with a tumor mass significantly ($p < 0.01$) below that of the controls. In the following, these two subgroups will be called the progressor group and the regressor group, respectively.

Table 2 shows that no tumor cell cytotoxic antibodies could be detected in sera from control mice. A weak cytotoxic activity was seen in sera from BCG-treated mice, but the activity was without relation to the tumor mass.

Table 2. TC-CDCA in sera from individual mice. The values indicate in percent the mean tumor cell lysis ± SE of values from 3–8 mice

Days after tumor cell inoculation	Dilution of serum	Controls	BCG-treated	
			regressor[a]	progressor[b]
4	1:16	7% ± 3%	NT[c]	6% ± 3%
13	1:16	9% ± 2%	21% ± 5%	24% ± 7%
22	1:16	6% ± 4%	11% ± 4%	14% ± 5%

[a] Mice with a tumor mass significantly ($p < 0.05$) below controls.
[b] Mice with a tumor mass equal to controls.
[c] Regressor and progressor mice could not be distinguished on day 4.

In the DLC assay (Table 3), only some of the lymphoid cell suspensions could be tested against tumor cells, because some lymph nodes and spleens were heavily infiltrated with tumor cells at days 13 and 22, and the ratio TC:lymphoid cell was thus higher than 1:100. A weak DLC activity could be observed in lymphoid cell suspensions from both lymph nodes and spleens, but without correlation to the tumor mass.

In the ADLMC assay (Table 4), it was equally necessary to exclude some lymphoid cell suspensions due to a high number of tumor cells in the suspensions. The ADLMC activity was low in all groups on day 4, while a high activity was observed on days 13 and 22 in the regressor group, and only in this group.

The results of the cell kinetic analysis are shown in Table 5. It is seen that the kinetics as evaluated by MI and LI are identical for the controls and progressor mice, with a low proliferative activity on day 4, high proliferative activity on day 10, and again slow

Table 3. DLC assay. The tumor cell cytotoxicity of lymphoid cells from spleen and lymph nodes was tested in individual mice and given in percent as the mean ± SE of values from 3–8 mice

Days after tumor cell inoculation	TC:lymphocyte ratio	Lymphoid organ	Controls	BCG-treated	
				regressor[a]	progressor[b]
4	1:100	Spleen	37% ± 9%	NT[c]	35% ± 11%
		Lymph nodes	0		
13	1:100	Spleen	NT[d]	9% ± 4%	NT[d]
		Lymph nodes	0	8% ± 6%	5% ± 3%
22	1:100	Spleen	NT[d]	0	NT[d]
		Lymph nodes	NT[d]	0	NT[d]

[a] Mice with a tumor mass significantly ($p < 0/05$) below controls.
[b] Mice with a tumor mass equal to controls.
[c] Regressor and progressor mice could not be distinguished.
[d] TC:lymphocyte ratio $> 1:100$.

Table 4. ADLMC with lymphoid cells and sera from identical mice. The values are given in percent tumor cell lysis and represent the mean ± SE of the values from 3–8 mice

Days after tumor cell inoculation	TC:lymphocyte ratio	Dilution of serum	Lymphoid organ	Controls	BCG-treated	
					regressor[a]	progressor[b]
4	1:100	1:225	Spleen	22% ± 6%	NT[c]	21% ± 4%
			Lymph nodes	0	NT[c]	0
13	1:100	1:225	Spleen	NT[d]	72% ± 6%	NT[d]
			Lymph nodes	5% ± 3%	61% ± 10%	2% ± 1%
22	1:100	1:225	Spleen	NT[d]	64% ± 6%	NT[d]
			Lymph nodes	NT[d]	57% ± 9%	NT[d]

[a] Mice with a tumor mass significantly ($p < 0.05$) below controls.
[b] Mice with a tumor mass equal to controls.
[c] Regressor and progressor mice could not be distinguished.
[d] TC:lymphocyte ratio > 1:100.

proliferation on day 18. In contrast to this, regressor mice had high proliferative activity on day 18. A group of BCG-treated mice had on day 4 a higher proliferation rate when compared to controls and other BCG-treated mice. These mice were found in another study [10] to be regressor mice. In the regressor group, the MI is high and the LI low on day 10, and from the MI, the proliferation seems faster than in the controls, while the LI suggests the opposite. The cytophotometric measurements show a high number of cells in the G_2 phase and a low number of cells in G_1. The percentage of S phase cells is 24 and thus in agreement with the autoradiographic studies. Comparing the high MI value with the cytophotometric results, it is furthermore evident that the proliferation must be faster in the regressor group on day 10 than in the controls.

Table 5. Some cell kinetic parameters of the ascitic tumor cell population. The values are the means ± SE of values from 3–8 mice

Days after tumor cell inoculation	Cell kinetic parameter in %	Controls	BCG-treated	
			regressor[a]	progressor[b]
4	Mitotic index	3.2% ± 0.9%	5.7% ± 0.8%	3.0% ± 1.1%
	Labeling index	28.4% ± 2.9%	30.1% ± 1.7%	46.8% ± 2.3%
	G_1 cells	79%	64%	80%
	S cells	13%	32%	11%
	G_2 cells	8%	4%	9%
10	Mitotic index	5.8% ± 2.1%	8.8% ± 1.9%	6.1% ± 1.1%
	Labeling index	41.0% ± 5.1%	24.1% ± 3.1%	43.8% ± 4.7%
	G_1 cells	57%	17%	61%
	S cells	29%	24%	34%
	G_2 cells	14%	59%	5%
18	Mitotic index	0.5% ± 0.3%	6.1% ± 2.4%	0.6% ± 0.1%
	Labeling index	14.3% ± 3.4%	63.1% ± 6.7%	12.9% ± 1.8%
	G_1 cells	73%	22%	76%
	S cells	12%	57%	15%
	G_2 cells	15%	21%	9%

[a] Mice with a tumor mass significantly ($p < 0.05$) below controls.
[b] Mice with a tumor mass equal to controls.

Discussion

The survival curves and tumor growth curves confirm and extend earlier investigations on both the leukemia model used in this study and on L1210 leukemia [9]. In these studies, tumor regression first became apparent in the second phase of the gompertizian curve, whereas in the present study, differences in cell-cycle kinetic parameters could be observed in some BCG-treated mice compared to controls already in the transition from phase 1 to phase 2 of the gompertizian curve, indicating a very early tumor-reductive effect of BCG. The lack of correlation of CDAC and DLC activity with tumor regression suggests a minor role of these two immunologic mechanisms in the BCG-induced tumor-growth control. The rather weak DLC of lymphoid cells from the spleens of mice in all experimental groups and the complete absence of DLC activity in lymph node cells may indicate that a subpopulation of T-lymphocytes in the spleen is cytotoxic to tumor cells without prior stimulation. It is tempting to speculate that this cytotoxic cell belongs to the group of autoreactive lymphocytes that have been demonstrated in leukemic and adjuvant-treated mice.

ADLMC was only high in mice with a tumor cell number below that of the controls and was thus closely related to the ascitic tumor size. As, furthermore, the peritoneal fluid in mice with a low tumor cell number contained almost only lymphocytes [11], it seems reasonable to suggest that ADLMC in our model has an important role in the BCG-induced mechanisms that lead to tumor reduction. A similar importance of this immune mechanism has been suggested in other tumor systems of both mice and human beings [6, 12, 13].

The cell kinetic analysis is only preliminary in this study. It shows clearly, however, that the proliferative activity of the tumor in regressor mice is significantly higher than in control and progressor mice. The results furthermore suggest that the tumor cells are selectively killed in the G_1 and/or early S phase.

This has of course to be elaborated further. An important aspect seems to be whether the ADLMC mechanism has higher affinity for cells in the G_1 and early S phase compared to the other phases of the cell cycle. If it has, this will give further support to the hypothesis [11] that the ADLMC is important in BCG-induced tumor growth control.

References

1. AMIEL, J. L., BERARDET, M.: Induction d'une leucémie isogénique virale de Gross chez des C57B1/6 adultes par des injections répétées de cellules leucémique AkR. Rev. Franc. Etud. Clin. Biol. *14*, 587–589 (1969).
2. BOYSE, E. A., STOCKERT, E.: Improved complementation in the cytotoxicity test. Transplantation *10*, 446–449 (1970).
3. CALDER, E. A., IVINE, W. J., GHAFFER, A.: K-cell cytotoxic activity in the spleen and lymph nodes of tumour-bearing mice. Clin. Exp. Immunol. *19*, 393–397 (1975).
4. DEVLIN, R. G., McCURDY, J. C., BARONOWSKY, P. E.: Mixed lymphocyte reactivity against normal cells by splenic lymphocytes from tumour-bearing mice. II. Studies of auto-immune-like activity in completely syngeneic and semisyngeneic systems. J. Exp. Med. *139*, 230–237 (1974).
5. DUSTIN, P.: The quantitative estimation of mitotic growth in the bone marrow of rat by the stathmokinetic (colchinic) method. In: The Kinetics of Cellular Proliferation. Stohlman, F. (ed.). New York: Grune and Stratton, 1959, pp. 50–57.
6. JONES, J. T., McBOIDE, W. H., WEIR, D. W.: The in vitro killing of syngeneic cells by peritoneal cells from adjuvant-stimulated mice. Cell. Immunol. *18*, 275–283 (1975).
7. KLEIN, G., RÉVÉSZ, H.: Quantitative studies on the multiplication of neoplastic cells in vivo. I. Growth curves of the Ehrlich and MCIM ascites tumors. J. Natl. Cancer Inst. *14*, 229–272 (1953).
8. MATHÉ, G.: Introduction to active immunotherapy of cancer. It's immunoprophylaxis and immunorestoration. Berlin–Heidelberg–New York: Springer-Verlag, 1976, Vol. I, pp. 400.

9. Mathé, G., Pouillart, P., Lapeyraque, E.: Active immunotherapy of L1210 leukemia applied after the graft of tumor cells. Brit. J. Cancer 23, 814–824 (1969).
10. Olsson, L., Mathé, G.: The effect of BCG on the growth of a murine leukemia: a cytokinetic analysis. Cancer Res 37, 1743–1749, 1977.
11. Olsson, L., Florentin, I., Kiger, N., Mathé, G.: The effects of BCG on the growth of a mouse leukemia: various cellular and humoral parameters of the effect of antibodies and lymphoid cells to tumor cells and their correlation to tumor growth in vivo. In press, J. Natl. Cancer Inst.
12. O'Toole, C., Stejskal, V., Perlmann, P. et al.: Lymphoid cells mediating tumor-specific cytoxicity to carcinoma of the urinary bladder. J. Exp. Med. 139, 457–465 (1974).
13. Pollack, S., Heppner, G., Brown, R. J. et al.: Specific killing of tumor cells in vitro in the presence of normal lymphoid cells and sera from host immune to the tumor antigens. Int. J. Cancer 9, 316–323 (1973).

4. Monitoring

Biochemical Aids to Cancer Management

E. H. COOPER

The clinical biochemist has an important role to play in the evaluation of new strategies for the improvement of the immediate and long-term end results of cancer management. In the past, clinicians relied on the laboratory to help in the recognition and treatment of the gross disturbances of metabolic balance that arose as the result of mechanical obstruction of the major systems by cancer, such as the uretus, bile ducts and intestinal tract. Equally, it has long been known that cancer may produce a variety of paraneoplastic syndromes and disturbances of normal regulatory mechanisms. Fever, cachexia, dermatomyositis, hypertrophic pulmonary arthropathy, neuropathy, defects of bone marrow cell production and coagulation. Some of the mechanisms of these complications can be explained biochemically, others cannot; if we were able to identify the regulatory molecules, it might be an advance in medicine.

New techniques in biochemistry have resulted in specific sensitive tests for many hormones, and their advent has greatly enriched contemporary knowledge of the tumours of endocrine origin as well as tumours that can mimic endocrine tissue by inappropriate hormone production. This has given the clinician powerful tools for studying the evolution of a few cancers, the level of circulating β human chorionic gonadotrophin (HCG) in choriocarinoma being the classical example of how a specific test can guide the treatment plan, as the β HCG production is proportional to the number of viable tumour cells [1].

It was hoped that tumour-associated antigens (TAA), especially α-fetoprotein (AFP) and the carcinoembryonic antigen (CEA), might have changed our total approach to many common forms of cancer. However, as experience has built up, clinicians and laboratory scientists have adopted a more cautious attitude, whilst acknowledging that the TAAs are important as markers, they have become increasingly aware of their shortcomings (for recent reviews see [5, 6, 9].

To appreciate the nature of the problem, the clinician's requirements must be clearly identified and then we can see if tests presently available fulfill these needs.

The research on tumour markers has coincided with reappraisal of the treatment of solid tumours to find the right combination of treatment modalities to deal with both the local tumour and its distant metastases. The most difficult part of this strategy is to appreciate the behaviour of the metastases when they are too small to detect clinically, or without procedures such as laparotomy that usually occur once in a planned sequence of treatment. Consequently, there are three major situations in which cancer monitoring tests should be valuable:

1. In the earlier detection of metastases
2. In the evaluation of the effects of therapy on the recurrence of a metastatic cancer
3. To aid in the assessing of the prognosis undergoing a potentially curative treatment

This argument can be illustrated by considering colorectal, bladder cancer. Several of the points are applicable to other common types of cancer, though the logic has to take into account the behaviour patterns of the individual tumours, especially their favoured sites for metastatic growth.

Colorectal Cancer

The hope that CEA would be a valuable test for the primary diagnosis of cancer has not been fulfilled. Dukes A and B tumours may not be associated with a raised CEA and an inflammatory disease of the bowel often produces moderate increases of CEA. On the other hand, serial measurements of the level of CEA in the blood after resection of a primary tumour can provide the clinician with evidence of recurrence of metastases many months ahead of their detection clinically. As the liver is a common site of metastases in colorectal cancer, it is expedient and informative to combine the measurement of CEA with a sensitive marker of liver function. A rise of serum gamma glutamyl transpeptidase (GGT) is more of a sensitive indicator of hepatic metastases than alkaline phosphatase, 5'nucleotidase or the transaminases [3, 8]. However, in our experience, a rise of CEA will tend to precede the rise of GGT, sometimes by a few months.

Compared to the surgeon's assessment of the abdomen at laparotomy, the combined CEA and GGT tests are still relatively insensitive. His eye can detect small metastases in liver or in the peritoneum which may remain undetectable biochemically for several months after resection of the primary tumour. Once these tests show a *rising* value, it is probable that the tumour is well-established. A rising CEA alone gives no clue as to the site of the metastases. Recently, MILFORD WARD et al. [7] have investigated the possibilities of using disturbances of the individual proteins in the α_1 and α_2 globulin group, the acute phase reactant proteins, as aids in monitoring large bowel cancer. They suggest that a raised CEA with a disproportionate increase of haptoglobin might indicate a recurrence involving the bowel wall. For a series of 70 patients, they have evidence that the preoperative levels of CEA, α_1 antitrypsin and α_1 acid glycoprotein can be combined to provide a discriminant to identify patients who will eventually develop metastases after a "curative resection". The combination appears to be a better discriminant than the preoperative CEA titres alone, only time will tell if it is reliable when used in larger trials.

The experience of colorectal cancer has focussed our attention on the possibility of devising simple multiparametric tests to monitor other types of cancer. The test battery is well-known in clinical biochemistry in which a group of parameters are measured for the individual levels as well as the pattern of their change collectively; liver and renal function tests and the electrolytes are typical examples. Immense experience has gone into the ultimate choice of tests included in the battery—in cancer, this approach was used as an attempt to improve diagnosis and generally abandoned, due to lack of specificity. Now it is here revived in the context of monitoring where serial observations and detailed knowledge can narrow the probability of interpretation of the results.

Bladder Cancer

This is a typical example of a cancer in which assessment is largely clinical, repeated cystoscopy being the crucial investigation backed up by occasional urography and possibly cytology. The problem is to assess the extent of the local invasion and the distant metastases which will occur in about 30% of bladder cancer deaths [4]. CEA is of limited value for surveillance due to cross-reacting CEA-like substances in infected urine but the blood levels may be helpful in those advanced cancers that produce this antigen.

The identification of hepatic metastases can be made from a rising serum GGT, and invasion of bone can cause elevation of the alkaline phosphatase (ALP) level above 60 Iu/l; as ALP is an indicator of both bone and hepatic metastases, it is uncertain from a raised

GGT and ALP whether this indicates liver or liver and bone metastases. However, analysis of the ALP by electrophoresis and heat stability may help to resolve this question, particularly if the ALP is above 100 Iu/l.

In common with many forms of cancer, invasive bladder cancer is associated with significant uses of haptoglobin, α_1 antitrypsin and α_1 acid glycoprotein. Members of the EORTC urological group are attempting to develop a multiparametric system for monitoring invasive bladder cancer, the parameters mentioned above have emerged as the most likely constituents of the system. This is more than an academic exercise as spread of the tumours outside the pelvis means that standard combinations of surgery and radiotherapy are only palliative. The recent studies of BROSS et al [2] suggest that metastases may be a cascade process with the liver and lung acting as critical forces from which tumours disseminate to distant organs and tissues. Biochemically, there are moderately good systems to detect tumours in the liver; there are no specific organ markers for lung, and bone metastases produce valuable disturbances of the blood phosphatases and hydroxyproline excretion depending on their osteolytic or osteosclerotic properties.

We still have need for simple tests for tumour cells in sites such as the lung or peritoneal cavity. Two well-known markers of cancer, increased phosphohexose isomerase activity in the blood [10] and the reversal of the lactic dehydrogenase isoenzyme patterns, are worth careful longitudinal studies; perhaps these systems were abandoned too soon in the past. The interest needs to focus on an asymptomatic patient who has a tumour burden— unfortunately, earlier studies are plagued with a surfeit of data on the hopeless terminal case, which produce dramatic biochemical changes but virtually no impact on the clinician's decision making process.

References

1. BAGSHAWE, K. D.: Tumour associated antigens. Brit. Med. Bull. *30*, 68 (1974).
2. BROSS, I. D. J., VIADANA, E., PICKREN, J.: Do generalized metastases occur directly from the primary? J. Chronic Diseases *28*, 149 (1975).
3. COOPER, E. H., TURNER, R., STEELE, L., NEVILLE, A. M., MACKAY, A. M.: The contribution of serum enzymes and carcinoembryonic antigens to the early diagnosis of metastatic colorectal cancer. Brit. J. Cancer *31*, 111 (1975).
4. COOPER, E. H., WILLIAMS, R. E.: The biology and clinical management of bladder cancer. Oxford: Blackwells (1975).
5. GALEN, R. S.: Multiphasic screening and biochemical profiles: state of the art. Prog. in Clin. Pathol. *6*, 83 (1975).
6. GO, V. L. M.: Cancinoembryonic antigen. Cancer *37*, 562 (1976).
7. MILFORD WARD, A., COOPER, E. H., TURNER, R., ANDERSON, J. A., NEVILLE, A. M.: Acute phase reactant protein profiles: an aid to the monitoring of large bowel cancer by carcinoembryonic antigen and serum enzymes. Brit. J. Cancer *35*, 170 (1977).
8. MUNJAL, D., CHAWLA, P. L., LOKICH, J. J., ZAMCHECK, N.: Carcinoembryonic antigen and phosphexose isomerase, gamma glutamyl transpeptidase and lactate dehydrogenase levels in patients with and without liver metastases. Cancer *37*, 1800 (1976).
9. NEVILLE, A. M., COOPER, E. H.: Biochemical monitoring of cancer. Ann. Clin. Biochem. *13*, 283 (1976).
10. SCHWARTZ, M. K.: Laboratory aids to diagnosis—enzymes. Cancer *37*, 542 (1976).

Laboratory Testing for Cancer

L. H. REES

Introduction

For many years innumerable claims have been made for blood tests capable of detecting the presence of clinically occult cancer, but none of the many 'cancer tests' has withstood detailed evaluation. However, some are available with potential use in screening for neoplasia, for making the initial diagnosis, for localisation of occult neoplasia and monitoring response to therapy, and for early detection of tumour recurrence. The whole field has recently been critically reviewed by NEVILLE and COOPER [54]. Cancer testing can be divided into observations on (1) immunological phenomena associated with cancer, (2) substances produced in response to tumours, (3) tumour-derived products and (4) miscellaneous tests.

Immunological Phenomena Associated with Cancer (Table 1)

Table 1. Immunological phenomena associated with neoplasia

1. Macrophage electrophoretic mobility (MEM)
2. Structuredness of the cytoplasmic matrix
3. Microcytotoxicity
4. Leucocyte migration inhibition
5. Leucocyte adherence inhibition

1. Macrophage Electrophoretic Mobility (MEM) Test

This test has attracted considerable attention as a possible diagnostic procedure in patients with malignant disease and has been reviewed elsewhere [9, 27].

The MEM test originated from the observation that patients with multiple sclerosis were sensitised to myelin basic protein (MBP), a constituent of nerve and brain tissue. Peripheral lymphocytes obtained from the patient are incubated with MBP and the supernatant fluid from the reaction added to guinea pig peritoneal macrophages. The macrophage electrophoretic mobility is measured in a cytopherometer before and following this incubation [28]. Slowing of the macrophages indicates a positive response and the observation is presumed to depend upon lymphokine production caused by the interaction between the MBP and the lymphocytes, subsequently reducing the negative electrostatic charge on their surface [28]. The MEM test was applied to sera from a variety of patients with carcinomatous neuropathies and spinocerebellar degeneration; all showed lymphocyte sensitisation. However, a 'control' group (cancer patients without carcinomatous neuropathy) was observed to be sensitised. Subsequently, a cancer antigen extracted from tumour tissue, cancer basic protein (CBP) [24], was observed to give better discrimination and this was employed in all future tests.

However, the method has limitations as a 'test' for the presence of cancer. Thus, false positives occur in patients with a variety of neurological and inflammatory diseases. In contrast, false negatives may be recorded in patients with very advanced or rapidly growing neoplasia [29], and it is of interest that once a test is positive it will remain so for many years, despite complete tumour resection or apparent 'cure'.

The technical problems associated with the MEM test have limited its widespread application. However, improvements in the design of the cytopherometer may mean that the MEM test could be applied to particular populations at special risk.

2. Structuredness of the Cytoplasmic Matrix (SCM)

The development of this test followed observations made during studies of the cell reproductive cycle using a measurement of the degree of polarization of fluorescent light production by cells in the presence of a nonfluorescent substrate, (fluorosceindiacetate), during exposure to polarized light [16, 48]. When CBP is added to the lymphocytes, cancer and control patients are more easily discriminated. It is proposed that the basis of the test is an alteration in the structuredness of the lymphocyte cytoplasmic matrix soon after contact with a previously encountered antigen.

Addition of phytohaemagluttinin (PHA) to the same test system allows even greater discrimination between the cancer and noncancer groups [17].

However, in contrast to the MEM test, the SCM test becomes negative after complete eradication of the tumour.

3. Microcytoxicity

The basis of this test is a simple one. Target tumour cells are grown in multiwell plates in the presence of lymphoid cell populations, and growth inhibition or 'death' of the cells is measured by counting the number of adherent cells remaining at the end of the test [38]. This test has been extensively investigated in experimental tumours such as those caused by the murine sarcoma virus (MSV), and both macrophages and T-lymphocytes have been shown to kill such target cells in these assays [56]. However, it is difficult to employ the use of the microcytoxicity test in human cancer for several reasons. Firstly, suitable target tumour cells are difficult to obtain and although transplanted cell lines have been employed, these may have lost the relevant antigen or have acquired a new antigen, possibly associated with virus infection. Secondly, it is difficult to establish the specificity of any observed cytotoxic reaction, since lymphocytes from normal healthy individuals have also been observed to elicit cytotoxic reactions [40, 56, 72]. Until these problems are resolved, the clinical value of the microcytoxicity test remains unclear.

4. Leucocyte Migration Inhibition and Adherence Inhibition Tests

Various other in vitro tests have been investigated [20, 22, 36]; thus, the leucocyte migration inhibition test is used to assay lymphokines released from sensitised T-lymphocytes in patients with cancer [22], but these tests are also difficult to evaluate, since adequate controls have not been included in most of the studies.

From this brief account of the in vitro immunological tests currently employed in assessing cellular immunity in patients with cancer, it is clear that although data obtained from animal tumours appear promising, studies in the human are far from complete. If immunotherapy is to be of more value in cancer treatment, then well-established in vitro tests are imperative in the assessment of response to therapy.

Substances Produced in Response to Neoplasia (Table 2)

Table 2. Substances produced in response to neoplasia

---

1. Hydroxyproline
2. Ferritin
3. Polyamines
4. Nucleosides and nucleotides

---

1. Urinary Hydroxyproline

Hydroxyproline is a constituent of collagen, most of which is found in bone, and metabolic studies have shown that urinary excretion of hydroxyproline is related to bone matrix turnover. Increased excretion of hydroxyproline will occur in patients with many bone diseases, including those with metastatic bone cancer, and it occurs also in some patients with malignant disease who have only nonosseous metastases [37]. However, the ratio of urinary hydroxyproline to creatinine (OHP/C) is more sensitive than the measurement of urinary OHP alone, and it has been shown to be raised before bony metastases are apparent clinically, radiologically or by bone scanning [59]. The OHP/C ratio is also more sensitive than measurement of serum alkaline phosphatase or urinary calcium in the detection of bony metastases and is also useful in the assessment of therapeutic response in patients with established metastases [57].

2. Ferritin

A fetal ferritin-like α_2 globulin called α_2H has been detected in the sera of 80% of 452 children with cancer [15], and its measurement used to monitor recurrence of childhood hepatoma, where it appears to be a more sensitive marker than α-fetoprotein (AFP). Similarly, in adults, it has been shown to have potential value as an indicator of recurrent head, neck and colorectal cancer [54].

3. Polyamines

Raised levels of urine and serum polyamines (spermine and spermidine) occur in association with a variety of neoplasia [23], usually in an advanced stage. These substances play a regulatory role in cell growth by influencing nucleic acid biosynthesis and function [69]. Thus, polyamine levels will rise concomitantly with increased protein synthesis [67] and, since they are not metabolised rapidly, high levels will be observed in patients with cancer. Unfortunately, high levels are also seen in those with active inflammatory or regenerative diseases. As with the other techniques described above, because of lack of specificity, the measurement of polyamines may be of little value in initial diagnosis but is still useful in the assessment of response to treatment.

4. Nucleosides and Nucleotides

In recent years, sensitive techniques such as radioimmunoassay and gas-liquid chromatography-mass spectrometry have become available for the measurement of the methylated nucleosides and nucleotides, in particular pseudouridine and the methylated bases, N^2-dimethylguanosine and 1-methylinosine. A raised urinary excretion of these substances has been shown in patients with a wide variety of neoplasia including the leukaemias and Hodgkin's disease as well as carcinomas of bronchus, breast, ovary and testis and levels tend to be higher with the more advanced diseases [2, 25, 73]. Again, high levels may be observed in patients with chronic inflammatory disease [25].

Tumour-Derived Products

1. Pregnancy-Specific β_1 Glycoprotein (SP$_1$ or PSβG) and Pregnancy-Associated α_2 Glycoprotein (PAM)

This protein can be detected in plasma of pregnant women; levels rise during gestation and reach a plateau in the last 4 weeks. SP$_1$ has been measured in patients with trophoblastic neoplasia and serial determinations may prove of value in assessment of this disease. More recently, localisation of SP$_1$ by immunostaining of tumour tissue from patients with breast cancer has been used to predict prognosis [42]. This substance has also been detected in other tumours [43]. However, criticisms of these studies [32, 41] have mainly been directed at the specificity of the antisera employed as well as at the lack of inclusion of adequate controls. PAM can be detected in pregnancy plasma, levels rising during gestation and falling within 6 weeks post partum. PAM has been measured in patients with a variety of neoplasia and used to monitor therapy, levels falling after successful surgery and rising before the appearance of overt metastases [70, 71].

These are listed in Table 3.

Table 3. Tumor-derived products

---

1. Pregnancy specific proteins
2. Products normally specific to the fetus, e.g. CEA, AFP
3. Products normally specific to the placenta, e.g. HCG,
   β-HCG subunit, HPL, placental alkaline phosphatase
4. Products normally specific to the lactating women, e.g.
   human milk casein and other milk proteins
5. Other hormones
   Ectopic: ACTH, ADH, thyrocalcitonin, etc.
6. Other enzymes

CEA = carcinoembryonic antigen; AFP = α-fetoprotein;
HCG = human chorionic gonadotrophin;
HPL = human placental lactogen;
ACTH = adreno corticotropic hormone;
ADH = antidiuretic hormone.

2. Fetal Products

a) Carcinoembryonic antigen (CEA)
This glycoprotein was first detected in the liver, pancreas and gut of the human fetus during the middle trimester of intrauterine life. Later, high concentrations were detected in primary and metastatic neoplasia arising in the colon and rectum [35]. However, following

the development of more sensitive radioimmunoassay techniques for its measurement, CEA-like immunoreactivity was detected in normal adult tissues and in a wide variety of neoplasia as well as in the plasma of patients with inflammatory diseases (Table 4).

Table 4. Incidence of raised plasma CEA levels in various neoplastic and nonneoplastic disorders[a]

	Disorder	Incidence (%) of raised plasma CEA levels
Neoplastic		
	Colon	73
	Pancreas	92
	Liver	67
	Bronchus	72
	Breast	52
	Uterus	53
	Ovary	36
Nonneoplastic		
	Ulcerative colitis and Crohn's disease	21
	Cirrhosis and alcoholic disease	42
	Chronic bronchitis and emphysema	25
	Fibroadenosis	7

[a] Data from LAURENCE and NEVILLE (1972), BARRALET and MACH (1975) and NEVILLE and COOPER (1976).

Nonetheless, since plasma CEA levels may relate to the site and extent of tumour tissue spread [49], sequential CEA measurements in individuals can be employed in early detection of tumour recurrence. Thus, in a large series of patients with colorectal cancer followed in a collaborative, multicentre study [54], CEA was measured at each outpatient attendance. In 53 of the 220 patients studied, recurrence of tumour occurred during the 2-year study, and 36 of these had raised CEA levels (>40 ng/ml). Twenty-six of these did not have clinicallly overt disease when plasma CEA levels were first raised, and the authors conclude that about 75% of their patients will have developed rising CEA levels postoperatively either at the same time as clinical recurrence but usually before. Rising CEA titres tend to occur when metastases are hepatic [19] and this measurement combined with a rise in γ-glutamyl transpeptidase (γGT) is strongly suggestive of the liver as the recurrent site. By contrast, when the metastases are in other sites, CEA levels usually rise alone. However, while serial CEA measurements are of value in the follow-up of patients after colorectal resection, similar studies of other neoplasia (for example bronchus and breast) have been less rewarding.

Many groups have studied the potential value of CEA measurements in patients undergoing chemo- or radiotherapy. Although CEA levels may fall, the actual CEA concentration does not necessarily reflect the tumour mass, and transient elevations of CEA levels may be observed shortly after the institution of antitumour therapy [8], presumably reflecting cell death with CEA release. On the other hand, disease may spread without any alteration in CEA concentration [19]. Despite these deficiences, sequential CEA determinations do give the clinician some indication of the effectiveness of therapy.

b) Alpha-fetoprotein (AFP)

This α_1-globulin is a normal product of fetal liver, gut and yolk sac [1], and its measurement had found its greatest clinical potential in the diagnosis of neural tube defects in utero [50, 51]. However, with the introduction of more sensitive techniques, AFP (like CEA) can be detected in plasma from normal people [58]. Originally, high circulating concentrations in the adult were believed to be associated only with primary hepatic neoplasia [65], but with improved techniques, raised immunoreactive AFP levels have even been found in patients with other types of malignancy as well as in regenerative and inflammatory diseases (Table 5). Although most hepatomas do secrete AFP, levels do not appear to relate well to tumour cell mass, and extensive studies have failed to detect raised AFP levels before clinical tumour recognition [58].

Table 5. Incidence of raised AFP levels in various neoplastic and nonneoplastic disorders

Disorders	Incidence of raised AFP levels (%) [a]
Neoplasia	
Liver	89
Biliary tract	25
Pancreas	24
Stomach	15
Colorectal	5
Lung	7
Malignant teratoma	86
Nonneoplastic	
Viral hepatitis	31
Alcoholic cirrhosis	14
Chronic active hepatitis	31
Extrabiliary obstruction	0
Pancreatitis	0
Ulcerative colitis	16
Crohn's disease	7
Peptic ulceration	0

[a] Data from RUOSLAHTI et al. (1974), PURVES et al. (1973), SILVER et al. (1974) and NEVILLE and COOPER (1976).
Adapted from NEVILLE and COOPER (1976).

However, monitoring of AFP levels has proven of exceptional value in one field, in the management of male patients with testicular teratomas [47].

In these patients, AFP concentrations correlate well with the clinical response to both radiotherapy and chemotherapy and can be used to predict relapse in some patients. Certainly both AFP and human chorionic gonadokrophin (HCG) should be measured in all patients either with testicular neoplasia or suspected of having testicular neoplasia [55].

3. Placental Products

The use of HCG assays in clinical management of women with gestational choriocarcinoma has long served as an excellent model for the use of a placental hormone as a biochemical marker of malignancy. Thus, using fully automated immunoassays for HCG and HCGβ, BAGSHAWE [6, 7] has calculated that 10^{-12} g of HCG is secreted by each choriocarcinoma cell in a 24 h period and that approximately 1 mm^3 tumour (1 $\times$ 10^6 cells) can be detected by measuring circulating HCG whilst only 1 cm^3 (1 $\times$ 10^9) can be detected radiologically or clinically [7].

A variety of placental hormones and enzymes are known to be secreted by nontrophoblastic neoplasia and thus constitute 'ectopic' hormone secretion [14, 18, 31, 63]. Thus, about 5% of tumours (mainly of lung, stomach, pancreas, ovary and liver) make human placental lactogen (HPL) and 12% HCG or its free α- or β-subunit. HCG subunits may be secreted without the intact molecule [64]. The efficacy of HCG measurements in patients with metastasised neoplasia undergoing treatment has been assessed [53], and in some instances, HCG levels appear to correlate well with clinical response. However, it is obvious that the close relationship between cell mass and hormone concentration displayed by gestational choriocarcinoma does not, unfortunately, hold true for most ectopic hormone secretion.

Raised alkaline phosphatase levels occur in patients with two main types of carcinoma, hepatic and osseous. It should be noted that metastatic hepatic carcinoma is more often associated with raised levels than is primary hepatoma. In contrast, some primary neoplasia of bone (e.g. osteogenic sarcoma) may often cause greatly elevated alkaline phosphatase levels.

Studies on the placental isoenzymes of alkaline phosphatase [Regan isoenzyme [30]] in patients with cancer have shown that several different phenotypes exist and indeed any one may be unique to each individual patient [44]. However, the actual incidence is in dispute and this may result from the different technologies employed in their measurement [45]. Similarly, there is considerable disagreement about the relationship between the circulating isoenzyme activity and tumour mass [11].

4. Products Normally Specific to the Pregnant or Lactating Woman

Some evaluation of the measurement of two milk proteins, lactoferin and casein in women with mammary carcinoma have been undertaken. Unfortunately, lactoferin lacks specificity because it is a normal constituent of circulating monocytes. By contrast, human milk casein is a normal constituent of human milk and circulates in detectable amounts in a small number of normal males and pregnant females and in high concentrations in lactating women. Using a radioimmunoassay for human milk casein, HENDRICK and FRANCHIMONT [39] demonstrated raised levels in women with carcinoma of the breast although as yet there are few data correlating serum concentrations with the stage of the disease or its response to therapy.

5. Other Hormones

The overall incidence of ectopic hormone secretion is not known and estimates differ widely depending whether they are based on clinical or biochemical criteria (Table 6). Thus, in a group of 43 patients with oat cell carcinoma of the lung, plasma cortisol levels in excess of 10 μg/100 ml were recorded at midnight in 51% and at 9 a.m. following dexamethasone in 49% although only three patients were regarded as having the overt ectopic ACTH syndrome [34]. Similarly, using simultaneous urinary and plasma osmolality measurements, 32% of 56 patients with oat cell lung cancer were found to have inappropriate antidiuretic hormone secretion.

More recently GEWIRTZ and YALOW [33] found immunoreactive ACTH in 93% of primary lung tumours from patients without evidence of overt ectopic ACTH secretion although their afternoon plasma ACTH levels lay above the normal range. Similarly, in a study of 14 unselected lung tumours from patients without evidence of ectopic ACTH secretion, high

Table 6. Incidence of endocrine abnormalities in patients with neoplasia

Syndrome	Incidence (%)	Tumor
Cushing's syndrome	0–2.0	Lung cancer
	2.8	Oat cell carcinoma of lung
	7	Oat cell carcinoma of lung
	49	Oat cell carcinoma of lung
Inappropriate antidiuresis	0.9–2.0	Lung cancer
	8	Oat cell carcinoma of lung
	12	Oat cell carcinoma of lung
	35	Oat cell carcinoma of lung
Nonmetastatic hypercalcaemia	1.0–7.5	Lung cancer
	14	Unselected cancers
	15	Squamous lung cancer
Gynaecomastia	0.5–0.9	Lung cancer
	2.0	Oat cell carcinoma of lung
Hyperthyroidism	0–1.4	Lung cancer

Data taken from Locks (1962), Azzopardi and Whittaker (1969), Kato et al. (1969), Azzopardi et al. (1970), Anderson (1973), Azzopardi, J. G. (personal communication, 1973), Eagan et al. (1974) and Gilby et al. (1975).

tumour concentrations of ACTH were found in the oat cell carcinomas and carcinoids and significantly lower levels in squamous cell and adrenocarcinomas [12].

Several important factors appear to operate which will tend to obscure the true incidence of ectopic hormone secretion (Table 7), and it is more than likely that with the more frequent use of sensitive radioimmunoassay techniques this phenomenon will eventually be shown to be very common [62]. Thus, the measurement of hormones, as well as the substances mentioned earlier, can be used in screening, tumour localisation by differential venous catheterisation, or in the assessment of the response to treatment [60, 61, 63].

In this regard, ACTH measurements have recently been successfully employed to localise two occult neoplasia, one a thymic carcinoid tumour and the other an adrenal phaeochromocytoma and both were successfully resected (L. H. Rees, personal observations). In these patients, ACTH measurements are used at follow-up for the detection of early recurrence. Similarly, ACTH measurements have been employed as a marker of response to chemotherapy in a patient with oat cell carcinoma of the lung, therapy being introduced as ACTH levels rose. Excellent quality of life was achieved for a much longer time than is usual in patients with oat cell lung cancer and ectopic ACTH secretion.

Undoubtedly, the ectopic hormones are easier to study as tumour markers, partly because the secretion of some produces a clearly recognisable clinical syndrome, and much more specific and sensitive techniques are available for their measurement than for the other substances mentioned earlier.

6. Other Enzymes

A detailed assessment of the importance of the wide variety of enzymes found to be present in increased amounts in patients with carcinoma is beyond the scope of this paper. However, studies have been made of sialyltransferase, prolyl hydroxylase, 5'-nucleotide phosphodiesterase, adenosine deaminase and acid phosphatase in a variety of tumours. Unfortunately, either alone or in combination, these enzyme changes can rarely be

Table 7. Factors tending to obscure the true incidence of ectopic hormone secretion

Cause	Examples
1. Inadequate clinical follow-up	Higher incidence of hypercalcaemia (15%) when patients are followed to death
2. Production of a hormone without an easily recognisable clinical effect	HPL, oxytocin, calcitonin
3. Production of a biologically inactive precursor of the hormone	'Big' ACTH, ProPTH
4. Production of a biologically inactive subunit of the hormone	α-glycoprotein hormone subunits
5. Short duration of the illness preventing development of clinical syndrome	GH
6. Operation of normal physiological feedback mechanisms suppressing normal hormone production	ACTH
7. Multiple ectopic hormone secretion	The ectopic secretion of ACTH obscuring the clinical sequelae of simultaneous ectopic ADH secretion
8. The bias of the investigator and his laboratory facilities	

Data of REES (1975).

HPL = human placental lactogen; ACTH = adrenocorticotropic hormone; ADH = antidiuretic hormone; ProPTH = proparathyroid hormone.

considered specific for cancer. However, once the diagnosis of cancer has been made, such enzyme measurements can contribute to the overall spectrum of tests which may be used to monitor the progress of the patient's disease [21].

Miscellaneous Tests

Mathematical Analysis of Biochemical Profiles Although individual tumours may secrete a particular hormone or be associated with a particular biochemical change, the production of multiple hormones and/or proteins by a simple neoplasm is well-recognised [62] and each may be the product of a different cell within the tumour mass [13]. Thus, in some instances, multiple biochemical determinations may summate towards producing a more accurate and earlier diagnosis. For example, large cell bronchial neoplasia can be detected by the measurement of HCG, HCG subunits, HPL and placental alkaline phosphatase [14, 53] hepatomas by the measurement of prolyl hydroxylase with AFP, the presence of liver metastases from large bowel cancer by the simultaneous measurement of γGT and CEA. The secretion of HCG and AFP by testicular teratomas has already been mentioned. TORMEY and colleagues [73] report that 97% of patients with metastatic breast cancer have simultaneously raised levels of CEA, HCGβ and nucleoside N^2,N^2-dimethylgluanosine, observations which undoubtedly have important bearings on prognosis for the patient as well as guiding the physician towards a more rational introduction of chemotherapy and immunotherapy regimes.

Obviously, the use of multiple analyses of this nature requires special high capacity analyzers, facilities for data handling and statistical analysis [68], all of which are still in their infancy.

Conclusions

We must conclude that at this time no 'cancer test' exists. Most of the available tests produce false positives and false negatives so that the use of a multiplicity of tests will give greater discrimination. However, their use in monitoring changes in the disease process, either in detection of tumour recurrence or in response to particular therapy may be of value. Nevertheless, the continued study of the biochemical changes discussed are important in furthering our understanding of the metabolic responses to and consequences of human neoplasia.

References

1. ABELEV, G. I.: α-fetoprotein as a marker of embryo-specific differentiations in normal and tumor tissues. Transplant. Rev. 20, 3–37 (1974).
2. ADAMS, W. C., DAVIS, F., NAKATANI, M.: Purine and pyrimidine excretion in normal and leukemic subjects. Amer. J. Med. 28, 726–734 (1960).
3. ANDERSON, G.: The incidence of paramalignant syndromes. In: Paramalignant Syndromes In Lung Cancer. London: William Heinemann, 1973, p. 4.
4. AZZOPARDI, J. G., FREEMAN, E., POOLE, G.: Endocrine and metabolic disorders in bronchial carcinoma. Brit. Med. J. IV, 528–530 (1970).
5. AZZOPARDI, J. G., WHITTAKER, R. S.: Bronchial carcinoma and hypercalcaemia. J. clin. Path. 22, 718–724 (1969).
6. BAGSHAWE, K. D.: The clinical biology of the trophoblast and its tumours. In: Choriocarcinoma. London: Edward Arnold, 1969.
7. BAGSHAWE, K. D.: Tumour associated antigens. Brit. med. Bull. 30, 68–73 (1974).
8. BAGSHAWE, K. D., ROGERS, G. T., SEARLE, F., WILSON, H.: Blood carcinoembryonic antigen, Regan isoenzyme, and human chorionic gonadotrophin in primary mediastinal carcinoma. Lancet (1973) I, 210–211.
9. BALDWIN, R. W., EMBLETON, M. J.: Assessment of cell-mediated immunity to human tumour associated antigens. Int. Rev. exp. Path. 17, 49–95 (1977).
10. BARRALET, V., MACH, J-P.: Variations of the carcinoembryonic antigen level in the plasma of patients with gynecologic cancers during therapy. J. Amer. Obstet. Gynec. 121, 164–168 (1975).
11. BELLIVEAU, R. E., YAMAMOTO, L. A., WASSELL, A. R., WIERNIK, P. H.: Regan isoenzyme in patients with haematopoietic tumors. Amer. J. Clin. Path. 62, 329–334 (1974).
12. BLOOMFIELD, G. A., HOLDAWAY, I. M., CORRIN, B., RATCLIFFE, J. G., REES, G. M., ELLISON, REES, L. H.: Lung tumours and ACTH secretion. Clin. Endoc. 6, 95–104 (1977).
13. BRAUNSTEIN, G. D., MCINTIRE, K. R., WALDMANN, T. A.: Discordance of human chorionic gonadotrophin and alpha-fetoprotein in testicular teratocarcinomas. Cancer 31, 1065–1068 (1973a).
14. BRAUNSTEIN, G. D., VAITUKAITIS, J. L., CARBONE, P. P., ROSS, G. T.: Ectopic production of human chorionic gonadotrophin by neoplasms. Ann. Int. Med. 78, 39–45 (1973b).
15. BUFFE, D., RIMBAUT, C., LEMERLE, J., SCHWEISGUTH, P., BURTIN, P.: Presence d'une ferroproteine d'origine tissulaire, L'α₂H dans le sérum des enfants porteurs de tumeurs. Int. J. Cancer 5, 85–87 (1970).
16. CERCEK, I., CERCEK, B., FRANKLIN, C. I. V.: Biophysical differentiation between lymphocytes from healthy donors, patients with malignant diseases and other disorders. Brit. J. Cancer 29, 345–358 (1970).
17. CERCEK, B., CEREK, L.: Changes in the structuredness of cytoplasmic matrix, SCM, in human lymphocytes induced by PHA and cancer basic protein as measured in single cells. Brit. J. Cancer 33, 539–543 (1976).

18. CHARLES, M. A., CLAYPOOL, R., SCHAAF, M., ROSEN, S. W., WEINTRAUB, B. D.: Lung carcinoma associated with production of three placental proteins. Arch. Int. Med. *132*, 427–431 (1973).
19. CHU, T. M., NEMOTO, T. J.: Evaluation of carcinoembryonic antigen in human mammary carcinoma. J. Nat. Cancer Inst. *51*, 1119–1122 (1972).
20. COCHRAN, A. J., GRANT, R. M., SPILG, W. G., MACKIE, R. M., ROSS, C. E., HOYLE, D. E., RUSSELL, J. M.: Sensitization to tumour-associated antigens in human breast carcinoma. Int. J. Cancer *14*, 19–25 (1974).
21. COOPER, E. H.: The nature of cancer. Ann. clin. Biochem. *13*, 467–470 (1976).
22. CHURCHILL, W. H.: Nat. Cancer Inst. Monogr. *35*, 237 (1972).
23. DENTON, M. D., GLAZIER, H. S., WALLE, T., ZELLNER, D. C., SMITH, F. G.: Clinical application of new methods of polyamine analysis. In: Polyamines in Normal and Neoplastic Growth. Russell, D. H. (ed.). New York: Raven Press 1973, pp. 373–380.
24. DICKINSON, J. P., CASPARY, E. A., FIELD, E. J.: Common tumour specific antigen. I. Restriction in vivo to malignant neoplastic tissue. Brit. J. Cancer *27*, 99–105 (1973).
25. DLUGAJCZYK, A., EILER, J. J.: Studies on 5-ribosyluracil in man. Proc. Soc. exp. Biol. (N.Y.) *123*, 453–457 (1966).
26. EAGAN, R. T., MAURER, L. H., FORCIER, R. J., TULLOH, M.: Small cell carcinoma of the lung: staging, paraneoplastic syndromes, treatment and survival. Cancer *33*, 527–532 (1974).
27. FIELD, E. J.: The immunological diagnosis of human malignant disease. Ann. clin. Biochem. *13*, 495–502 (1976).
28. FIELD, E. J., CASPARY, E. A.: Lymphocyte sensitisation: an in vitro test for cancer? Lancet (1970) II, 1337–1341.
29. FIELD, E. J., CASPARY, E. A.: Lymphocyte sensitisation in advanced malignant disease: a study of serum lymphocyte depressive factor. Brit. J. Cancer *26*, 164–173 (1972).
30. FISHMAN, W. H., INGLIS, N. R., GREEN, S., ANSTISS, C. L., GHOSH, N. K., REIF, A. E., RUSTIGIAN, R., KRANT, M. J., STOLBACH, L. L.: Immunology and biochemistry of regan isoenzyme of phosphatase in human cancer. Nature *219*, 697–699 (1968).
31. GASPARD, U., HENDRICK, J. C., REUTER, A. M., FRANCHIMONT, P.: Dosage radioimmunologique de l'hormone chorionique sommatamammotrope humaine (HCS) par lés immunoadsorbant anticorps. Ann. Biol. Clin. (Paris). *31*, 447–454 (1973).
32. GAU, G., CHARD, T.: Pregnancy proteins in breast cancer. Lancet (1976) II, 627.
33. GEWIRTZ, G., YALOW, R. S.: Ectopic ACTH production in carcinoma of the lung. J. clin. Invest. *53*, 1022–1023 (1974).
34. GILBY, E. D., REES, L. H., BONDY, P. J.: Ectopic hormones as markers of response to therapy in cancer. In: Biological Characterization of Human Tumours. Amsterdam: Excerpta Medica, 1975, pp. 132–138.
35. GOLD, P., FREEDMAN, S. O.: Demonstration of tumor-specific antigens in human colonic carcinomata by immunological tolerance and adsorption techniques. J. exp. Med. *121*, 439–462 (1965).
36. GROSSER, N., THOMSON, D. M. P.: Cell-mediated anti-tumor immunity in breast cancer patients evaluated by antigen-induced leukocyte adherence inhibition in test tubes. Cancer Res. *35*, 2571–2579 (1975).
37. GUZZO, C. E., PACHAS, W. N., PINALS, R. S., KRANT, M. J.: Urinary hydroxyproline excretion in patients with cancer. Cancer *24*, 382–387 (1969).
38. HELLSTROM, I., HELLSTROM, K. E.: Colony inhibition studies on blocking and non-blocking effects of cellular immunity to Moloney sarcomas. Int. J. Cancer *5*, 195–201 (1970).
39. HENDRICK, J. C., FRANCHIMONT, P.: Radioimmunoassay of casein in the serum of normal subjects and of patients with various malignancies. Europ. J. Cancer *10*, 725–730 (1974).
40. HEPPNER, G., HENRY, E., STOLBACH, L., CUMMINGS, F.: Problems in the clinical use of the microcytotoxicity assay for measuring cell-mediated immunity to tumor cells. Cancer Res. *35*, 1931–1937 (1975).
41. HEYDERMAN, E., NEVILLE, A. M.: Immunoperoxidase localisation of pregnancy protein. Lancet (1976) II, 744.
42. HORNE, C. H. W., REID, I. N., MILNE, G. D.: Prognostic significances of inappropriate production of pregnancy proteins by breast cancers. Lancet (1976) II, 279–282.
43. HORNE, C. H. W., REID, I. N., TOWLER, C. M., MILNE, G. D.: Production of pregnancy specific β_1 glycoprotein by non-trophoblastic tumours. Protides of Biological Fluids *24*, 567–570 (1976).
44. INGLIS, N. R., KIRLEY, S., STOLBACH, L. L., FISHMAN, W. H.: Phenotypes of the Regan isoenzyme and identity between placental D-variant and the Nagao isoenzyme. Cancer Res. *33*, 1657–1661 (1973).
45. JACOBY, B., BAGSHAWE, K. D.: A radioimmunoassay for placental-type alkaline phosphatase. Cancer Res. *32*, 2413–2420 (1972).

46. KATO, Y., FERGUSON, T. B., BENNETT, D. E., BURFORD, T. H.: Oat cell carcinoma of the lung. A review of 138 cases. Cancer 23, 681–686 (1969).
47. KOHN, J., ORR, A. H., McELWAIN, T. J., BENTALL, M., PECKHAM, M. J.: Serum alpha fetoprotein in patients with testicular tumours. Lancet (1976) II, 433–436.
48. LAJTHA, L. G.: Fluorescence probe and biochemical characterization of leukaemic cells. Blood Cells 1, 63–65 (1975).
49. LAURENCE, D. J. R., NEVILLE, A. M.: Foetal antigens and their role in the diagnosis and clinical management of human neoplasms: a review. Brit. J. Cancer 26, 335–355 (1972).
50. LEEK, A. E., RUOSS, C. F., KITAU, M. J., CHARD, T.: Raised alpha fetoprotein in maternal serum with anencephalic pregnancy. Lancet (1973) II, 385.
51. LEIGHTON, P. C., GORDON, Y. B., KITAU, M. J., LEEK, A. E., CHARD, T.: Levels of alpha-fetoprotein in maternal blood as a screening test for fetal neural-tube defect. Lancet (1975) II, 1012–1019.
52. LOCKS, M. O.: Incidence of hypercalcaemia in patients with proved carcinoma of the lung. Lancet (1962) II, 165–167.
53. MUGGIA, F. M., ROSEN, S. W., WEINTRAUB, B. D., HANSEN, H. H.: Ectopic placental proteins in non-trophoblastic tumors. Cancer 36, 1327–1337 (1975).
54. NEVILLE, A. M., COOPER, E. H.: Biochemical monitoring of cancer. Ann. clin. Biochem. 13, 283–305 (1976).
55. NEWLANDS, E. S., DENT, S., KARDANA, A., SEARLE, F., BAGSHAWE, K. D.: Serum α_1-feto protein and HCG in patients with testicular tumours. Lancet (1976) II, 744–745.
56. OWEN, J. J. T.: Cellular Immunity. Ann. Clin. Biochem. 13, 485–487 (1976).
57. POWLES, T. J., LEESE, C. L. BONDY, P. K.: Hydroxyproline excretion in patients with breast cancer and response to treatment. Brit. Med. J. 2, 164–166 (1975).
58. PURVES, L. R., BRANCH, W. R., GEDDES, E. W., MANSO, E., PORTUGAL, M.: Serum alpha-fetoprotein VII. The range of apparent serum values in normal people, pregnant women and primary liver cancer high risk populations. Cancer 31, 578–587 (1973).
59. RADOM, S., ZULAWASKI, M., GOLEBIOWSKA, D.: Urinary hydroxyproline, serum alkaline phosphatase calcium and phosphorus in patients with bone neoplasms. Polish Med. J. 11, 810–814 (1972).
60. REES, L. H.: The biosynthesis of hormones by non-endocrine tumours—a review. J. Endocr. 67, 143–175 (1975).
61. REES, L. H.: Concepts in ectopic hormone production. Clin. Endocr. 5, (Suppl.), 363s–372s (1976).
62. REES, L. H., BLOOMFIELD, G. A., REES, G. M., CORRIN, B., FRANKS, L. M., RATCLIFFE, J. G.: Multiple hormones in a bronchial tumor. J. clin. Endocr. Metab. 38, 1090–1097 (1974).
63. REES, L. H., LANDON, J.: Biochemical abnormalities of some human neoplasms. In: Scientific Foundations of Oncology. Symington, T., Carter, R. L. (eds.). London: William Heinemann, 1976, pp. 107–116.
64. ROSEN, S. W., WEINTRAUB, B. D.: Ectopic production of the isolated alpha subunit of the glycoprotein hormones. New Eng. J. Med. 290, 1441–1447 (1974).
65. RUOSLAHTI, E., PIHKO, H., SEPPÄLÄ, M.: α-fetoprotein: immunochemical purification and chemical properties. Expression in normal state and in malignant and non-malignant liver disease. Transplant. Rev. 20, 38–60 (1974).
66. SILVER, H. K. B., DENEAULT, J. GOLD, P., THOMPSON, W. G., SHUSTER, J., FREEDMAN, S. O.: The detection of alpha 1-fetoprotein in patients with viral hepatitis. Cancer Res. 34, 244–247 (1974).
67. SNYDER, S. H., RUSSEL, D. H.: Polyamine synthesis in rapidly growing tissues. Fed. Proc. 29, 1575–1582 (1970).
68. SOLBERG, H. E.: Discriminant analysis in clinical chemistry. Scand. J. Clin. Lab. Invest. 35, 705–712 (1975).
69. STEVENS, L.: The biochemical role of naturally occurring polyamines in nucleic acid synthesis. Biol. Rev. 45, 1–27 (1970).
70. STIMSON, W. H.: Correlation of the blood-level of a pregnancy-associated macroglobulin with the clinical course in cancer patients. Lancet (1975) I, 777–779.
71. STIMSON, W. H., SINCLAIR, J. M.: An immunoassay for a pregnancy-associated alpha-macroglobulin using antibody-enzyme conjugates. Febs. Letts. 47, 190–192 (1974).
72. TAKASUGI, M., MICKEY, M. R., TERESAKI, P. I.: Reactivity of lymphocytes from normal persons on cultured tumor cells. Cancer Res. 33, 2898–2902 (1973).
73. TORMEY, D. C., WAALKES, T. P., AHMANN, D., GEHRKE, C. W., ZUMWATT, R. W., SNYDER, J., HANSEN, H.: Biological markers in breast carcinoma. I. Incidence of abnormalities of CEA, HCG, three polyamines and three minor nucleosides. Cancer 35, 1095–1100 (1975).

II. General Strategy

The Strategy of Cancer Treatment: Introduction

S. K. CARTER

There are many approaches to treating a patient with cancer. Cancer is not a single disease but a multiplicity of diseases with the variation being dependent on the organ system involved. Each type of cancer has its own diagnostic problems and its potential responsiveness to a wide range of therapeutic interventions. Each disease requires its own therapeutic strategy which is a unique blend of the various modalities available for usage. The development of this strategy requires a multidisciplinary input from surgical oncologists, radiation oncologists, medical oncologists, and pathologists. In the past, the various modalities have tended to function as independent units which were welded together in a sequential therapeutic flow for the patient. Each of the therapeutic modalities has developed independently and the thrust and the momentum of their development has led to the situation in which there are more therapeutic research opportunities available than there are therapeutic research resources available. Even with the needed expansion of therapeutic research resources, it is unlikely that more than a small fraction of the available modality-oriented research thrusts can be adequately evaluated. When contemplating this relative embarassment of riches, it must not be forgotten that the final common pathway of modality-oriented development is disease-oriented therapy. What we are faced with today is an inherent conflict in cancer therapy research; the conflict between modality-oriented development and disease-oriented strategy. For any given stage, of any given tumor type, the surgical oncologist offers the potential of more or less radical and innovative procedures. The radiation oncologist offers a range of new fractionation schedules and new delivery systems. The chemotherapist offers an endless mix of new drugs and drug combinations while the immunologist offers a wide range of approaches to immune modulation. Clearly some priorities need to be set, especially when one considers the unlimited numbers of interactions which can occur with combined modality studies. The priorities which have to be set should ideally be worked out within a disease-oriented strategy which takes into consideration the exigencies of the natural history of the disease under various classical therapeutic maneuvers. The id of modality-oriented development has to be tempered by the superego of disease-oriented strategy to most fully develop the ego of maximum therapeutic research benefit to the cancer patient.

One of the most important developments that has impacted on the strategy of cancer treatment has been the full flowering of the combined modality approach into the area of adult solid tumor therapy [5]. The pediatric oncologist has known for a long time the value of a multimodal therapeutic attack because of the results achieved in Wilm's Tumor [9, 17, 18], embryonal rhabdomyosarcoma [14, 15, 19], and Ewing's Sarcoma [11, 13]. This potential is now being appreciated by the clinical oncologists treating breast cancer [1, 10] and the other major cancer killers [3, 6, 8].

Experimentally it has been known for a long time that the control of tumors requires eradication of the last neoplastic cell [16]. Clinically, it has been obvious for many years that surgical removal or radiotherapeutic ablation of "localized" masses has not achieved the desired cancer control in a large number of patients. The oncologists have come to realize that many tumors which are apparently localized are in truth microscopically disseminated.

We do not have the diagnostic tools available to us today to diagnose this, but it is proven when the microscopic dissemination ultimately is manifested as recurrent or clinically evident metastatic diseases. Intensive study of the "natural history" of relapses after surgical or radiotherapeutic curative intent approaches have indicated groups in whom dissemination can be assumed to have occurred at the time of diagnosis in a large percentage of cases. Such groups include breast cancer patients with positive axillary lymph nodes, large bowel cancer cases with disease penetrating through the entire bowel and/or involving the regional lymph nodes, and all curative resection gastric cancer, pancreatic cancer, and lung cancer patients.

If disseminated disease exists at the time of diagnosis, then some therapeutic approach is needed which has the ability to control tumor cells anywhere in the body. The therapeutic modalities which have this potential include chemotherapy, endocrinotherapy, and immunotherapy. Chemotherapy is at this time the master candidate for adjuvant usage to local therapy because of its proven cell kill potential in a wide range of human malignancies. As with surgery or radiotherapy, chemotherapy can be curative or palliative in varying degrees depending upon the individual tumor. By "cure" is meant that the life expectancy of the treated cancer patient is the same as "normal" life expectancy. Specifically, the same as that of a matched cohort in the general population. Cures from drugs alone have been obtained in such diseases as acute lymphocytic leukemia, Hodgkin's disease, diffuse histiocytic lymphomas, tecticular cancer, choriocarcinoma, and Burkitt's tumor [2]. Chemotherapy achieves a high rate of objective tumor regression and enhanced survival in acute myelocytic leukemia, non-Hodgkin's lymphomas, multiple myeloma, adenocarcinomas of the breast and ovary, and the chronic leukemias.

It has long been known experimentally that chemotherapy is more effective when tumor masses are small than when the tumor cell burden is high. The concept of first order kinetic cell kill by drugs (fixed percentage kill rather than fixed number kill per effective dose) means that, with a small tumor burden, total cell kill can be achieved with a reasonable number of repetitive doses which with a large tumor cell burden would still leave residual cells which would eventually develop "resistance" and start to grow again. The assumption underlying the adjuvant chemotherapy trials of today is that the drug regimens which can give objective regressions (greater than 50% shrinkage of measurable tumor mass) in advanced diseases will be able to achieve total cell kill when applied to the microscopic residual disease remaining after surgical removal of the great mass of tumor bulk. The validity of this assumption is borne out by the results of FISHER et al. and BONADONNA et al. [1, 10] in breast cancer and the results of JAFFE et al. and CORTES et al. [7, 12] in osteogenic sarcoma. As indicated earlier, the pediatric oncologist has long seen evidence that this assumption is a correct one.

One of the critical questions that still remains to be determined is what level of activity against advanced disease is required for chemotherapy before successful adjunctive application can be assumed. It is encouraging that L-PAM [4] which causes objective regressions in only 19% of advanced disease patients has been successful in stage II breast cancer. On the other hand, 5-fluorouracil [3] which has equivalent activity in advanced large bowel cancer has not been shown to be successful in Dukes C curative resection cases when utilized after surgery. The explanation probably lies with either the greater residual tumor cell burden in Dukes C colorectal cancer as compared to stage II breast cancer or in a mix of kinetic differences between the tumor types and drug availability at the critical tumor cell sites. Since we do not have the ability to measure any of this at the present time, our explanations must remain hypothetic and our correlations must be made with the available clinical data. At this time, a wide range of single and combination drug regimens are being utilized in combined modality trials (Table 1), and when the data are all available for analysis, perhaps a greater correlation can be made.

The utilization of immunotherapy as an adjuvant to surgery and/or radiotherapy rests on

Table 1. Advanced disease activity and adjuvant study correlation

Optimal activity in advanced disease		Drugs	In adjuvant studies
Breast	50–70%	"CMF"—Cytoxan, methotrexate, 5-FU "CFP"—Cytoxan, 5-FU, prednisone "AC"—Adriamycin + cytoxan "CMFVP"—Cytoxan, methotrexate, 5-FU, vincristine, prednisone	Yes
Colon	40%	Methyl CCNU + 5-FU	Yes
Lung (small cell)	100%	CCNU + cytoxan + MTX	No
Lung (squamous	30%	"BACON"—Bleomycin, adriamycin, CCNU, nitrogen mustard, vincristine	No
Pancreas	20%	5-FU	No
Stomach	40–50%	Methyl CCNU + 5-FU	Yes
Ovary	50%	L-phenylalanine mustard	Yes
Cervix	25%	Cytoxan, bleomycin	No
Endometrium	25%	Progestins	No
Testicle	75–100%	Velban + bleomycin ±platinum ± actinomycin D	No
Prostate	20%	Cytoxan, adriamycin	No
Bladder	30%	Adriamycin, platinum	No
Kidney	10–15%	Velban, progestins	No
Melanoma	20%	DTIC, methyl CCNU	Yes
Head and neck	50%	MTX	Yes
Sarcoma	50–60%	Adriamycin + DTIC + vincristine + cytoxan	Yes
Osteosarcoma	25%	High dose methotrexate—leucovorin rescue, adriamycin	Yes
Esophagus	10%	Bleomycin	Yes

many of the same assumptions outlined for chemotherapy. The critical differences between immunotherapy and chemotherapy at this point in time within the framework of this strategy are as follows: (1) immunotherapy is postulated to kill tumor cells by zero order kinetics (fixed number); (2) immunotherapy is postulated to be able to control only small cell numbers, therefore, (3) regression of advanced disease cannot be utilized as a predictor for adjuvant choice; (4) the correlation of tests, which measures immune response enchancement with immune modulation, and tumor cell control is still not established; and (5) the question of disease specificity with various tools for immune modulation remains to be established. Despite these differences the data of BEKESI and HOLLAND in acute myelocytic leukemia and of MORTON in malignant melanoma presented at this symposium show evidence that immune modulation can be effective in achieving increased control in a combined modality setting.

As we attempt to develop our therapeutic strategies, the importance of adequately staging all patients is easily evident. We need to strike for total international agreement on staging approaches and staging nomenclatures so that we can correlate the massive data which are being reported each year. We need to approach each tumor with clinical staging initially and pathologic staging wherever possible. The conflicts between clinical and pathologic staging systems need to be resolved recognizing that each tumor will have to be staged with an individualized mix of clinical and pathologic techniques as available within the location patterns of spread for each type.

An approach to the therapeutic flow for a tumor and its integration with staging can be shown with breast cancer. The clinical staging determines operability and the potential for making a curative intent therapeutic attack with surgery (clinical stage 1 and 2). The pathologic staging determines the group which will be at a high risk for recurrence (pathologic stage 2) and therefore should be entered in adjuvant protocols as against the good risk group (pathologic stage 1) which would probably best be closely observed and not treated in the postsurgical situation. For each tumor, there will need to be a balance of the recurrence risk with the potential tools for adjuvant therapy (on a disease-oriented basis) as one develops the priorities for combined modality therapeutic research.

We are in an exciting period of therapeutic research in which the potential to increase the control rate of major tumor types is high. If we are to fulfill this potential, we will need to develop even more fully the multidisciplinary input to disease-oriented strategy where it is occurring today in many cancer centers. No longer can any therapeutic modality isolate itself and claim certain tumors and stages for their own. Multimodal cooperation will be the routine of the future.

References

1. BONADONNA, G., BRUSAMALINO, E., VALAGUSSA, P., et al: Adjuvant study with combination chemotherapy in operable breast cancer. Proc. Amer. Ass. Cancer Res. *16*, 254 (Abstract) (1975).
2. CARTER, S. K.: The chemical therapy of breast cancer. Semin. Oncol. *1*, 131–144 (1974).
3. CARTER, S. K.: Large bowel cancer—the current status of treatment. JNCI *56*, 3–10 (1976).
4. CARTER, S. K., SLAVIK, M.: Chemotherapy of Cancer. Ann. Rev. Pharmacol. *14*, 157–183 (1974).
5. CARTER, S. K., SOPER, W. T.: Integration of chemotherapy into combined modality treatment of solid tumors. I. The overall strategy. Cancer Treat. Rev. *1*, 1–13 (1974).
6. COMIS, R. L., CARTER, S. K.: Integration of chemotherapy into a combined modality treatment of solid tumors. III. Gastric cancer. Cancer Treat. Rev. *1*, 221–238 (1974).
7. CORTES, E. P., HOLLAND, J. F., WANG, J., et al: Amputation and adriamycin in primary osteosarcoma. New Engl. J. Mcd. *291*, 998–1000 (1974).
8. DEVITA, V. T., WASSERMAN, T. H., YOUNG, R. C., et al: Perspectives on research in gynecologic oncology. Cancer (1976) (in press).
9. FARBER, S.: Chemotherapy in the treatment of leukemia and Wilms' tumor. J. Am. Med. Assoc. *198*, 826–836 (1966).
10. FISHER, B., CARBONE, P., ECONOMOU, S., et al: L-Phenylalanine mustard (L-PAM) in the management of primary breast cancer—a report of early findings. New Eng. J. Med. *292*, 117–122 (1975).
11. HUSTU, H. O., HOLTEN, C., JAMES, P., et al: Treatment of Ewing's sarcoma with concurrent radiotherapy and chemotherapy. J. Pediatrics *73*, 249–251 (1968).
12. JAFFE, N. J., FREI, E., TRAGGIS, D., et al: Adjuvant methotrexate and citrovorum-factor treatment of osteoseric sarcoma. New Engl. J. Med. *201*, 994–997 (1974).
13. JOHNSON, R. E., POMEROY, T. C.: Integrated therapy for Ewing's sarcoma. Am. J. Roentgenol. *114*, 532–535 (1972).
14. PINKEL, D., PRATT, C.: Embryonal rhabdomyosarcoma. In: Cancer Medicine. Holland, J., Frei, E. (eds.). Philadelphia: Lea and Febiger, 1973, pp. 1900–1907.
15. PRATT, C. B., HUSTU, H. O., FLEMING, I. P., et al: Coordinated treatment of childhood rhabdomyosarcoma with surgery, radiotherapy and combination chemotherapy. Cancer Res. *32*, 606–610 (1972).
16. SKIPPER, H. E., SCHABEL, F. M., WILCOX, W. S.: Experimental evaluation of potential anticancer agents. XIII. On the criteria and kinetics associated with "curability" of experimental leukemia. Cancer Chemotherapy Reports *35*, 1–111 (1964).
17. SULLIVAN, M. P., SUTOW, W. W.: Successful therapy for Wilms' tumor. Texas Med. *65*, 46–51 (1969).

18. Sutow, W. W., Gehan, E. A., Heyn, R. M. et al: Comparison of survival curves 1956 versus 1962 in children with Wilms' tumor and neuroblastoma. Pediatrics *45*, 800–811 (1970).
19. Wilbur, J., Sutow, W., Sullivan, M., et al: Successful treatment of rhabdomyosarcoma with combination chemotherapy and radiotherapy (Abstract). Proceedings American Society of Clinical Oncology, Inc., Chicago, 1971.

1. Leukemias and Hematosarcomas

Treatment of Murine EAkR Lymphosarcoma by Surgery Combined With Systemic or Local Active BCG Immunotherapy Applied Repeatedly

F. Economides, M. Bruley-Rosset, and G. Mathé

Summary

A combined treatment modality incorporating surgery plus BCG immunotherapy was administered to (C57Bl/6 × DBA/2)F1 mice grafted with EAkR lymphosarcoma. A single preoperative local or postoperative systemic BCG administration cured 20–30% of the animals, but did not prolong the survival time of these groups. Repeated s.c. injections of BCG resulted in a significant increase in survival time compared to the group submitted to surgery alone.

In contrast, multiple i.v. injections of BCG before and after surgery were no more effective than surgery alone and were less effective than a single postsurgical i.v. injection in producing cures.

We have concluded that for local BCG therapy, multiple injections before and after surgery are more effective than a single injection. However, for systemic therapy, multiple injections are less effective than a single injection applied postoperatively.

Introduction

It has previously been shown [12] that nonspecific active immunotherapy with BCG is not effective in curing tumor-bearing animals if the number of tumor cells in them exceeds 10^5. It therefore seems logical to apply it for the treatment of residual disease as adjuvant therapy to other procedures capable of reducing the volume of the tumor, e.g., chemotherapy [1, 14, 18], surgery [2, 11, 20], or radiotherapy [15, 22]. Treatment of the tumor by surgery alone does not usually cure the animals since it cannot eliminate adjacent or distant microscopic foci of tumor cells already present at the time of excision.

A treatment modality, however, combining surgery and BCG immunotherapy together has recently been demonstrated to be more effective than either procedure alone [21, 19]. Besides, Morton et al. have reported [16] that local BCG application as adjuvant therapy to surgery increased the duration of remission and the time of survival of his patients suffering from stage II melanoma.

We could show in a previous study [4] that active immunotherapy was more effective if applied systemically after surgery whereas local application yielded better results only if performed before surgical removal of the tumor.

The present work was undertaken to develop further the knowledge that this previous data yielded, by showing the effect of repeated i.v. or s.c. applications of BCG at the site of tumor inoculation before and after surgery.

Materials and Methods

Inbred female (C57Bl/6 × DBA/2)F1 mice of 8–10 weeks of age were purchased from Iffa Credo Laboratories and were grafted with EAkR lymphosarcoma. EAkR lymphosarcoma was induced in C57Bl/6 mice by injecting leukemic cells obtained from AkR mice in which leukemia grew spontaneously. The tumor was kept in ascitic form by weekly i.p. inoculations of 5×10^6 cells. For our study, the (C57Bl/6 × DBA/2)F1 mice were used, in which s.c. injections of 5.10^5 leukemic cells into the right inguinal area resulted in solid tumor growth. This cell concentration had been found to be the minimal dose of tumor cells required to kill 100% of the animals [4].

Surgery
Resection of tumor plus regional lymph node (RLN) was performed 8 days after inoculation since we have shown that at this time, its effect on survival is significantly beneficial over the controls no matter whether the RLN is spared or not [5]. At this stage, no distant metastases were evident and the contralateral lymph node was not infiltrated as shown histologically.

Immunotherapy
Fresh living BCG from the Pasteur Institute at the dose of 1 mg/mouse (5×10^6–10^7 viable u) was injected i.v. or locally (s.c. at the site of inoculation of tumor cells) on days 2 or 10 after inoculation, that is, 6 days before and 2 days after surgery. A second group of animals received two injections of 1 mg of BCG (on days 2 and 8) and a third one three repeated injections (on days 2, 8, and 10) of the same dose. These three groups were compared to those submitted to surgery or immunotherapy alone. Statistical analysis was performed by the nonparametric Wilcoxon test.

Results

Figs. 1 and 2 illustrate the results of our previous experiments on tumor resection plus s.c. or i.v. BCG immunotherapy. It can be seen that while surgery alone failed to cure the animals, the *intravenous* administration of BCG on day 10, that is 2 days *after* operation, cured 30% of the mice (Fig. 1). Similar results were obtained when BCG was given s.c. 6 days *before* operation (on day 2) as is shown in Figure 2, where 30% of the mice survive free of the disease, although survival is not significantly prolonged. It can also be seen that i.v. BCG administration before surgery did not modify its effect (Fig. 2) yielding no prolongation in survival. Even worse results are observed with s.c. BCG *after surgery* (Fig. 1, BCG s.c. on day 10). It seems that this modality caused enhancement of tumor growth and decreased the survival time as compared with the results obtained from surgery alone.
The results of our recent experiments are shown in Figures 3 and 4. Local administration of two injections of BCG (one on day 2, that is 6 days before surgery, and another on the day of tumor excision) cures 20% of animals and prolongs the survival time ($p < 0.05$, Fig. 3). The same is true in Figure 4 which illustrates that the result of three s.c. injections of BCG (days 2, 8, and 10) yields even better results in survival ($p < 0.02$) and cure.
It appears that multiple i.v. injections for systemic active immunotherapy as adjuvant therapy on days 2 and 8 (Fig. 3) and days 2, 8, and 10 (Fig. 4) are no more effective than surgery alone and less effective than a single i.v. injection 2 days after surgery (day 10, Fig. 1) in producing absolute survival.

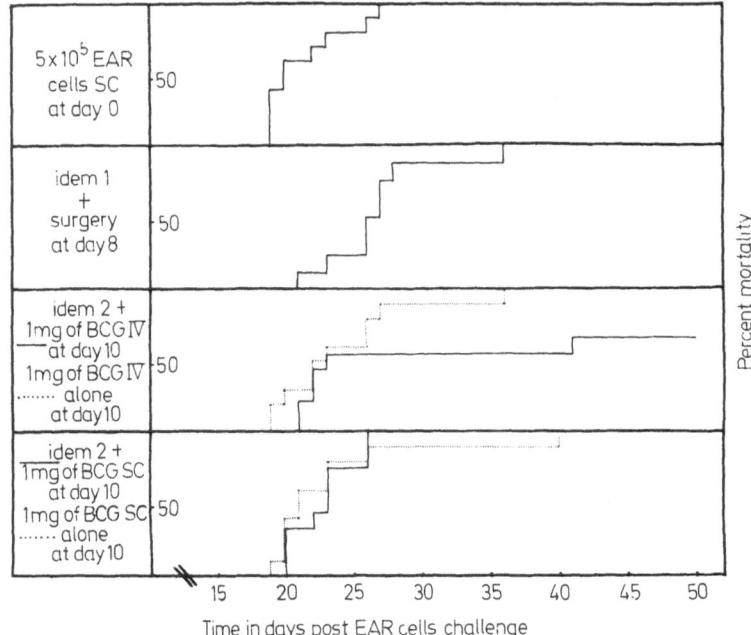

Fig. 1 Effect of BCG immunotherapy and surgery on the survival of (C57Bl/6 × DBA/2)F1 mice bearing EAkR lymphosarcoma.
(———) 1 mg of BCG i.v. or s.c. 2 days after operation (day 8).
(· · · ·) BCG immunotherapy without operation.
Results expressed as mortality in relation to time

Discussion

From the above-mentioned results, we may conclude that, in the case of local (s.c.) active immunotherapy, the multiple injection modality of BCG administration over a period lasting 6 days before operation to 2 days afterward is more effective than a single injection of one dose of BCG (1 mg/mouse). On the other hand, in the case of systemic (i.v.) active immunotherapy, this modality is less effective than a single postoperative injection, and does not yield better results than those obtained with surgery alone. These differences in results could be ascribed to the mode of action of BCG, which, depending on dose and route of administration, causes an antitumor or an enhancement effect, [20, 13, 3, 9, 23], as has been shown in various models. It was interesting to find that one preoperative s.c. injection of BCG (6 days before surgery) and a second injection on the day of operation caused a remarkable antitumor effect, whereas a single postoperative s.c. injection was found to enhance tumor growth.

In preliminary experiments, we found that this enhancement phenomenon after postoperative s.c. BCG was abolished if mice had also been injected with the same dose soon after the tumor excision on day 8 (unpublished results). To have an antitumor effect, an additional dose was needed, as shown in the present work. This could be due to the stimulation of the host immune mechanisms, which prevented the dissemination of the tumor. KHALIL et al. [10] have shown the presence of an histocytic reaction in the site of

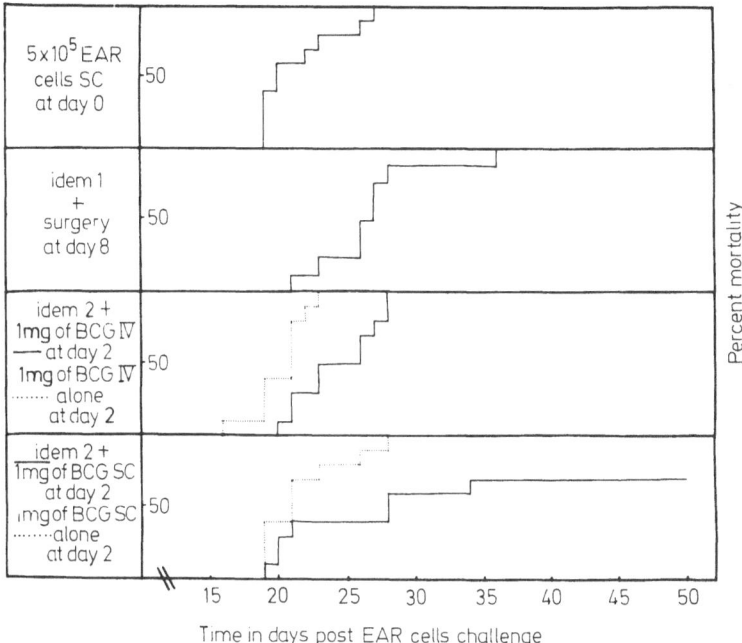

Fig. 2. Effect of BCG immunotherapy and surgery on the survival of (C57Bl/6 × DBA/2)F1 mice bearing EAkR lymphosarcoma.
(————) 1 mg of BCG i.v. or s.c. 6 days before operation (day 8).
(· · · ·) BCG immunotherapy without operation.
Results expressed as mortality in relation to time

BCG injection and in regional lymph nodes where increased trapping of lymphocytes was also seen [24]. Moreover, lymphocytes derived from tumor-draining nodes exhibited a more intense reactivity to mitogens in in vitro stimulation tests [7].

The presence of a "blocking mechanism" produced by BCG administered at a dose causing tumor enhancement could explain why three i.v. injections for systemic immunotherapy did not bring about an antitumor effect superior to surgery. This accumulated dose may have provoked a condition of immunodepression similar to that described by HALLE-PANNENKO [8] and FLORENTIN et al. [6], who demonstrated a decreased number of PFC (Jerne's test) and an induction of suppressor cell activity in the spleens of mice treated with high doses of BCG (3 mg).

References

1. AMIEL, J. L., BERARDET, M.: An experimental model of active immunotherapy preceded by cytoreductive chemotherapy. Europ. J. Cancer 6, 557 (1970).
2. BALDWIN, R. W., PIMM, M. V.: BCG immunotherapy of local subcutaneous growths and post-surgical pulmonary metastases of a transplanted rat epithelioma of spontaneous origin. Int. J. Cancer 12, 420 (1973).
3. BARILETT, G. L., ZBAR, B., RAPP, H. S.: Suppression of murine tumor growth by immune reaction to the Bacillus Calmette-Guérin strain of mycobacterium bovis. J. Nat. Cancer Inst. 48, 245 (1975).

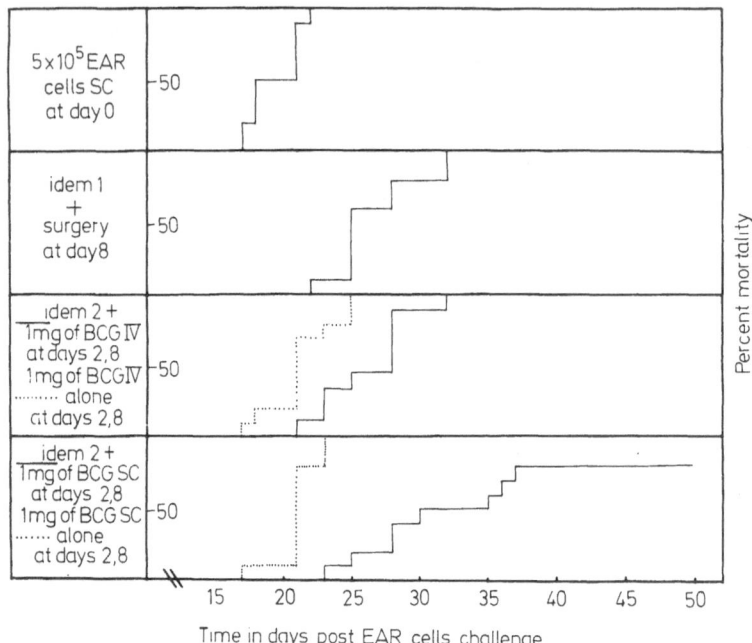

Fig. 3. Effect of repeated BCG injections combined or not to surgery on the survival of (C57Bl/6 × DBA/2)F1 mice bearing EAkR lymphosarcoma.
(———) 1 mg of BCG i.v. or s.c. 6 days before and on the day of operation (day 8).
(· · · ·) BCG immunotherapy on the same days as before but without operation.
Results expressed as mortality in relation to time

4. ECONOMIDES, F., BRULEY-ROSSET, M., MATHÉ, G.: Effect of pre and post surgical active BCG immunotherapies on murine EAkR lymphosarcoma. Biomedicine 25, 372 (1976).
5. ECONOMIDES, F., BRULEY-ROSSET, M., MATHÉ, G.: Effects of the removal of the regional lymph nodes on the survival of mice bearing B16 melanoma or EAkR tumour. Biomedicine 25, 390 (1976).
6. FLORENTIN, I., HUCHET, R., BRULEY-ROSSET, M., HALLE-PANNENKO, O., MATHÉ, G.: Studies on the mechanisms of action of BCG. Cancer Immunol. Immunother. 1, 31 (1976).
7. GOLDFARB, P. M., HARDY, M. A.: The immunologic responsiveness of regional lymphocytes in experimental cancer. Cancer 35, 778 (1975).
8. HALLE-PANNENKO, O.: Comparison of various preparation of BCG in the experimental screening of the EORTC-ICIG. Cancer Immunol. Immunother. 1, 41 (1976).
9. HANNA, M. G., PETERS, L. C.: Efficacy of intralesional BCG therapy in guinea pigs with disseminated tumor. Cancer 36, 4 (1975).
10. KHALIL, A., BOURUT, C., HALLE-PANNENKO, O., MATHÉ, G., RAPPAPORT, H.: Histologic reactions of the thymus, spleen, liver and lymph nodes to intravenous and subcutaneous BCG injections. Biomedicine 22, 112 (1975).
11. LACOUR, F., SPIRA, A., LACOUR, J., PRADE, M.: Polyadeneic-polyuridylic acid, an adjunct to surgery in the treatment of spontaneous mammary tumors in C3H-H mice and transplantable melanoma in the hamster. Cancer Res. 32, 648 (1972).
12. MATHÉ, G.: Immunothérapie active de la leucémie L1210 appliquée après la greffe tumorale. Rev. Franç. Etud. Clin. Biol. 13, 881 (1968).
13. MATHÉ, G., KAMEL, M., DEZFULIAN, M., HALLE-PANNENKO, O., BOURUT, C.: An experimental screening for "systemic adjuvants of immunity" applicable in cancer immunotherapy. Cancer Res. 33, 1987 (1973).
14. MATHÉ, G., HALLE-PANNENKO, O., BOURUT, C.: Immune manipulation by BCG administered before or after cyclophosphamide for chemo-immunotherapy of L1210 leukaemia. Europ. J. Cancer 10, 661 (1974).

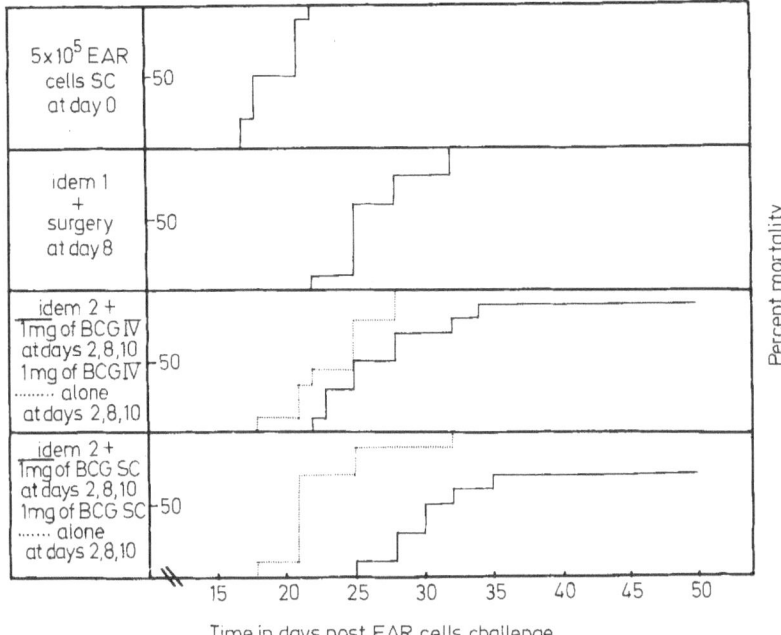

Fig. 4. Effect of repeated BCG injections combined or not to surgery on the survival of (C57Bl/6 × DBA/2)F1 mice bearing EAkR lymphosarcoma.
(————) 1 mg of BCG i.v. or s.c. 6 days before operation, on the day of operation (day 8) and 2 days afterward.
(· · · ·) BCG immunotherapy on the same days as before but without operation.
Results expressed as mortality in relation to time

15. MARTIN, M., BOURUT, C., HALLE-PANNENKO, O., MATHÉ, G.: BCG immunotherapy of Lewis tumor residual disease left by local radiotherapy. Biomedicine 23, 337 (1975).
16. MORTON, D. L., EILBER, F. R., MALMIGREN, R. A., WOOD, W. C.: Immunological factors which influence response to immunotherapy in malignant melanoma. Surgery 68, 158 (1970).
17. NATHANSON, L.: Regression of intradermal malignant melanoma after intralesional injection of mycobacterium bovis strain BCG. Cancer Chemoth. Rep. 56, 659 (1972).
18. PEARSON, J. W., CHAPARAS, S. D., CHIRIGOS, M. A.: Effect of dose and route of Bacillus Calmette-Guérin in chemo-immunostimulation therapy of a murine leukemia. Cancer Res. 33, 1845 (1973).
19. PENDERGRAST, W. J., DRAKE, W. P., MARDINEY, M. R.: A proper sequence for the treatment of B16 melanoma chemotherapy, surgery and immunotherapy. J. Nat. Cancer Inst. 57, 539 (1976).
20. SPARKS, F. C., O'CONNELL, T. X., LEE, Y. T. N.: Adjuvant pre-operative and post-operative immunochemotherapy for mammary adenocarcinoma in rats. Surg. Forum 24, 118 (1973).
21. SPARKS, F. C., BREEDING, J. H.: Tumor regression and enhancement resulting from immunotherapy with "Bacillus Calmette-Guérin" and neuraminidase. Cancer Res. 34, 3262 (1974).
22. YRON, I., COHEN, D., ROBINSON, E., HARBER, M., WEISS, D. W.: Effects of MER and therapeutic irradiation against established isografts and stimulated local recurrence of mammary carcinomas. Cancer Res. 35, 1779 (1975).
23. ZBAR, B., BERNSTEIN, I. D., RAPP, H. J.: Suppression of tumor growth at the site of infection with living Bacillus Calmette-Guérin. J. Nat. Cancer Inst. 46, 831 (1971).
24. ZATZ, M. M.: Effects of BCG on lymphocyte trapping. J. of Immunol. 116, 1587 (1976).

Interspersion of Cyclophosphamide and BCG in the Treatment of L1210 Leukemia and Lewis Tumor

G. Mathé, O. Halle-Pannenko, and C. Bourut

Summary

The therapeutic value of interspersing cyclophosphamide (CPM) chemotherapy and BCG immunotherapy was investigated in two tumor models: L1210 leukemia and Lewis solid tumor (LLT). In the case of L1210 leukemia, the antileukemic effect of CPM was enhanced by subsequent BCG administration where a single cycle of combined treatment was applied; treatment by repeated doses of CPM interspersed with BCG was no more effective than CPM chemotherapy alone. In the case of LLT tumor, the effect of one cycle of combined CPM-BCG treatment was not different from CPM administered alone but treatment by repeated doses of CPM interspersed with BCG immunotherapy was less effective than CPM chemotherapy alone. These results indicate that, while the effect of BCG immunotherapy may be favorable or nil when BCG is applied after cell-reducing chemotherapy, it may be nil or unfavorable when applied repeatedly in interspersed chemoimmunotherapy treatments.

Introduction

Our first experiments on active immunotherapy of L1210 murine leukemia revealed the efficacy of this form of treatment in eradicating the disease only when a small number ($\leqslant 10^5$) of neoplastic cells were present [2]. However, subsequent experiments [3] demonstrated that, even when this necessary condition is fulfilled, individuals may respond in three different ways: (1) complete tumor regression, (2) a "plateau" in tumor growth (lasting as long as 60 days) followed by relapse with a new phase of rapid tumor growth, and (3) no perceptible alteration of tumor growth. A cell kinetic study of the "plateau phenomenon" suggested that the number of "new" cells being produced by the tumor is, in this case, equal to the number of cells being destroyed by immunotherapy, so that an equilibrium is maintained [1]. We wondered if, in such cases, chemotherapy interspersed with immunotherapy might reduce the volume of the tumor enough to enable immunotherapy to eradicate the tumor.

Interspersion of chemotherapy and immunotherapy represents a tempting strategy for tumor therapy. Such interspersion has already been used in clinical trials [7]. We are, nevertheless, reluctant to intersperse chemotherapy and immunotherapy, as we previously showed that, while BCG applied after cyclophosphamide (CPM) is able to cure mice carrying L1210 leukemia not cured by CPM alone, BCG applied before CPM adversely affects the antineoplastic action of the latter [4] and induces a strong immunodepression demonstrated by allogeneic skin graft experiments [5]. Thus, the experiments reported here were devoted to an investigation of the value of interspersing chemo- and immunotherapy.

Materials and Methods

1. In experiments using *L1210 leukemia*, the mice were inoculated i.v. with 10^3 live leukemia cells on day 0. BCG was injected i.v. at the optimal immunostimulating dose of 1 mg/mouse [6], and CPM was injected i.p. at the suboptimal dose of 80 mg/kg [4]. Mice were given one, two, or three cycles of CPM-BCG therapy, one cycle essentially being defined as a single treatment with CPM followed 5 days later by a single injection of BCG. Thus, CPM was administered either on day +1 only or on days +1 and +21, or on days +1, +21, and +41. Similarly, BCG was administered either on day +6 only, or on days +6 and +26, or on days +6, +26, and +46.

2. In experiments using the *Lewis lung tumor (LLT)*, which grows as a solid tumor with lung metastases, 2×10^6 live LLT cells were injected i.m. on day 0. BCG and CPM treatments were identical with the protocol used for the L1210 experiments, except that mice were given only one or two cycles of CPM-BCG therapy.

Mortality was recorded daily and autopsies were made. Differences between groups in the same experiment were analyzed either by the X^2 test (L1210 leukemia) or by Wilcoxon's assigned rank nonparametric test (LLT). Each group contained 16–20 mice.

Results

The results are presented in Figs. 1 and 2. In the treatment of L1210 leukemia (Fig. 1), CPM-BCG combination therapy is more efficient than CPM alone only when the leukemic mice were given a single cycle of treatment. When the animals receive two or three cycles of combined therapy, their survival does not differ significantly from that of control mice treated with CPM alone.

While two injections of CPM are effective in prolonging survival of animals carrying the Lewis tumor (Fig. 2), two cycles of combined CPM-BCG therapy are not effective.

Discussion

These observations confirm (1) the effectiveness of BCG applied as an immunotherapy agent in the treatment of L1210 leukemia and (2) that BCG is more efficient against this disease when applied after CPM chemotherapy than alone [4], at least with an interval of 5 days.

However, the experiment clearly demonstrates that two or three CPM-BCG sequential combinations are much less effective than one such combination.

As BCG induces a powerful antileukemic effect when applied after CPM chemotherapy given only once, one is tempted to wonder if the reduced effect of the repeated administrations of both agents is not due to the deteriorative effect of the interspersed sequence: CPM-BCG-CPM. Indeed, we previously showed that the sequence BCG-CPM, when given once, is less effective than BCG or CPM alone [4]. Moreover, we demonstrated that this sequence is a powerful means of inducing immunosuppression as demonstrated by allogeneic skin graft experiments [5].

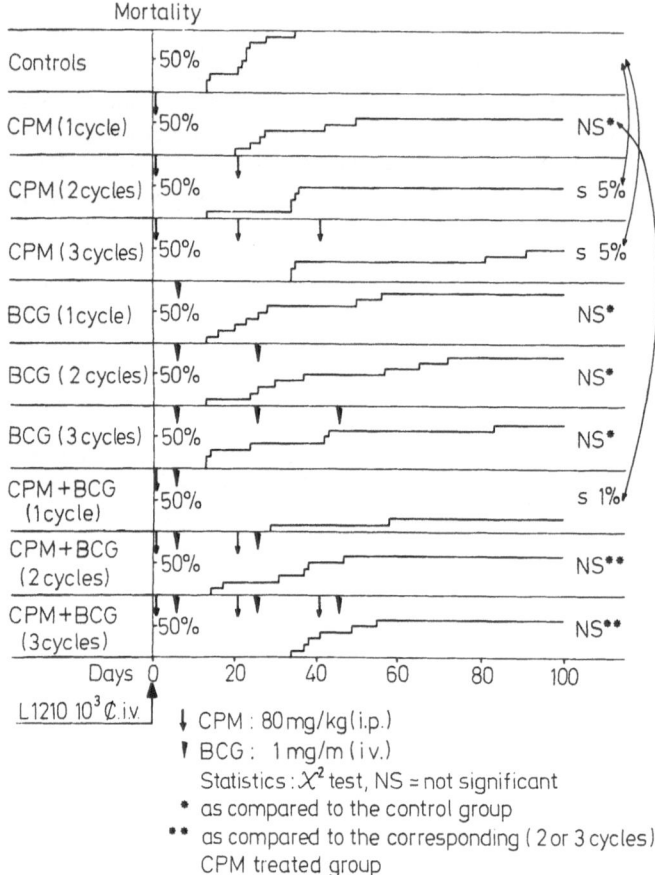

Fig. 1. Interspersion of CPM and BCG for treatment of L1210 leukemia; when their sequential combination is given 2–3 times, the effect is poorer than that obtained by one injection of CPM followed by one administration of BCG

The effects observed on solid Lewis tumors are more complex to explain. A single application of BCG given after a single injection of CPM is no more active than CPM alone; more interesting is the fact that the mice submitted to two sequences of combined CPM-BCG treatment have a significantly shorter survival than those treated by two injections of CPM. This may be due either to the same phenomenon as that observed on L1210 leukemia, namely that BCG applied before CPM adversely affects the effect of the CPM or to a possible growth enhancing effect of BCG on this tumor, which we have already observed [6].

It should be emphasized that such a result, observed when using an immunosuppressive drug such as CPM, may not be found when using a nonimmunosuppressive drug; a later paper will confirm this hypothesis, reporting on an experiment in which the nonimmunosuppressive RFCNU[(chloro-2-ethyl)-1-ribofuranosyl-2'-3' paranitrobenzoate-5')3 nitrosourea)] (unpublished data) was used.

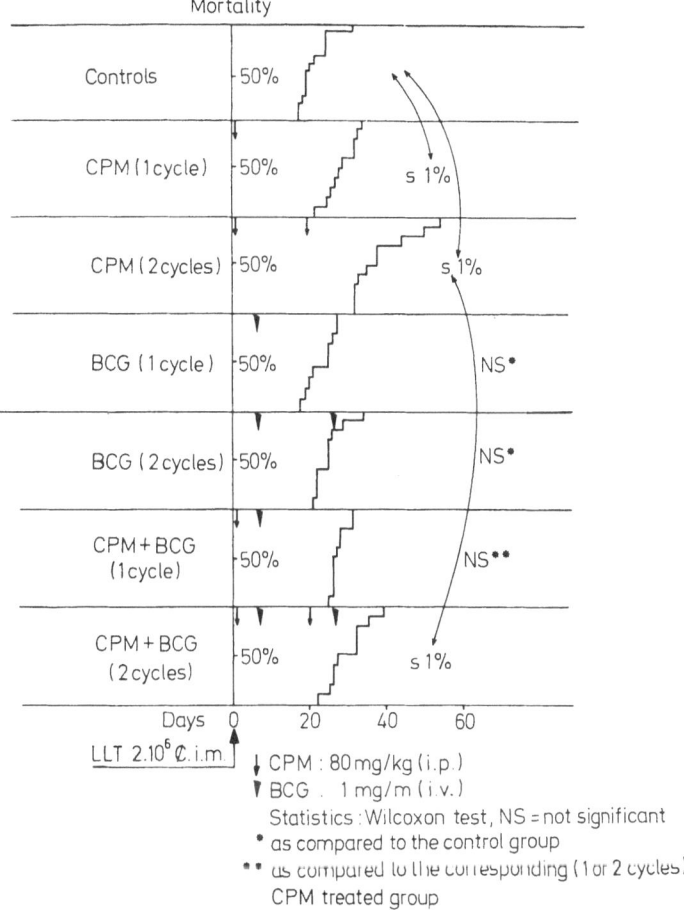

Fig. 2. Interspersion of CPM and BCG for treatment of Lewis tumor; BCG given after CPM does not improve its effect. When applied twice and interspersed with two injections of CPM, it weakens their effect

References

1. LHERITIER, J.: Personal communication.
2. MATHÉ, G.: Immunothérapie active de la leucémie L1210 appliquée après la greffe tumorale. Rev. Franc. Etud. Clin. Biol. 9, 881 (1968).
3. MATHÉ, G., AMIEL, J. L., SCHWARZENBERG, L., SCHNEIDER, M., CATTAN, A., SCHLUMBERGER, J. R., HAYAT, M., DE VASSAL, F.: Active immunotherapy for acute lymphoid leukemia. Lancet (1969) I, 697.
4. MATHÉ, G., HALLE-PANNENKO, O., BOURUT, C.: Immune manipulation by BCG administered before or after cyclphosphamide for chemoimmunotherapy of L1210 leukemia. Europ. J. Cancer 10, 661 (1974a).
5. MATHÉ, G., HALLE-PANNENKO, O., BOURUT, C.: Potentiation of a cyclophosphamide-induced immunodepression by the administration of BCG. Transplantation Proceedings 6, 431 (1974b).

6. MATHÉ, G., KAMEL, M., DEZFULIAN, M., HALLE-PANNENKO, O., BOURUT, C.: An experimental screening for systemic adjuvants of immunity applicable in cancer immunotherapy. Cancer Res. *33*, 1987 (1973).

7. POWLES, R., KAY, H. E. M., McELWAIN, T. J., ALEXANDER, P., CROWTHER, D.: HAMILTON-FAIRLEY, G., PIKE, M.: Immunotherapy of acute myeloblastic leukemia in man. In: Investigation and Stimulation of Immunity in Cancer Patients. Mathé, G., Weiner, R. (eds.). Heidelberg: Springer Verlag, 1974.

Results in Children of Acute Lymphoid Leukemia: Protocol ICIG-ALL 9 Consisting of Chemotherapy for Only 9 Months Followed by Active Immunotherapy

Comparison With the Results of More Prolonged Chemotherapy Protocols

Recognition of Two Groups of Acute Lymphoid Leukemias from Prognostic Parameters

G. Mathé, F. De Vassal, L. Schwarzenberg, M. A. Gil, M. Delgado, R. Weiner, J. Pena-Angulo, D. Belpomme, P. Pouillart, D. Machover, J. L. Misset, J. L. Pico, C. Jasmin, M. Hayat, M. Schneider, A. Cattan, J. L. Amiel, M. Musset, and C. Rosenfeld

In 1962, we started a controlled study (the principle of which was based on our experimental data) [19] to compare active systemic immunotherapy (AI) with no treatment for patients with acute lymphoid leukemia (ALL) after stopping their remission chemotherapy. The difference in remission duration and survival in favor of AI became significant so rapidly [21] that, for obvious ethical and juridical reasons, we were not authorized to introduce more patients than the 30 already in the trial, nor to perform another trial with controls left without treatment. We recently published two critical discussions of this trial [20, 22].

Since then, we have conducted several trials on AI, the overall results of which indicate: (1) the absence of late relapse, the remission curve forming a plateau of cure expectancy after 4 years, (2) the absence of lethal toxicity of immunotherapy, in contrast to the high lethality in remission due to maintenance chemotherapy (4–28%) [see 29], and (3) the possibility of making a prognosis at the beginning of the disease on three parameters: the WHO Reference Center cytologic type [26, 27], the immune (T or null) cell type [2, 3], and the volume of the neoplasia [23].

In 1970, we established a protocol, ICIG-ALL 9, with a *short* duration of remission chemotherapy (9 months) followed by AI; the results after 3–5 years are now available. We can thus: (1) compare these results with those of other protocols conducted by us with more prolonged remission chemotherapy given before the AI or studies conducted by other groups applying only prolonged maintenance chemotherapy [1, 4, 6, 11, 15, 17, 38] and (2) estimate the value of the prognostic parameters mentioned above.

Patients and Methods

Protocol ICIG-ALL 9 is described in Fig. 1, along with protocol 10, for comparison. This Figure shows that protocol 9 comprises only 9 months of remission chemotherapy before immunotherapy, while protocol 10 has a much longer maintenance chemotherapy for 25 months including a combination of 6-mercaptopurine (6-MP), methotrexate (MTX), and cyclophosphamide (CPM) for the latter 18 months of this period.

Thus, we can compare the effect of AI applied between the 9th and the 25th months in protocol 9, with one of the best maintenance chemotherapy programs applied during this period in protocol 10. This is valid comparison as the age and sex ratios and the proportions of children with the two poor prognostic parameters (the incidence of the prolymphoblastic

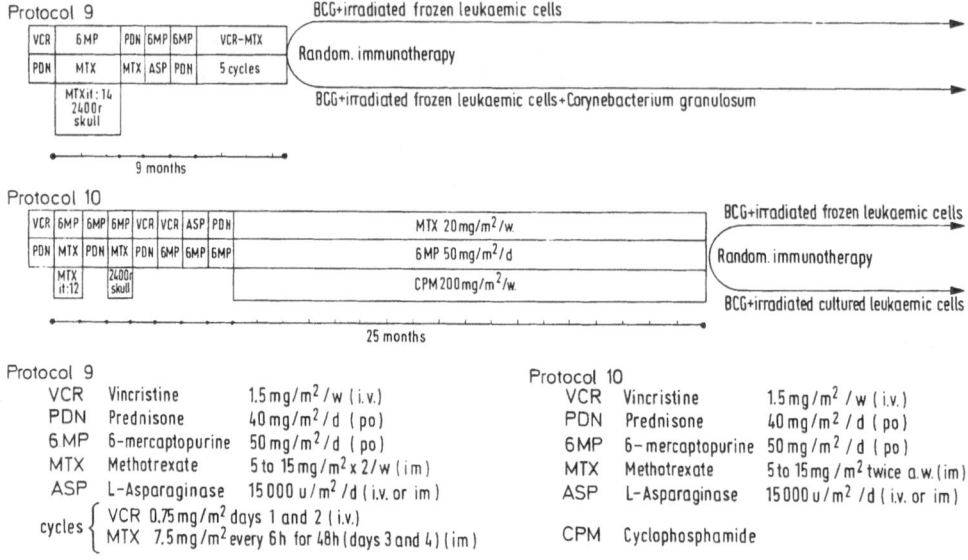

Fig. 1

type and the incidence of the V+ forms [23, 26]) do not differ in these two studies (see Table 1) (see significance of V+ and V− below).

Partial results of the comparison of these protocols in patients of all ages have recently been published [29].

Other conditions allowing this comparison are the absence of differences in the present results between the two branches of AI of the respective protocols: (1) in protocol 9 the addition of *C. granulosum* to BCG and leukemic cells does not improve their effect [29], and (2) in protocol 10, the results of the groups receiving BCG and pooled leukemic cells taken from the patients at the beginning of their diseases and preserved at −196° do not differ from those of the group receiving BCG and leukemic cells of the cultured "Reh" line [28], the cells of which present three markers (including the tumor associated antigen(s)) characteristic of the fresh leukemic cells used for initiating the culture of this line [35].

Comparison of the toxicities of immunotherapy and complementary chemotherapy will be confined to deaths other than from leukemia. A comparison of the results of sperm, lymphocyte chromosome, and bone marrow stem cell investigations carried out on patients submitted to short chemotherapy protocols or to long chemotherapy protocols is under study [30].

We attempted to make a prognosis at the beginning of the disease based on the two parameters mentioned above: (1) the cytologic types of the WHO International Reference Center for the histologic and cytologic classification of the neoplastic diseases of the hematopoietic and lymphoid tissues [27] (prolymphoblastic, macrolymphoblastic, micro-lymphoblastic, and prolymphocytic), and (2) the volume of the neoplasia (we call V+, the cases in which the number of leukemic cells in the blood is $\geq 10,000/mm3$ and/or with spleno-adenomegaly, and V−, the cases in which the number of leukemic cells is $\leq 10,000/mm3$ and/or without spleno-adenomegaly). From our previous work [19, 23], we considered that the microlymphoblastic, V− macrolymphoblastic, and prolymphocytic types were of good prognosis, and that the prolymphoblastic, V+ macrolymphoblastic, and prolymphocytic types of poor prognosis. In 1970, when we started protocol 9, the immune marker study [2, 3] was not yet operational for all patients.

Table 1. Repartition of the patients in protocols ICIG-ALL 9 and 10 according to ages, sex, and prognostic parameters

Protocols	Number of cases	Age	Sex		Cytologic types					Prognostic factors		
			F	M	PLB[a]	PLC[b]	MLB[c]	mLB[d]	Unclassified	MLB and V− MLB and PLC	PLB and V+ MLB and PLC	Unclassified
9	31	2–13 years <5 years: 12 (39%) ⎫ 5–10 years: 14 (45%) ⎬ 84% >10 years: 5 (16%) ⎭	9 29%	22 71%	7 23%	13 42%	4 13%	2 6%	5 16%	10 32%	16 52%	5 16%
10	14	1–13 years <5 years: 8 (57%) ⎫ 5–10 years: 4 (29%) ⎬ 86% >10 years: 2 (14%) ⎭	5 36%	9 64%	3 21%	3 21%	5 36%	1 7%	2 14%	4 29%	7 50%	3 21%

[a] PLB = prolymphoblastic.
[b] PLC = prolymphocytic.
[c] MLB = macrolymphoblastic.
[d] mLB = microlymphoblastic.

Results

1. Overall Results of Protocol ICIG-ALL 9

Of the 31 children under the age of 15 years introduced into the trial, 29 (94%) entered so-called "complete remission" (the two failures were two patients whose disease was of the prolymphoblastic types). Twenty-two children were submitted to immunotherapy and randomized between AI with *C. granulosum* (ten patients) and AI without *C. granulosum* (12 patients).

Fig. 2 gives a curve made according to the direct method [36] of the cumulative duration of first remission. One observes that this curve is broken to form a plateau at the 2nd year for 14 patients out of 29; 13 subjects out of 25, the follow-up of whom is now 50 months, are still in first remission.

Fig. 3 gives the "direct method" curve [36] of the cumulative survival. One sees that 18 out of 30 patients were alive at the 36th month, 17 out of 27 at the 50th month (no deaths occurred between these two dates).

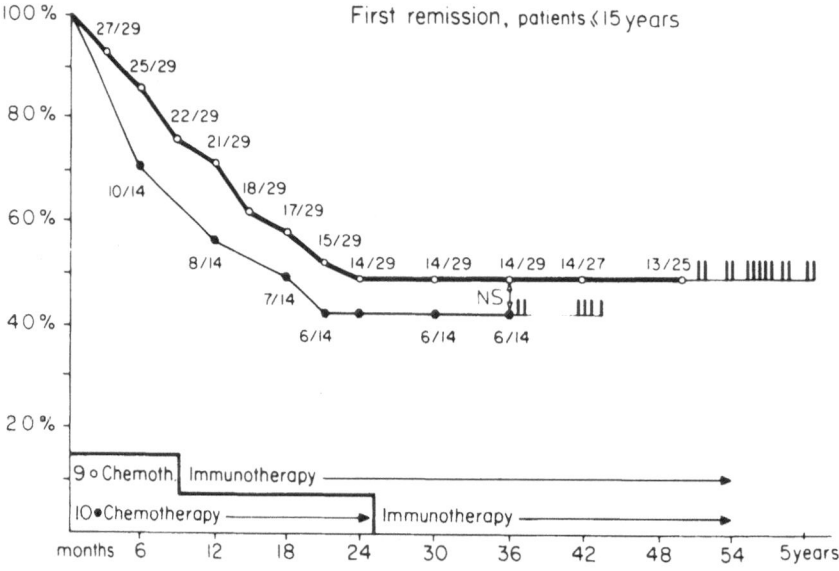

Fig. 2. First remission, patients ≤15 years

2. Comparison of the Results of Protocol ICIG-ALL 9, With Short Preimmunotherapy Chemotherapy, With the Results of Protocol ICIG-ALL 10, With Long Preimmunotherapy Chemotherapy

The comparison of the results of protocol 9 comprising a short postremission chemotherapy (9 months) followed by AI, with those of protocol 10, comprising a 25-month chemotherapy, does not show any significant difference in the proportion of patients belonging to the plateaux of the cumulative remission duration curves (Fig. 2) and the cumulative survival curves (Fig. 3).

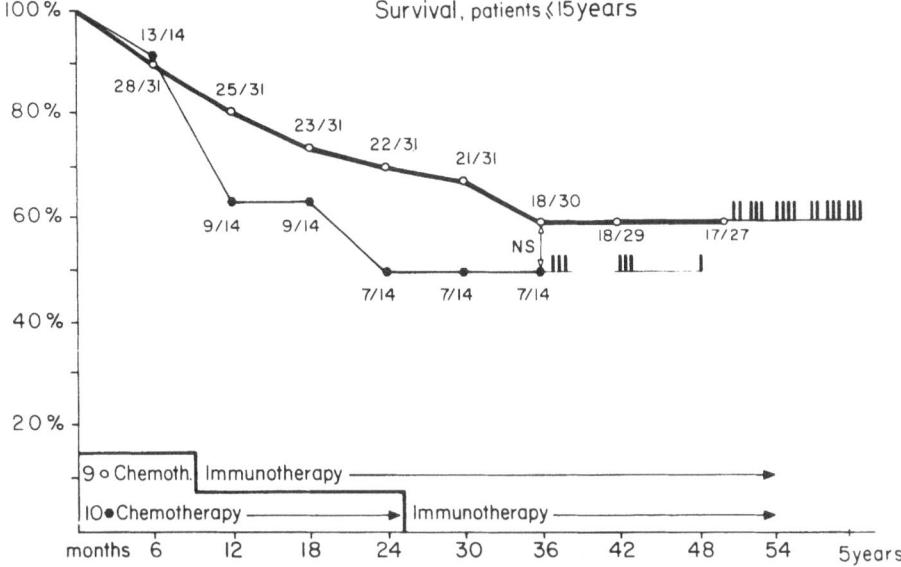

Fig. 3. Survival, patients ⩽ 15 years

3. Results According to the Classification of the Patients on the Prognostic Parameters Available in 1970

Fig. 4 shows a very significant difference between the cumulative remission duration curves of the "good prognostic group" (all microlymphoblastic V− macrolymphoblastic, and prolymphocytic types), and the "poor prognostic group" (V+ macrolymphoblastic, prolymphocytic, and all prolymphoblastic types) of protocol 9: the curve of the first group forms a plateau, expressing cure expectancy, for eight out of ten patients between the 20th and the 50th month, while the curve of the other group only forms plateau for two out of 14 patients (the difference is significant $p < 10^{-4}$).

Fig. 5 shows a similar difference, significant at $p < 0.01$, between the respective curves of cumulative survival of these two groups: the curve of the good prognostic group forms a plateau for nine out of ten patients between the 6th and the 50th month, while the curve of the poor prognostic group forms a plateau for only five out of 15 patients and only between the 42nd and the 50 month.

4. Comparison of Active Immunotherapy Toxicity With Postremission Chemotherapy Toxicity

We regret that there were six deaths during protocols 9 and 10 during the 611 months chemotherapy, in contrast to no deaths during the same length of AI.

The above deaths during chemotherapy were due to chest infections in five cases and a gastrointestinal hemorrhage in one case.

No side effects of AI for protocol 9 have been noted except a slight fever < 38°C the day of BCG application. We do not consider this to be a manifestation of toxicity, but an expression of the BCG bacteriemia which, from our experimental data [14, 34], we regard

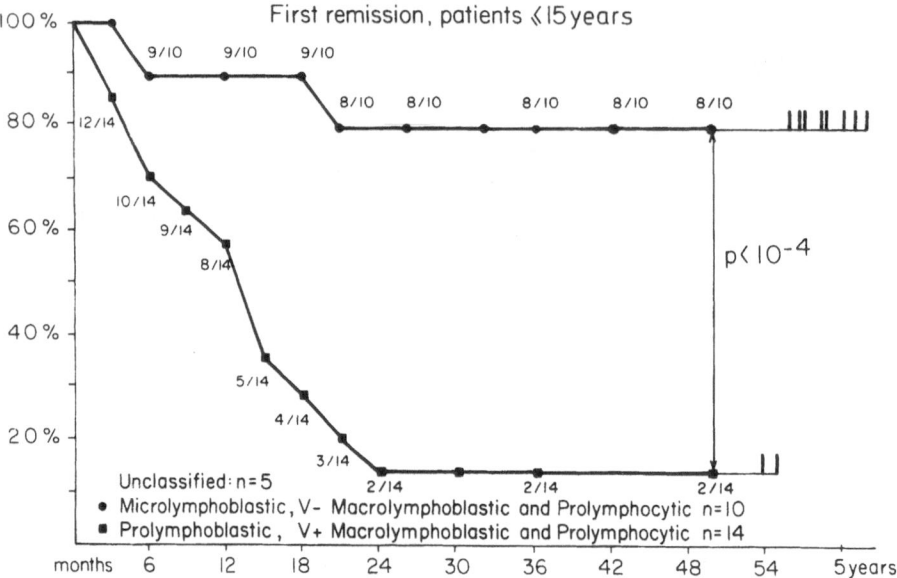

Fig. 4. First remission, patients ≤ 15 years

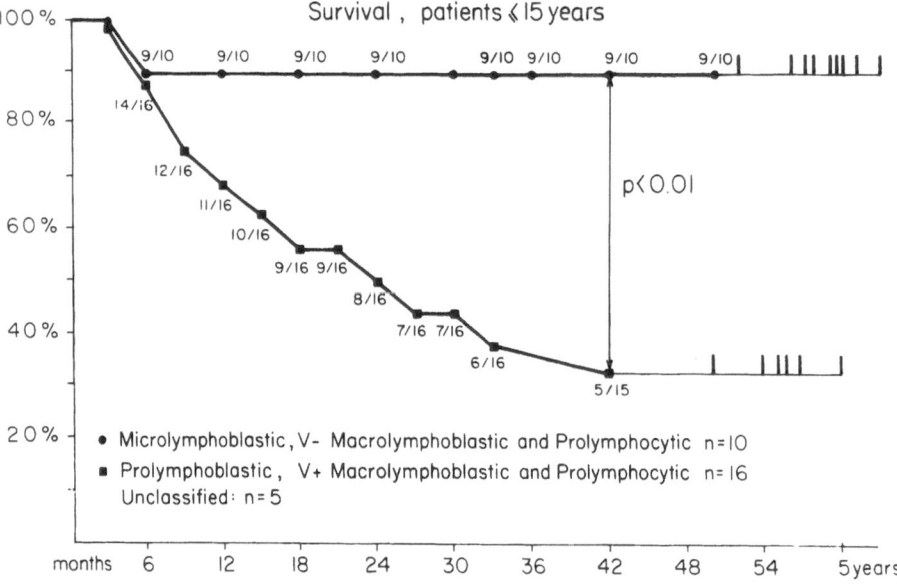

Fig. 5. Survival, patients ≤ 15 years

as necessary for immunotherapy efficacy [18], and which is, therefore, an indication of the correct BCG application.

The comparison of the data on sperm, lymphocyte chromosome, and bone marrow stem cell investigations of the patients submitted, respectively, to short and long chemotherapies will be published later [30].

Discussion

1. Overall Results: Cure Expectancy

The results in children <15 years of age for the ICIG-ALL protocol 9 are remarkable for three features: (1) the break in the curve of first remissions to form a plateau between the 2nd and the 5th year, a plateau which, from other studies, can be considered as a high probability of cure expectancy, (2) the high percentage of all patients treated who are in this plateau of first remission, *about 50% of all children submitted to the trial*, and (3) the still higher proportion (about 60%) of patients who are in the plateau of survivors, with no death between the 3rd and the 5th year.

2. Comparison of the Results of Protocol 9, With Short Preimmunotherapy Chemotherapy, With Those of Protocols With Long Preimmunotherapy Chemotherapy and Those Published in the Literature With Long Maintenance Chemotherapy

a) Protocol 9 Versus Protocol 10: First Remission and Cure Expectancy
Fig. 2 shows that for protocols 9 and 10, the children of which are strikingly comparable for age, sex, and prognostic factors, there is no difference in the percentage of children belonging to each of the remission curve plateaux; in other words, both have a high probability of cure expectancy.
From this comparison, we can deduce that from the 9th to the 25th month, active immunotherapy is as efficient as one of the best maintenance chemotherapies (6-MP, MTX, and CPM).
Survival
Fig. 3 shows that, while the median survival time for protocol 10 patients is 2 years, this median has still to be attained for protocol 9 patients between the 4th and the 5th year. However, the respective proportions of patients belonging to each of the plateaux between the 4th and 5th year are not significantly different.

b) Protocol 9 Results Versus Results of Another Protocol (ICIG-ALL 11), With Long Preimmunotherapy Chemotherapy
We have conducted another protocol, ICIG-ALL 11, with long preimmunotherapy chemotherapy (19 months of 6-MP, MTX, and CPM), but without an initial postremission chemotherapy similar to that of protocols 9 and 10 [24, 25]. Because of this difference, we did not include it in the above comparison. However, it should be mentioned that the proportions of the patients belonging to the first remission and survival plateaux (being 54% and 71%, respectively) are not significantly different from those in protocol 9.

c) Protocol 9 Results Versus Results of Long Maintenance Chemotherapy Protocols Obtained From the Literature
Efficiency
We have also compared the results of protocol 9, comprising short chemotherapy followed by AI, with those of protocols composed of only long maintenance chemotherapy, which are already published or are under publication, and have a follow-up >4 years [1, 4, 6, 11, 15, 17, 38].
From this comparison, it seems reasonable to conclude that a protocol comprising a short complementary cell-reducing chemotherapy followed by AI is as effective as the most efficient branch of the comparable Memphis photocol called "total therapy study VII-1970–1971," comprising a 3-year maintenance chemotherapy [38]; in this branch, 43% of the patients are on the plateau (which is less than for protocol 9, but not significantly

different), while the proportions are 32%, 23%, and 18% for the other branches. It is superior to the other maintenance chemotherapy protocols or branches of protocols published in the literature [4, 6, 11, 17, 38].

With regard to the acute leukemia group B results [1, 15] it appears that, among the numerous branches of protocols 6307–6311, 6313, 6601, 6801, and 7111, two present a survival plateau after 6 years; one branch of protocol 6601 has a plateau for 25% of the patients and one branch of protocol 6801 has a plateau for 65% of the patients, which is no different to the plateau of survival of protocol 9 patients.

The EORTC Hemopathy Working Party [10] has compared maintenance chemotherapy and AI between the 12th and the 24th month after first remission in a randomized trial. They observed no significant difference between the maintenance chemotherapy and immunotherapy branches for remission and survival durations. This observation supports our observation on the comparison of the results of protocol 9 with those of protocols 10 and 11, and allows us to conclude that AI is as active as the best maintenance chemotherapy between the 1st and the 2nd year after remission induction, a period during which no chemotherapist would leave an ALL patient without maintenance chemotherapy.

This conclusion, as well as the results of the study by EKERT et al. [8, 9] showing that chemoimmunotherapy is more active than chemotherapy, can be added to the result of our first pilot trial [20, 21, 22] and to the data presented in this paper, to argue in favor of the efficiency of AI in ALL.

We will only comment briefly on the negative results of three attempts at AI of ALL [12, 16, 31]; these have been discussed more fully elsewhere [20, 22]. Briefly, a negative result does not prove that the method is not effective, but that its application in the given trial was not efficient. Negative results have been registered in immunotherapy trials of other diseases on which the results of most trials have shown the efficiency of this therapeutic weapon [39], and furthermore, negative results have been reported in chemotherapy trials on diseases in which its efficiency has been demonstrated by many other trials [see 7].

Considering the absolute, as well as the comparative results of protocol 9, we can conclude not only that a protocol comprising a short cell-reducing complementary chemotherapy followed by AI is of great efficiency, but also that immunotherapy of ALL is indicated on both scientific and ethical bases.

Toxicity

The above recommendation is not only justified by the efficiency of AI, but also by the differences in the toxicities of AI and maintenance chemotherapy. In over 300 patients who have been submitted to it [19, 37], immunotherapy has not induced a single death in protocols 9, 10, or 11, whereas the lethal toxicity of maintenance chemotherapy varies from 4 to 28% in the literature [see 29].

The EORTC Hemopathy Working Party [10] has confirmed this important fact, registering four deaths out of 29 randomized maintenance chemotherapy patients and none out of 29 immunotherapy patients.

In addition, one must inquire about late side effects and to this end, we are conducting an investigation on sperm, lymphocyte chromosomes, and bone marrow stem cells.

3. Correlation Between Early Prognosis Typing and Disease Evolution

The very marked differences observed between patients submitted to protocol 9 and distinguished at the beginning of their disease on the WHO Reference Center cytologic typing [26, 27] and the volume of the neoplasia [23], as belonging to either the "good prognosis group" (microlymphoblastic, V− macrolymphoblastic, and prolymphocytic types) or the "poor prognosis group" (prolymphoblastic, V+ macrolymphoblastic, and prolymphocytic types) (Figs. 4 and 5) confirm our previous observations [19, 22].

The value of these parameters for prognosis has been confirmed by some research groups treating patients by maintenance chemotherapy only [15, 33] but not by others [13, 32]. Similarly, whereas BROUET et al. [5] do not find any prognostic difference between the T and null cell types of Jean Bernard ALL patients submitted to maintenance chemotherapy, we find that, in the immunotherapy patients, the T type Leukemias relapse rapidly, while the null cell leukemias have a high cure expectancy [2, 3].

Hence, the discrepancies between the different research groups as to the value of prognostic parameters, whether they be due to differences in the populations of treated patients or to differences in the diagnostic criteria used on identical patients in different treatment centers, may also be due to differences in treatments: cytologic and immune parameters do not permit the prognostic groups to be distinguished in Jean Bernard's patients who were submitted to maintenance chemotherapy [5, 13], whereas they do in our patients who were submitted to immunotherapy [2, 3, 23, 26].

This leads us to search for new drugs, treatments combinations, and modalities of applications in order to treat the poor prognosis patients with a more intensive therapy, even if this treatment involves a certain risk. Taking such a risk for the good prognosis patients (with a cure expectancy of 80%) is obviously unethical. Treating the poor prognosis patients with a more intensive therapy than the good prognosis ones has already improved the overall prognosis for patients in our protocol ICIG-ALL 12 compared to protocols 9, 10, and 11.

Summary

Protocol ICIG-ALL 9 with only 9 months remission chemotherapy followed by active immunotherapy has given a cure expectancy (the proportion of the patients on a plateau of first remission) of about 50%, while 60% of the children are on the plateau of survival.

These results do not differ from those of another protocol (ICIG-ALL 10) conducted on an identical population of patients and comprising a 25-month remission chemotherapy before immunotherapy.

This observation, confirmed by a randomized trial of the EORTC Hemopathy Working Party, indicates that, between the 9th and the 25th month, active immunotherapy is as efficient as maintenance chemotherapy.

The overall results of this protocol with short chemotherapy followed by active immunotherapy have been compared with those of another prolonged maintenance chemotherapy before immunotherapy protocol (ICIG-ALL 11) and with published protocols comprising only long maintenance chemotherapy; protocol 9 is, as far as the first remission plateau (cure expectancy) and the survival plateau are concerned, superior to most of these protocols (or their branches).

Lethal toxicity of active immunotherapy is nil, in contrast to the proportion of deaths (4–28%) occurring during remission in the patients submitted to maintenance chemotherapy.

Thus, active immunotherapy is scientifically and ethically indicated in ALL treatment.

However, not all patients with so-called ALLs should be treated identically: our early prognosis parameters (WHO cytologic types and volume of the tumor, in this study) allow us to distinguish a good prognosis group in which protocol 9 gave an 80% cure expectancy. The patients with a poor prognosis should be the object of further research for a more efficient therapy. Even if this should be more intensive, the risk is justified in this group, while it is not so for the good prognosis group. Research in this direction has already led to improved prognosis for ALL patients submitted to the protocol we apply at present.

Acknowledgements

The authors would like to thank Dr R. POWLES for his valuable assistance in the preparation of the text.

References

1. Acute Leukemia Group B (James Holland): Introduction to the acute lymphoid leukemias session. In: Symposium on Immunotherapy of Cancer: Present Status of Trials in Man. 27–29th October 1976, Bethesda. New York: Raven Press, 1977 (in press).
2. BELPOMME, D., DANTCHEV, D., DU RUSQUEC, E., GRANDJON, D., HUCHET, R., POUILLART, P., SCHWARZENBERG, L., AMIEL, J. L., MATHÉ, G.: T and B lymphocyte markers on the neoplastic cell of 20 patients with acute and 10 patients with chronic lymphoid leukemia. Biomedicine 20, 109 (1974).
3. BELPOMME, D., MATHÉ, G., DAVIES, A. J. S.: Clinical significance and prognostic value of the T—B immunological classification of human primary acute lymphoid leukemias. Lancet I, 555 (1977).
4. BERNARD, J., WEIL, M., JACQUILLAT, C.: Treatment of acute lymphoblastic leukemia. Wadley Medical Bulletin 5, 1 (1975).
5. BROUET, J. C., VALENSI, F., DANIEL, M. T., FLANDRIN, G., PREUD'HOMME, J. L., SELIGMANN, M.: Immunological classification of acute lymphoblastic leukemias: evaluation of its clinical significance in a hundred patients. Brit. J. Haematol. 33, 319 (1976).
6. CLARKSON, B. D., DOWLING, M. D., GEE, T. S., CUNNINGHAM, I. B., BURCHENAL, J. H.: Treatment of acute leukemia in adults. Cancer 36, 775 (1975).
7. CLARYSSE, A., KENIS, Y., MATHÉ, G.: Cancer chemotherapy. Its role in the treatment strategy of hematologic malignancies and solid tumors. Heidelberg-New York: Springer-Verlag, 1976.
8. EKERT, H., JOSE, D. G.: Chemotherapy and BCG in acute lymphocytic leukaemia. Lancet (1975) II, 713.
9. EKERT, H., JOSE, D. G., WATERS, K. D., SMITH, P. J., MATHEWS, R. N.: Intermittent chemotherapy and BCG in continuation therapy of children with acute lymphocytic leukemia. In: Symposium on Immunotherapy of Cancer: Present Status of Trials in Man. 27–29th October 1976, Bethesda. New York: Raven Press, 1977 (in press).
10. E.O.R.T.C. Hemopathy Working Party: Immunotherapy versus chemotherapy as maintenance treatment of acute lymphoblastic leukemia. In: Symposium on Immunotherapy of Cancer: Present Status of Trials in Man. 27–29th October 1976, Bethesda. New York: Raven Press, 1977 (in press).
11. FERNBACH, D. J., GEORGE, S. L., SUTOW, W. W., RAGAB, A. H., LANE, D. M., HAGGARD, M. E., LONSDALE, D.: Long-term results of reinforcement therapy in children with acute leukemia. Cancer 36, 1552 (1975).
12. HEYN, R., JOO, P., KARON, M., NESBIT, M., SHORE, N., BRESLOW, N., WEINER, R., REED, A., SATHER, H., HAMMOND, D.: BCG in the treatment of acute lymphocytic leukemia. In: Symposium on Immunotherapy of Cancer: Present Status of Trials in Man. 27–29th October 1976, Bethesda. New York: Raven Press, 1977 (in press).
13. JACQUILLAT, C., WEIL, M., GEMON, M. F., BOIRON, M., BERNARD, J.: Acute lymphoblastic leukemia in adults. In: Therapy of Acute Leukemias. Mandelli, F., Amadori, S., Mariani, G. (eds.). Rome: Minerva Medica, 1975, p. 113.
14. KHALIL, A., RAPPAPORT, H., BOURUT, C., HALLE-PANNENKO, O., MATHÉ, G.: Histologic reactions of the thymus, spleen, liver, lymph nodes to i.v. and s.c. BCG injections. Biomedicine 22, 121 (1975).
15. LEE, S. L., KOPEL, S., GLIDEWELL, O.: Cytomorphological determinants of prognosis in acute lymphoblastic leukemia of children. Seminars in Oncology 3, 209 (1976).
16. LEVENTHAL, B. G.: Immunotherapy of acute lymphoid leukaemia. In: Symposium on Immunotherapy of Cancer: Present Status of Trials in Man. 27–29th October 1976, Bethesda. New York: Raven Press, 1977 (in press).
17. LONSDALE, D., GEHAN, E. A., FERNBACH, D. J., SULLIVAN, M. P., LANE, D. M., RAGAB, A. H.: Interrupted vs. continued maintenance therapy in childhood acute leukemia. Cancer 36, 341 (1975).
18. MATHÉ, G.: Surviving in company of BCG. Cancer Immunol. Immunoth. 1, 3 (1976).
19. MATHÉ, G.: Cancer active immunotherapy: immunoprophylaxis and immunorestoration. An introduction. Heidelberg-New York: Springer-Verlag, 1976.

20. Mathé, G.: Human models for cancer active immunotherapy. Biomedicine 26, 1 (1977).
21. Mathé, G., Amiel, J. L., Schwarzenberg, L., Schneider, M., Cattan, A., Schlumberger, J. R., Hayat, M., De Vassal, F.: Active immunotherapy for acute lymphoblastic leukaemia. Lancet (1969) I, 697.
22. Mathé, G., Amiel, J. L., Schwarzenberg, L., Schneider, M., Cattan, A., Schlumberger, J. R., Hayat, M., De Vassal, F.: Follow-up of the first (1962) pilot trial on active immunotherapy of acute lymphoid leukaemia. A critical discussion. Biomedicine 26, 29 (1977).
23. Mathé, G., De Vassal, F., Delgado, M., Pouillart, P., Belpomme, D., Joseph, R., Schwarzenberg, L., Amiel, J. L., Schneider, M., Cattan, A., Musset, M., Misset, J. L., Jasmin, C.: 1975 current results of the first 100 cytologically typed acute lymphoid leukemia submitted to BCG active immunotherapy. Cancer Immunol. Immunoth. 1, 77 (1976).
24. Mathé, G., De Vassal, F., Schwarzenberg, L., Delgado, M., Pena-Angulo, J., Belpomme, D., Pouillart, P., Machover, D., Misset, J. L., Pico, J. L., Jasmin, C., Hayat, M., Schneider, M., Cattan, A., Amiel, J. L., Musset, M., Rosenfeld, C.: Results of acute lymphoid leukaemia protocol ICIG-ALL 11 (in preparation).
25. Mathé, G., De Vassal, F., Schwarzenberg, L., Delgado, M., Pena-Angulo, J., Belpomme, D., Pouillart, P., Machover, D., Misset, J. L., Pico, J. L., Jasmin, C., Hayat, M., Schneider, M., Cattan, A., Amiel, J. L., Musset, M., Rosenfeld, C.: Comparison of the results of children acute lymphoid leukaemia protocols with short chemotherapy (protocol 9) or long chemotherapies (protocols 10 and 11) followed by active immunotherapy predictable prognosis and therapeutic incidence. Biomedicine 26 (1977) (in press).
26. Mathé, G., Pouillart, P., Sterescu, M., Amiel, J. L., Schwarzenberg, L., Schneider, M., Hayat, M., De Vassal, F., Jasmin, C., Lafleur, M.: Subdivision of classical varieties of acute lymphoid leukemias. Correlation with prognosis and cure expectancy. Europ. J. Clin. Biol. Res. 16, 554 (1971).
27. Mathé, G., Rappaport, H.: Histological and cytological typing of neoplastic diseases of haematopoietic and lymphoid tissues. Geneva: World Health Organisation, 1976.
28. Mathé, G., Rosenfeld, C.: Use of cultured leukaemic cells for the specific stimulus in active immunotherapy. (in preparation).
29. Mathé, G., Schwarzenberg, L., De Vassal, F., Delgado, M., Pena-Angulo, J., Belpomme, D., Pouillart, P., Machover, D., Misset, J. L., Pico, J. L., Jasmin, C., Hayat, M., Schneider, M., Cattan, A., Amiel, J. L., Musset, M., Rosenfeld, C.: Chemotherapy followed by active immunotherapy (AI) in the treatment of acute lymphoid leukaemias (ALL) for patients of all ages. Results of ICIG-ALL protocols 1, 9 and 10. Prognostic factors and therapeutic implications. In: Symposium on Immunotherapy of Cancer: Present Status of Trials in Man. 27–29th October 1976. Bethesda. New York: Raven Press, 1977 (in press).
30. Mathé, G., Venuat, A. M., Rosenfeld, C., Pouillart, P.: Investigations on fertility lymphocyte chromosome and CFHa after a short or a long chemotherapy for acute lymphoid leukaemia. (in preparation).
31. Medical Research Council: Treatment of acute lymphoblastic leukaemia. Comparison of immunotherapy (BCG), intermittent methotrexate and no therapy after a five month intensive cytotoxic regimen (Concord trial). Brit. Med. J. 4, 189 (1971).
32. Murphy, S. B., Borella, L., Sen, L., Mauer, A.: Lack of correlation of lymphoblast cell size with presence of T-cell markers or with outcome in childhood acute lymphoblastic leukaemia. Brit. J. Haemat. 31, 95 (1975).
33. Necheles, T. F., Brenner, J. F., Bonacossa, I., Fristensky, R., Neurath, P. W.: The computer-assisted morphological classification of acute leukaemia. I. Preliminary results. Biomedicine 25, 241 (1976).
34. Rappaport, H., Khalil, A.: The immunoproliferative response of mice to intravenously or subcutaneously injected BCG. Cancer Immunol. Immunoth. 1, 45 (1976).
35. Rosenfeld, C., Venuat, A. M., Goutner, A., Guegand, J., Choquet, C., Tron, F., Pico, J. L.: An exceptional cell line established from a patient with acute lymphoid leukaemia. Proc. Amer. Assoc. Cancer Res. 16, 29 (Abstract 115) (1975).
36. Schwartz, D., Flamant, R., Lellouch, J.: L'essai thérapeutique chez l'Homme. Paris: Editions Médicales Flammarion, 1970.
37. Schwarzenberg, L., Simmler, M. C., Pico, J. L.: Human toxicology of BCG applied in cancer immunotherapy. Cancer Immunol. Immunoth. 1, 69 (1976).
38. Simone, J. V. Personal communication.
39. Symposium on immunotherapy of cancer: present status of trials in man, 27–29th October, 1976. Bethesda. New York: Raven Press, 1977 (in press).

Active Immunotherapy in Leukemia With Neuraminidase-Modified Leukemic Cells*

J. G. BEKESI and J. F. HOLLAND

Introduction

The enzymic cleavage of the terminal sugar residue from the plasma membrane of neoplastic cells by neuraminidase of vibrio cholerae origin causes a marked increase in immunogenicity of most experimental tumors [1–6, 8–16]. In a DBA/2 leukemia L1210 system, a single leukemic cell is capable of producing leukemia and the ultimate death of the host. However, mice which were immunized with neuraminidase-treated leukemia L1210 cells remained protected against a challenge of 100,000 untreated leukemic cells [1–3]. Repeated injections of neuraminidase-treated leukemia L1210 cells reduced the lethality rate and increased survival of mice with leukemia L1210 tumor grafts [15, 16]. Chemotherapy plus neuraminidase-treated L1210 cells administered in a sequence which preserves the host's immunobiologically competent cells resulted in the cure of a significant portion of immunized mice [4, 7, 9]. The immunoprotection evoked by the stimulation from the neuraminidase-treated tumor cells was specific for the particular tumor and could be transferred by sera or splenic lymphocytes into unimmunized syngeneic mice [5, 7, 15, 16]. Recently, considerable attention has been directed to combined modality therapy in spontaneous Gross virus-induced leukemia in AkR mice because in many respects AkR leukemia has similar characteristics to the human leukemias.

Our present work deals with the effectiveness of chemotherapy in combination with specific immunotherapy with neuraminidase-treated syngeneic and allogeneic cells in AkR mice. The effectiveness of preventive immunotherapy in MuLV-infected AkR mice was also tested. The experimental data led to successful clinical trial in acute myelocytic leukemia using neuraminidase-treated allogeneic myeloblasts as specific immunogen.

Materials and Methods

Eight-week-old female AkR mice and 5–7-month-old AkR female retired breeders were supplied by Jackson Laboratories, Bar Harbor, Maine. The mice were kept in a room thermostatically controlled at 20–23°C and allowed Purina chow (breeders) and tap water ad libitum. Leukemia L1210 tumor cells have been maintained by weekly intraperitoneal passage in DBA/2 Ha mice. Gross leukemia virus-induced E2G leukemia was maintained by weekly intravenous passage of 500,000–1 million viable cells in syngeneic C57BL mice. Spontaneous leukemic AkR mice were harvested from a colony of 3000–4000 AkR retired breeders. Animals were considered to be leukemic when the leukocyte counts were greater than 18,000 mm^3 and they had splenic and lymph node enlargement.

* This work was supported by contracts NCI Virus Cancer Program NO1-CP-43879 and NCI Immunotherapy Program NO1-CP-43225.

Incubation of Leukemic Cells with Neuraminidase

For all our studies, highly purified neuraminidase of vibrio cholerae was used.[1] Leukemic cells were incubated at 37°C in sodium acetate buffer (.05 M sodium acetate, .154 M sodium chloride, and .005 M calcium chloride) at pH 5.6–6.0 in the presence of 15–50 u of neuraminidase per 2.5×10^7 cells per ml. At the termination of incubation, the siliconized reaction flask was removed, cooled rapidly, and spun at $800–1000 \times g$ for 55 s in a clinical centrifuge. The final viability of leukemic thymocytes and E2G leukemic cells were 92 and 98% respectively as determined by the trypan blue exclusion method.

Prophylactic Therapy of MuLV-Infected AkR Mice With Neuraminidase-Treated Syngeneic and Allogeneic Leukemia Cells

Three-month-old female AkR mice were randomized into six groups of 40 mice each. Group I received saline injections every 15 days for a total of nine times. Group II received 2×10^7 neuraminidase-treated leukemia L1210 cells per injection i.d. Group III received 2×10^7 neuraminidase-treated allogeneic E2G cells per injection i.d. Group IV received 2×10^7 neuraminidase-treated normal AkR thymocytes per injection. Group V received 2×10^7 neuraminidase-treated leukemic AkR thymocytes i.p. while animals in group VI were immunized i.d. with the same number of untreated normal thymocytes per injection. The mice were checked daily for mortality until the termination of the study (450 days after the date of the birth). The thymus and spleens were removed from the mice which had died and the weights were recorded.

Chemoimmunotherapy in AkR Mice With Spontaneous Leukemia

Combination chemotherapy plus immunotherapy with neuraminidase-treated spontaneous leukemic thymocytes and allogeneic E2G leukemic cells in AkR mice with spontaneous leukemia were carried out after positive confirmation of the disease (palpation and white blood cell count). The combination chemotherapy consisted of vincristine plus 1-β-D-arabinofuranosylcytosine-5′-palmitate (palmO-ara-C) plus methyl CCNU [1-(2-chloroethyl)-3-(4-methylcyclohexyl)-1-nitrosourea]. Two to four days after termination of chemotherapy, the animals were randomly placed into the following groups: chemotherapy alone, chemotherapy followed by immunization with 2×10^7 neuraminidase-treated leukemic thymocytes or allogeneic E2G leukemic cells intradermally (i.d.) at the times indicates in the figures.

The MuLV titer in the experimental animals was determined by obtaining a 2% extract of a short section (4–6 mm) of mouse tails from ten individual animals in each group. The samples were obtained prior to treatment at the time of randomization, during and posttreatment. Each tail specimen was individually assayed by the XC focus forming assay as described by Rowe et al. The MuLV titer is expressed per ml of 2% extract of a 4–6 mm section of AkR mouse tail. Mice were checked for mortality rate daily. All animals were autopsied. Spleens, lymph nodes, and thymus glands were removed and the weights were recorded.

Chemoimmunotherapy of Acute Myelocytic Leukemia in Man

Chemotherapy
Previously untreated patients with acute myelocytic leukemia were induced into remission with Ara C (100 mg/m²) in a continuous i.v. infusion for 7 days plus daunorubicin at a dose

of 45 mg/m^2/day by direct injection on days 1, 2, and 3. These drugs induced approximately 70% of patients into complete remission. All patients were between the ages of 15–70. All received cyclic maintenance chemotherapy every 4 weeks. This consisted of 5-day courses of Ara C in addition to 6-thioguanine, cyclophosphamide, CCNU, or daunorubicin sequentially with each course repeated at 4-month cycles.

Collection of Allogeneic Myeloblasts

Separation of myeloblasts was achieved by leukophoresis on an AMINCO cell separator. The myeloblasts were collected in transfer bags containing acid citrate-dextrose solution. After cessation of leukophoresis, the myeloblasts were separated from contaminating red blood cells by sedimentation. The myeloblasts were mixed with special freezing media containing 15% autologous or AB plasma and 10% dimethylsulfoxide and were frozen in transfer bags by programmed freezing (Union Carbide biological freezer) at a temperature drop of 1°C per min until −38°C was reached and then rapidly to −90°C. The frozen cells were immediately stored in the vapor phase of liquid nitrogen.

Immunization with Neuraminidase-Treated Myeloblasts

Myeloblasts retrieved from liquid nitrogen storage prior to immunization were purified on albumin gradient to separate the viable from nonviable blast cells. After purification, the myeloblasts were incubated with vibrio cholerae neuraminidase. The incubation mixture contained 50 u of enzyme per 5×10^7 cells per ml in sodium acetate buffer at pH 5.6–6.0 for 60 min at 37°c. After incubation, the cells were washed three times with mixed salt and glucose media. Immunization with neuraminidase-treated allogeneic myeloblasts was performed by i.d. injections in approx. 48 sites selected for proximity to lymph node drainage areas (Fig. 1). Each inoculation site was injected with approx. $1.5–2 \times 10^8$ cells so that the total immunization load was about 10^{10} cells. In addition, as a control injection, heat-denatured neuraminidase (500 u per site), x-irradiated myeloblasts, and the supernatant of the incubation fluid were also injected in some patients. Delayed cutaneous hypersensitivity response to neuraminidase-treated myeloblasts was measured at 48 h and the induration in mm was recorded.

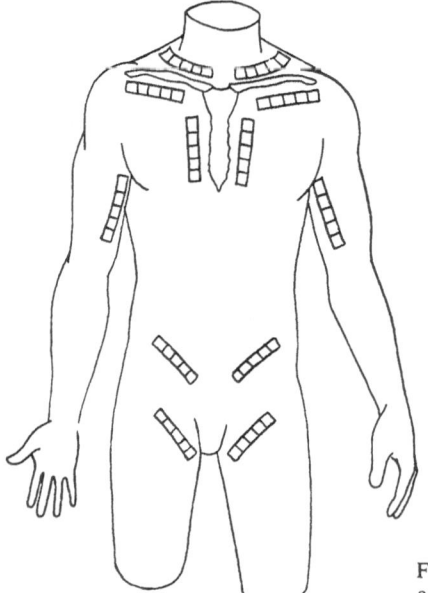

Fig. 1. Immunization diagram for neuraminidase-treated allogeneic myeloblasts

Immunologic Assessment of Patients

In Vivo The immunocompetence of patients in the protocol was measured by the delayed cutaneous hypersensitivity response to five recall antigens: PPD, dermatophytin "o", candida, streptokinase-streptodornase, and mumps. All recall antigens were applied in the volar forearm by i.d. inoculation in a volume of .1 ml through a 27 gauge needle. The delayed hypersensitivity response to antigens was read at 48 h in the same manner as for neuraminidase-treated myeloblasts. The skin tests were considered clinically positive if the diameter of the induration was 5 mm or greater.

In Vitro T- and B-lymphocyte function of peripheral blood lymphocytes was determined by monitoring the in vitro lymphocyte blastogenesis induced by selective T and B cell mitogens, e.g., phytohemagglutinin (PHA) for T cells and pokeweed mitogen (PWM) for B cells. The cells were cultured with .15–.3 μg/well of high purity of PHA (Burroughs Wellcome Co.) or with 30 μg/well of PWM (Grand Island Biological Co.). Lymphocyte blastogenesis was determined by measuring the level of DNA synthesis upon the addition of ^{3}H-thymidine.

The E-binding rosette technique was used for quantification of T-lymphocyte population before and during immunotherapy.

Biostatistics

Analysis of the remission duration of patients in the chemotherapy and chemoimmunotherapy groups was made by the generalized Kruskal-Wallis test proposed by BRESLOW [8].

Results and Discussion

Prophylactic Therapy of Gross Leukemia Virus-Infected AkR Mice With Neuraminidase-Treated Leukemic Cells

The vertically transmitted Gross leukemic virus is the etiologic agent for lymphoma in AkR mice. The virus remains dormant in the animals until they reach the age of 6 months, then they develop spontaneous lymphoma. By 12 months of age, about 95% of the AkR mice die from spontaneous leukemia. The efficacy of using allogeneic, nonvirally induced leukemia L1210 cells and the Gross leukemia virus-induced E2G leukemic cells treated with neuraminidase as an immunogen in prophylactic treatment in AkR mice was compared to the data obtained with neuraminidase-treated syngeneic normal leukemic thymocytes from AkR mice.

Leukemia L1210, E2G leukemia, and spontaneous AkR leukemia cells incubated in sodium acetate buffer alone maintained their viability well after 3 h of incubation and produced tumor when inoculated in syngeneic mice which had not been immunized. However, tumor cells incubated with 15–50 u of neuraminidase per 2×10^7 cells/ml showed no marked change in their permeability to trypan blue yet they produced no tumor when injected in normal immunologically competent syngeneic mice. In spite of the absence of any proteolytic activity in the neuraminidase preparation, higher conc of neuraminidase rapidly increased the permeability of leukemia L1210, E2G leukemia, and spontaneous AkR leukemia cells and at the same time decreased their immunogenicity (Fig. 2). Scanning microscopic studies appear to indicate that the rapid release of neuraminidase may lead to progressive structural disintegration of the surface membrane of the tumor cells. We have, therefore, determined and utilized the optimal enzyme conc for each tumor line.

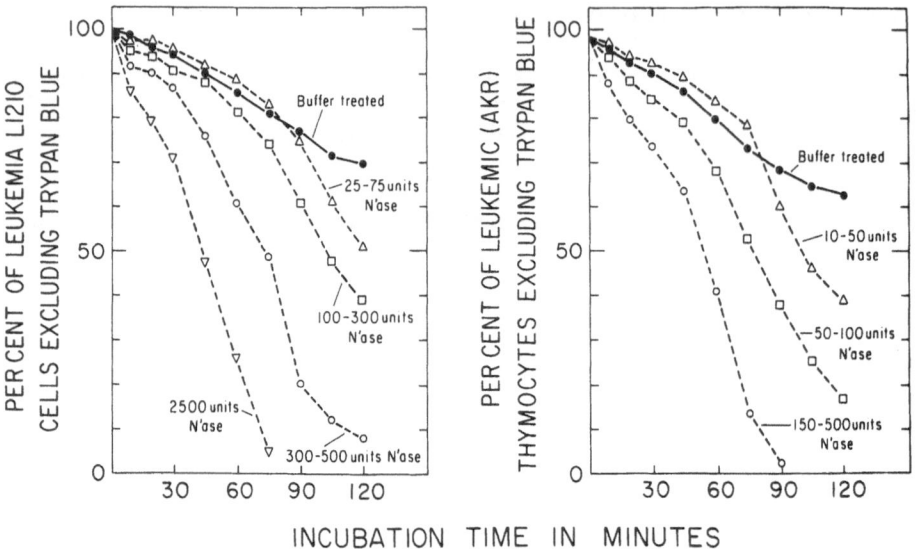

Fig. 2. Trypan blue exclusion of leukemia L1210 and spontaneous AkR leukemic thymocytes incubated with various concentrations of neuraminidase. Enzyme concentrations given as units per 2.5×10^7 cells per ml incubation media

Experimental results in Figure 3 and in Figure 4 show unequivocally that both neuraminidase-treated syngeneic leukemic AkR thymocytes and the allogeneic E2G leukemic cells were equally effective in delaying the appearance of primary lymphoma in AkR mice (p = .01). Immunization carried out with neuraminidase-treated leukemia L1210 cells or neuraminidase-treated normal AkR thymocytes was ineffectual and the treated mice died of leukemia at about the same rate as the control group. These pilot experiments clearly established the immunoprophylactic and therapeutic value of neuraminidase-treated Gross leukemia virus-induced spontaneous and allogeneic leukemic cells.

Chemoimmunotherapy in Spontaneous Leukemic AkR Mice

To extend our experience with chemoimmunotherapy in animals with transplantable tumor, we have investigated the effectiveness of cytoreductive therapy plus immunotherapy with neuraminidase-treated syngeneic and allogeneic leukemic cells in AkR mice. At the time of clinical diagnosis there are about 1.5×10^9 widely disseminated leukemic cells in AkR mice. Without chemotherapeutic intervention, AkR mice die after diagnosis of spontaneous leukemia at the rate of 50% by 16 days.

Spontaneous leukemic AkR mice treated with vincristine plus palmO-ara C followed by methyl CCNU sustained an increase in lifespan of about 180%. However, fewer than 5% of animals survived beyond 80 days. These mice died of lymphoma presumably as a result of reinduction of a second lymphoma cell population. When the same chemotherapy was followed by neuraminidase-treated syngeneic leukemic thymocytes as immunogenic stimulant, a significant percentage, about 35%, of leukemic AkR mice were apparently cured of the disease, only to relapse at a later time from a presumptively new leukemogenic event (Fig. 5).

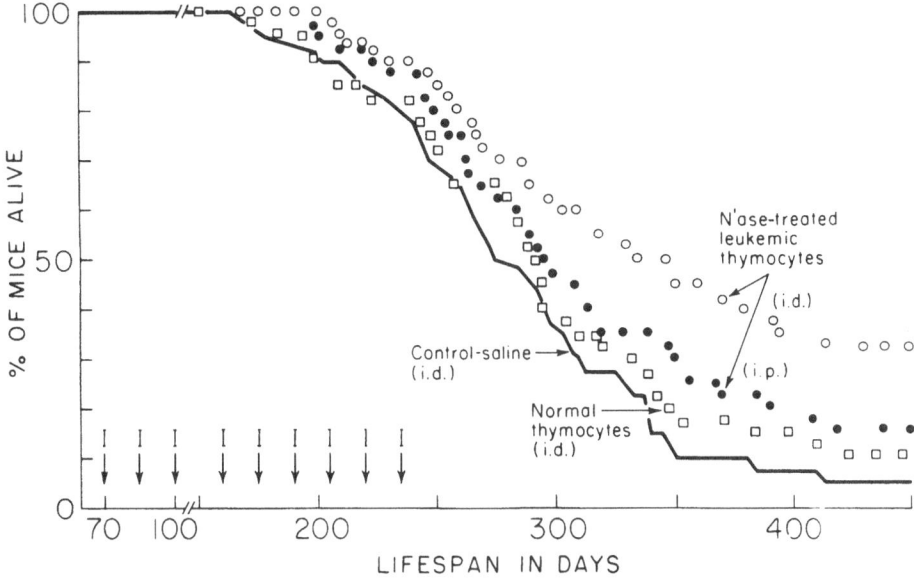

Fig. 3. Effect of immunotherapy with neuraminidase (N'ase)-treated normal and leukemic thymocytes on the appearance of primary leukemia in AkR mice. Mice were immunized at days indicated with 2×10^7 cells with normal thymocytes (□), leukemic thymocytes injected i.p. (●), leukemic thymocytes injected i.d. (○), control—saline, control—0.9% NaCl

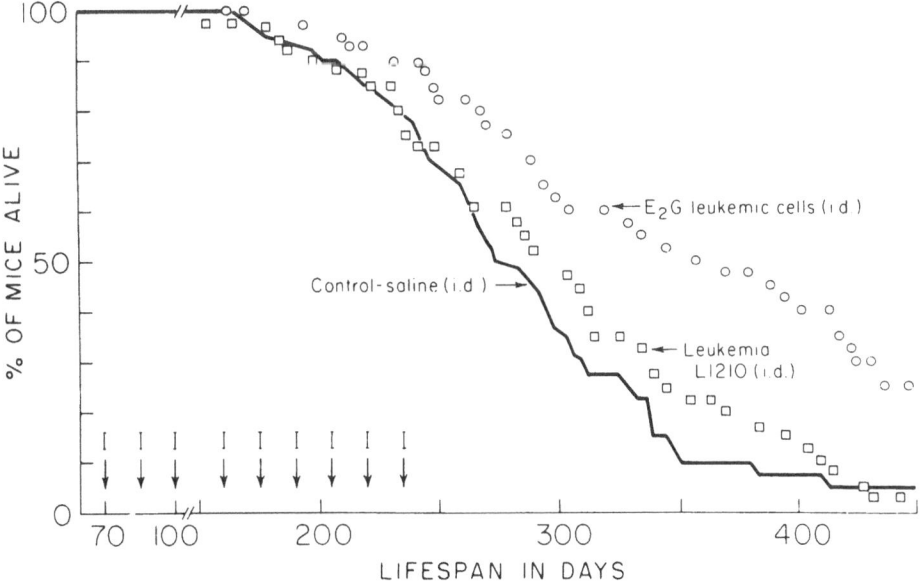

Fig. 4. Effect of preimmunization with neuraminidase-treated allogeneic E2G or L1210 leukemic cells on the appearance of spontaneous leukemia in AkR mice. Mice were immunized at days indicated with 2×10^7 cells with E2G leukemic cells i.d. (○) or leukemia L1210 cells i.d. (□). Control—saline, control—0.9% NaCl

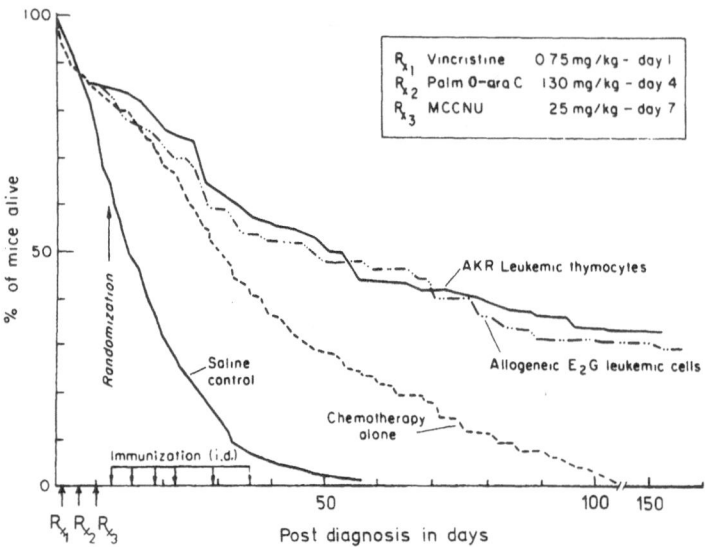

Fig. 5. Immunization of spontaneous leukemic AkR mice with neuraminidase-treated leukemic thymocytes or allogeneic E2G leukemia cells after cytoreductive therapy. AkR mice were randomized into the following three groups of 30 mice each after cytoreductive therapy: group I, chemotherapy alone, group II, immunization with 2×10^7 neuraminidase-treated syngeneic leukemic thymocytes i.d., group III, immunization with 2×10^7 neuraminidase-treated allogeneic E2G leukemia cells i.d. at the days indicated by arrows

Using the above experimental protocols, the relationship between the AkR virus titer and the type and clinical efficacy of the treatment was established. The results presented in Table 1 indicate that cytoreductive therapy alone did not significantly alter the viral titer in the treated AkR mice. Chemotherapy and immunotherapy with neuraminidase-treated leukemic thymocytes i.d. produced a noticeable decrease in viral titer after 13 days of the treatment, and this remained at a low level when tested at 45 days after the initiation of the treatment.

Combination of drug therapy plus i.d. immunization with neuraminidase-treated allogeneic E2G leukemia cells resulted in survival of up to 35% of the animals beyond 150 days without evidence of the disease (Fig. 5). It is particularly significant that the neuraminidase-treated E2G leukemic cells, which, like the AkR leukemia, are Gross virus-induced, but are completely different at the H_2 genetic locus from the AkR mice, were as effective as the syngeneic leukemic cells in prolonging the survival of leukemic AkR mice. This suggests the existence of a cross reacting common viral membrane antigen, and suggests that if similar etiology existed for human leukemia, it would not be essential to use autologous leukemic cells for immunization. These data provided the basis for using neuraminidase-treated allogeneic myeloblasts in human immunotherapeutic investigations.

Immunotherapy with Neuraminidase-Treated

Allogeneic Myeloblasts in Acute Myelocytic Leukemia (AML)

Based on our experimental data and on the improved remission duration attained with active immunotherapy using neuraminidase-treated allogeneic myeloblasts in a group of previously treated AML patients, a controlled clinical trial was initiated.

Table 1. Change of Gross leukemia virus titer in AkR mice after chemotherapy or chemotherapy + immunotherapy

Experimental groups	Virus titer[a]						
	Pretreatment	During treatment (R_X or R_X + immuR_X)					Posttreatment
Days:	0	4	8	13	17	21	45
Untreated leukemic AkR mice	1260	1317	1060	1520	1290	1620	
Chemotherapy + saline	1310	1020	890	756	1100	960	1390
Chemotherapy + immunotherapy				950	680	420	385

[a] Gross leukemia virus titer is expressed per 0.2 ml of 2% extract of a short section (4–6 mm) of mouse tails obtained from animals at days indicated using XC focus assay.

Fifty-eight previously untreated patients with AML were induced into complete remission by cytosine arabinoside and daunorubicin. Beginning on day 8 after the first sustaining course of chemotherapy and on day 15 of each cycle therafter, patients received either chemotherapy alone or chemotherapy plus neuraminidase-treated myeloblasts. Conc of $1.5–2 \times 10^8$ neuraminidase-treated myeloblasts were given i.d. in .2 ml of special media in at least 48 loci. Strong delayed cutaneous hypersensitivity reactions, often measuring 10–30 mm in diameter, were observed at each immunization site. Biopsies of cutaneous reactions showed extensive immunoblastic infiltration. No hypersensitivity reaction was noted at the site of heat-denatured neuraminidase or supernatant of the incubation.

The median remission duration of the chemotherapy group is 44 weeks while patients receiving neuraminidase-treated myeloblasts have not reached median remission at 120 weeks yet. The difference between the two groups is highly significant, $p = .003$. Nineteen of the 28 patients in the immunotherapy group are still in remission. Eleven of the 19 patients who received neuraminidase-treated tumor cells are still in remission at 108–234 weeks (Fig. 6).

The immunocompetence of patients was measured by the cutaneous hypersensitivity response to recall antigens: PPD, mumps, candida, varidase, and dermatophytin. Figure 7 summarizes the results of skin tests for five different test periods. About two-thirds of the patients studied gave positive response to candida and varidase at the time of randomization. Subsequent test periods show the delayed cutaneous hypersensitivity response after the third, sixth, ninth, and twelfth sustaining chemoimmunotherapy. Both quantitative and qualitative increase in response to recall antigens was noted among patients receiving neuraminidase-treated allogeneic myeloblasts.

Quantification of T-lymphocyte population of patients in the immunotherapy protocol was performed by using the E-binding rosette technique. Table 2 summarizes results for three test periods. Patients receiving combination of chemotherapy plus immunization with neuraminidase-treated tumor cells showed statistically significant increase of T-lymphocytes as compared to the value at the time of randomization both in terms of percentages and absolute numbers.

Fig. 8 summarizes the lymphoblastogenesis of normal and remission lymphocytes to PHA and PWM. Both mitogens show depressed stimulation of lymphocytes at the time of randomization as compared to normal subjects, and there is no apparent improvement in patients who received chemotherapy alone. Contrariwise, lymphocytes from patients who received chemotherapy plus neuraminidase-modified allogeneic myeloblasts showed progressively higher response to PHA and PWM approaching and surpassing the level of normal donors by the sixth cycle of chemoimmunotherapy.

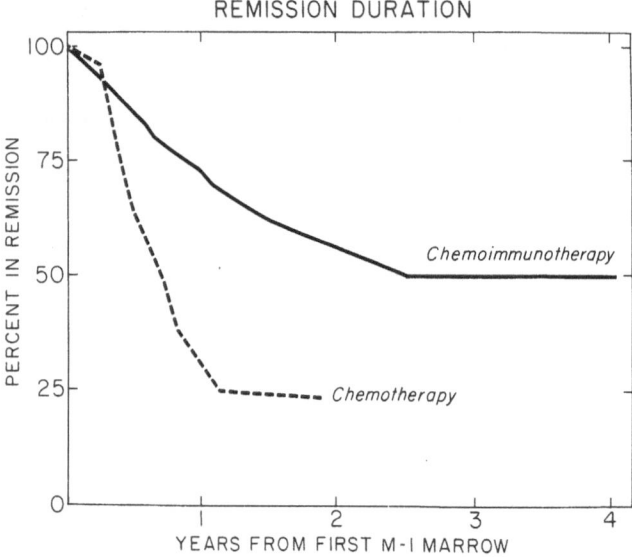

Fig. 6. Remission duration of patients with AML immunized with neuraminidase-modified allogeneic myeloblasts; 30 patients in the chemotherapy group; 28 patients in the chemoimmunotherapy group

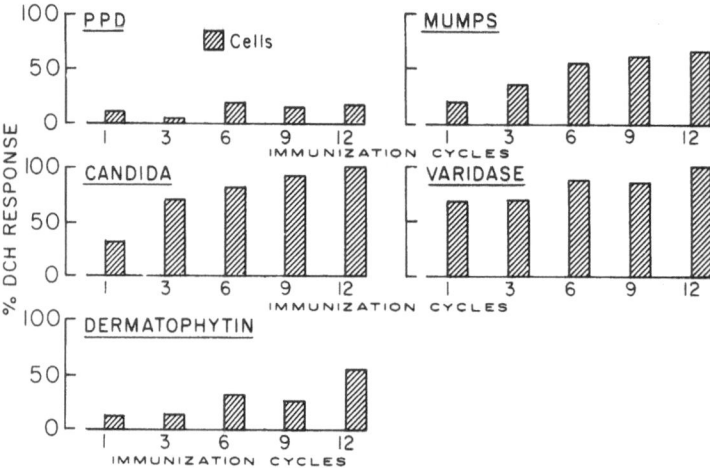

Fig. 7. Change of delayed hypersensitivity response to recall antigens during the course of immunotherapy. Skin test diameter at 48 h > 5 mm

Table 2. T-lymphocyte subpopulation in AML patients in the immunotherapy study

	At randomization		After 6 cycles		After 9 cycles	
	% T cells	T-lymphocytes[a]	% T cells	T-lymphocytes	% T cells	T-lymphocytes
Normal subjects N=69	74.4	1,986 ± 251				
Immunotherapy with neuraminidase myeloblasts N=15	53.31	483 ± 48	70.8	1,085 ± 111 $p=.00047$[b]	77.0	1,029 ± 93 $p=.00017$[b]

Determined by the E-binding rosette technique at 4°C with SRBC.
[a] ± SEM.
[b] Absolute T-lymphocytes at the time of randomization versus during therapy of AML patients.

AML: LYMPHOBLASTOGENESIS FROM PHA AND PW MITOGENS

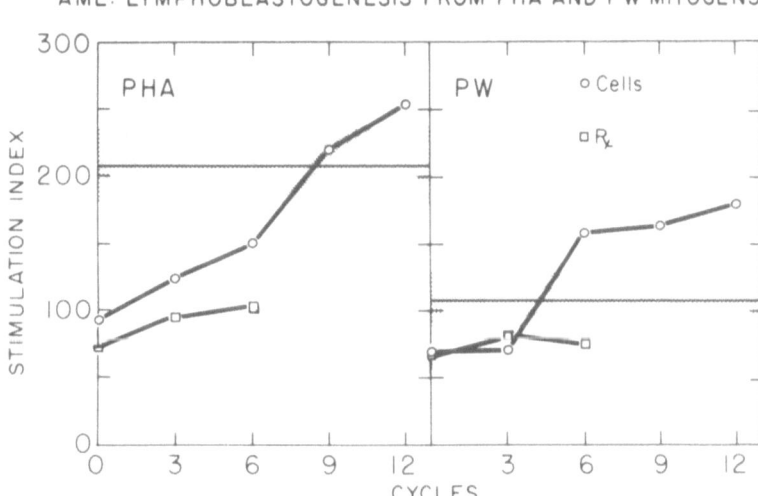

Fig. 8. Kinetics of PHA- and PWM-induced blastogenesis of peripheral lymphocytes from AML patients immunized with neuraminidase-modified myeloblasts

Summary

The AkR strain of mice are destined genetically to develop Gross leukemia virus-induced lymphatic leukemia. However, immunization with neuraminidase-modified spontaneous thymocytes and allogeneic (Gross virus-induced) E2G leukemia cells resulted in a significant delay in the appearance of primary lymphoma in AkR mice. This suggests the existence of cross reacting common viral membrane antigens. Immunization with untreated E2G leukemic cells or neuraminidase-modified leukemia L1210 cells and normal (AkR) thymocytes was ineffectual.

Comparable observations were made in AkR mice with diagnosed spontaneous leukemia. Without cytoreductive therapy, AkR mice die after diagnosis of spontaneous leukemia at the rate of 50% by day 16. Immunotherapy alone was ineffectual in experimental animals bearing florid leukemia. Combination of cytoreductive therapy plus active immunization with neuraminidase-treated spontaneous AkR leukemia thymocytes or with allogeneic (Gross virus-induced) E2G leukemic cells injected i.d. resulted in the survival of 35% of AkR mice beyond 150 days without evidence of disease. Immunotherapy in combination with cytoreductive therapy also significantly reduced the MuLV titer.

Based on experimental observations, a successful chemoimmunotherapy trial was conducted in patients with AML. Fifty-eight patients with AML were allocated in two groups following successful remission induction using cytosine arabinoside and daunorubicin. Patients designated to receive immunotherapy were injected i.d. in approximately 48 sites every 28 days with 10^{10} neuraminidase-treated allogeneic myeloblasts. For 30 of the 58 AML patients, the remission duration on chemotherapy alone was 44 weeks, whereas those receiving immunotherapy have not yet reached the median at 110 weeks. The difference between the groups is highly significant. The in vivo and in vitro immunodiagnostic tests indicate the restoration of normal immunocompetence in patients receiving immunotherapy versus the control patients treated with chemotherapy alone. Thus, the therapeutic effectiveness of immunotherapy with neuraminidase-treated allogeneic myeloblasts in combination with sustaining chemotherapy in patients with AML was positively established.

Acknowledgements

[1]We express our appreciation to the Behring Institute—Behringwerke AG Marburg, West Germany for supplying the highly purified neuraminidase for part of this study.
We also thank SUZAN SATTLER, RN, for the excellent assistance in performing the immunotherapy.

References

1. BAGSHAWE, K. D., CURRIE, G. A.: Immunogenicity of L1210 murine leukemia cells after treatment with neuraminidase. Nature (Lond) *218*, 1254 (1968).
2. BEKESI, J. G., ST. ARNEAULT, G., HOLLAND, J. F.: Increase of leukemia L1210 immunogenicity by *Vibrio cholerae* neuraminidase treatment. Cancer Res. *31*, 2130–2132 (1971).
3. BEKESI, J. G., ST. ARNEAULT, G., WALTER, L., HOLLAND, J. F.: Immunogenicity of leukemia L1210 cells after neuraminidase treatment. J. Natl. Cancer Inst. *49*, 107–118 (1972).
4. BEKESI, J. G., ROBOZ, J. P., WALTER, L., HOLLAND, J. F.: Stimulation of specific immunity against cancer by neuraminidase-treated tumor cells. Behring Inst. Mitt. *55*, 309–321 (1974).
5. BEKESI, J. G., ROBOZ, J. P., HOLLAND, J. F.: Characteristics of immunity induced by neuraminidase-treated lymphosarcoma cells in C3H (MTV+) and C3H (MTV−) mice. Israel J. Med. Sci. *12*, 288–303 (1976).
6. BEKESI, J. G., HOLLAND, J. F., FLEMINGER, R., YATES, J., HENDERSON, E. S.: Immunotherapeutic efficacy of neuraminidase-treated allogeneic myeloblasts in patients with acute myelocytic leukemia. In: Control of Neoplasia by Modulation of the Immune System. Chirigos, M. A. (ed.). New York: Raven Press, 1977, pp. 573–592.
7. BEKESI, J. G., ROBOZ, J. P., HOLLAND, J. F.: Therapeutic effectiveness of neuraminidase-treated tumor cells as an immunogen in man and experimental animals with leukemia. Annals of N.Y. Acad. Sci. *277*, 313–331 (1976).
8. BRESLOW, N. A.: Generalized Kruskal-Wallis test for comparing K samples subject to unequal patterns of censorship. Biometricka *57*, 579–594 (1970).

9. HOLLAND, J. F., BEKESI, J. G.: Immunotherapy of human leukemia with neuraminidase-modified cells. Med. Clinics of North America 60, 539–549 (1976).

10. LINDENMAN, J., KLEIN, P. A.: Immunological aspects of viral oncolysis. Recent advances in cancer research. Berlin: Springer-Verlag, 1967, Vol. IX, p. 66.

11. RIOS, A., SIMMONS, R. L.: Immunospecific regression of various syngeneic mouse tumors in response to neuraminidase-treated tumor cells. J. Natl. Cancer Inst. 51, 637–644 (1973).

12. RIOS, A., SIMMONS, R. L.: Active specific immunotherapy of minimal residual tumor: excision plus neuraminidase-treated tumor cells. Intern. J. Cancer 13, 71–81 (1974).

13. SANFORD, B. H.: An alteration in tumor histocompatability induced by neuraminidase. Transplantation 5, 1273 (1967).

14. SEDLACEK, H. H., MEESMANN, H., SEILER, F. R.: Regression of spontaneous mammary tumors in dogs after injection of neuraminidase-treated tumor cells. Int. J. Cancer 15, 409 (1975).

15. SETHI, K. K., BRANDIS, H.: Neuraminidase induced loss in the transplantability of murine leukemia L1210 induction of immunoprotection and the transfer of induced immunity to normal DBA/2 mice by serum and peritoneal cells. Br. J. Cancer 27, 106–113 (1973).

16. SETHI, K. K., TESCHNER, M.: Neuraminidase induced immunospecific destruction of transplantable experimental tumors. Postepy Hig. Med. Doswialdczaine 28, 103–120 (1974).

Chemotherapy and Immunotherapy Interspersion: Clinical Studies in Acute Myeloblastic Leukaemia

J. A. WHITTAKER

Introduction

The steady increase in complete remission rates for patients with acute myeloblastic leukaemia which was achieved in the 1960's with the advent of new cytotoxic agents has now reached a plateau. Major efforts have been devoted to attempts to prolong complete remission with immunotherapy, and several clinical trials using BCG as immunotherapy have shown encouraging results.

BCG has been given by scarification [1, 2] into the skin, by multiple skin puncture [3] or by the intravenous route [4]. We chose the intravenous route, and there are many reports showing that BCG given i.v. is effective in reducing the growth of a variety of antigenic transplanted tumours in animals. BCG suppresses the pulmonary metastases of a methylchlorothrene-induced rat sarcoma [5] when given i.v., and when *C. granulosum* and *C. parvum* were compared by i.v. and subcutaneous administration, the i.v. route was more effective in preventing pulmonary metastases [6].

The available evidence in animals suggests that a chemoimmunotherapy interval of about 12 days is optimal. This has been demonstrated both for *C. parvum* [7] and for BCG [8].

Patient Studies

In a 2-year period, 37 of 81 adults with acute myelogenous leukaemia (acute myeloblastic leukaemia or its variants acute myelomonocytic leukaemia, acute erythroleukaemia or acute promonocytic leukaemia) achieved complete remission after induction treatment with daunorubicin (DNR) and cytosine arabinoside (ARAC). They were randomised to maintenance treatment with monthly DNR/ARAC, or to identical chemotherapy plus intravenous BCG (Table 1). Eighteen BCG-treated patients had significantly longer survival times than 19 patients treated with chemotherapy only (Figs. 1 and 2) although no statistically significant difference can be seen in the remission duration of the two groups.

Table 1. Treatment Schedules

Remission induction	All patients	Daunorubicin 1.5 mg/kg i.v. × 1
		Cytosine arabinoside 1.0 mg/kg i.v. 12 h × 10
		(Five to nine treatments with intervals of 5–7 days between)
Maintenance treatment	Group A	Daunorubicin 1.5 mg/kg i.v. × 1 (or doxorubicin 1.0 mg/kg)
		Cytosine arabinoside 1.0 mg/kg: 8 h i.v. infusion in saline (given once each month)
	Group B	Maintenance treatment A
		plus i.v. BCG at day 14

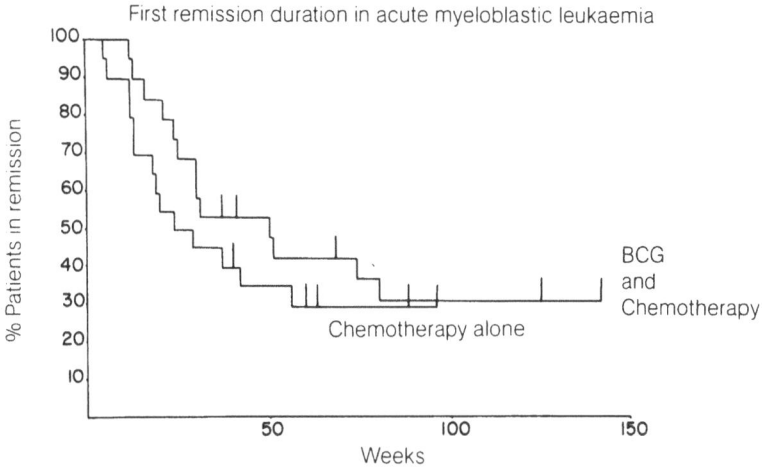

Fig. 1. Length of remission for acute myeloblastic leukaemia patients treated with chemotherapy and with chemotherapy—intravenous BCG. Vertical lines indicate patients still in complete remission. Difference in remission is not statistically significant

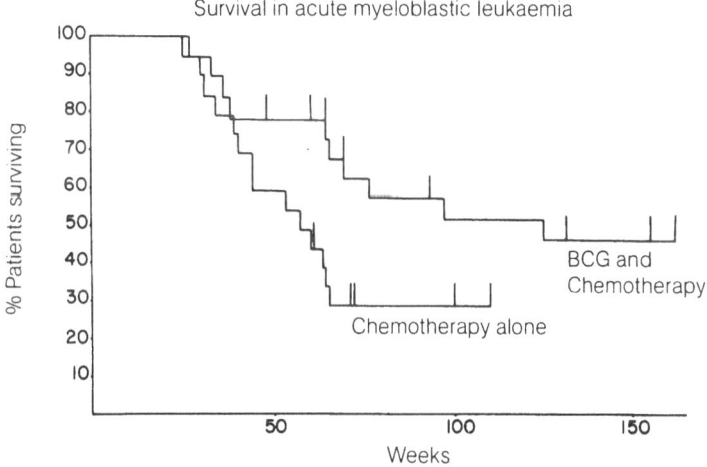

Fig. 2. Length of survival for acute myeloblastic leukaemia patients treated with chemotherapy and with chemotherapy—intravenous BCG. Vertical lines indicate patients still alive. Difference in survival $p < 0.02$ (log rank nonparametric analysis)

Thirteen patients in the BCG treatment group who have relapsed have received DNR/ARAC reinduction and six second and two third remissions have been obtained. Thirteen control group patients have relapsed and 11 have received further reinduction treatment with DNR/ARAC, but only one patient has entered a complete remission. Seven patients in the BCG-treated group who survived for 75 weeks or more (76, 93, 96, 125, 131, 155 and 162 weeks) were either positive to protein purified derivative (PPD) before treatment or converted to PPD positivity after BCG treatment (Table 2). By a battery of skin tests including PPD and Candida, similar results have been obtained with BCG administered by the subcutaneous route [2]. Our results suggest that i.v. BCG can restore immune reactivity in immunodepressed subjects and are contrary to results reported previously [9].

The BCG group had a total of 268 i.v. treatments. All patients had pyrexia 6–12 hours after injection lasting 12–72 hours and occasionally headaches and muscle pains. Two patients had nonfatal anaphylactic reactions which did not recur when BCG was subsequently readministered. Other complications of BCG therapy (Table 3) were not a problem, and we have not needed to withdraw treatment from any patient. Fatalities with BCG have been reported when using the intratumour route [10, 11], when BCG has presumably been injected inadvertently i.v. Dosages for intralesional injection have been considerably greater than the dose which we use and have been similar to the dosages which have caused severe reactions in animals [9, 12]. We have used i.v. BCG with great care and at the low dosage of less than 1×10^6 organisms. Initially, we have given diluted BCG as a precaution against unexpected patient sensitivity (Table 4).

Table 2. Skin testing before and after BCG treatment in adults with acute myeloblastic leukaemia in complete remission (16 of 18 patients)

Patient	Pretreatment		Posttreatment		1st remission duration (weeks)	Survival (weeks)
	Mantoux	Candida	Mantoux	Candida		
1	−	−	−	−	24	69
2	+	−	ND	ND	30	76
3	+	−	+	−	30	125
4	++	++	++	++	142[1]	162[1]
5	−	+	−	++	12	33
6	−	−	+	−	125[1]	131[1]
7	−	−	−	−	21	64
8	+	−	+	−	74	155[1]
9	−	−	ND	ND	51	65
10	−	−	++	+	80	96
11	−	−	ND	ND	25	36
13	−	−	+	−	68[1]	93[1]
14	+	−	++	−	50	64[1]
16	−	−	+	−	31	69[1]
17	−	−	+	+	41[1]	60[1]
18	+	−	+	−	38[1]	48[1]

+ = Positive; ++ = Strongly positive; ND = Not done; [1] = Remission (or survival) continues.

Table 3. Complications of intravenous BCG in adults with acute myeloblastic leukaemia

Anaphylactic reactions	2	
Headaches and muscle pains	3	
Transient jaundice	2	
Transient urticarial skin rash	1	
Epithelioid granulomas: Marrow	14	(18)
Liver	9	(10)
Lung	5	(6)
Spleen	2	(4)

(Figs. in brackets = total patients where biopsy or PM material available).

Table 4. BCG treatment schedule used to establish the dilution required to produce pyrexia

Day 1	1 ml freeze-dried BCG (4–9 × 10⁶ organisms/ml) diluted 1:100,000 with saline
	0.1 ml given in fast running i.v. saline drip
Day 2	0.1 ml 1:10,000 i.v.
Day 3	0.1 ml 1:1000 i.v.
Day 4	0.1 ml 1:100 i.v.
Day 5	0.1 ml 1:100 i.v.
Day 6	0.1 ml 1:1 i.v.

Similar results have been reported using BCG by scarification into the skin in the treatment of acute myeloblastic leukaemia by GUTTERMAN and his colleagues [2]. They treated a group of patients with a cytosine/vincristine/prednisone induction schedule, and those patients reaching remission were given a similar chemotherapy maintenance. Immunotherapy with Pasteur BCG (6×10^8 units) by scarification into the skin was given at 7, 14 and 21 days. Treatment cycles were repeated at 24–28 days. The experimental group showed a significantly longer remission duration than a group of patients treated with identical chemotherapy but not receiving BCG. These results have been confirmed by others [3] using BCG by multiple skin puncture.

Conclusion

BCG has increased remission and survival in acute myeloblastic leukaemia when administered interspersed with chemotherapy. Its route of administration does not appear to be critical although much work remains to be done concerning its dosage and frequency of administration. Skin testing with hypersensitivity skin test antigens suggests that a group of patients who are initially anergic but who convert following BCG treatment may have a good prognosis.

References

1. BALDWIN, R. W., PIMM, M. V.: B.C.G. immunotherapy of pulmonary growths from intravenously transferred rat tumour cells. Brit. J. Cancer 27, 48–54 (1973).
2. CURRIE, G. A., BAGSHAWE, K. D.: Active immunotherapy with corynebacterium parvum and chemotherapy in murine fibrosarcomas. Brit. Med. J. 1, 541–544 (1970).
3. GUTTERMAN, J. U., HERSH, E. M., RODRIGUEZ, V., McCREDIE, K. B., MAVLIGIT, G., REED, R., BURGESS, M. A., SMITH, T., GEHAN, E., BODEY, G. P., FREIREICH, E. J.: Chemoimmunotherapy of adult acute leukaemia; prolongation of remission in myeloblastic leukaemia with B.C.G. Lancet (1974) II, 1405–1409.
4. MATHÉ, G., AMIEL, J. L., SCHWARZENBERG, L., SCHNEIDER, M., CATTAN, A., SCHLUMBERGER, J. R., HAYAT, M., DE VASSAL, F.: Active immunotherapy in acute lymphoblastic leukaemia. Lancet (1969) I, 697–699.

5. Mathé, G., Schwarzenberg, L., Simmler, M. C., Jurczyk-Procyk, S.: Intravenous B.C.G. in monkey and man. Lancet (1976) I, 92.
6. McKhann, C., Gunnarsson, A.: In: Neoplasm Immunity. Crispen, R. G. (ed.). Illinois: Evanston, 1974, p. 31.
7. Milas, L., Gutterman, J. U., Bašić, I., Hunter, N., Mavligit, G. M., Hersh, E. M., Withers, H. R.: Immunoprophylaxis and immunotherapy for a murine fibrosarcoma with C. Granulosum and C. Parvum. Inter. J. Cancer *14*, 493–503 (1974).
8. Muggleton, P. W., Prince, G. H., Hilton, M. L.: Effect of intravenous B.C.G. in guineapigs and pertinence to cancer immunotherapy in man. Lancet (1975) I, 1353–1355.
9. Pearson, J. W., Pearson, G. R., Gibson, W. T., Chermann, J. C., Chirigos, M. A.: Combined chemoimmunostimulation therapy against murine leukaemia. Cancer Res. *32*, 904–907 (1972).
10. Spitler, L. E., Wybran, J., Lieberman, R., Levinson, D., Epstein, W., Hendrickson, C.: In: Neoplasm Immunity. Crispen, R. G. (ed.). Illinois: Evanston, 1974, p. 45.
11. Vogler, W. R., Chan, Y-K.: Prolonging remission in myeloblastic leukaemia by tice-strain bacillus calmette-guerin. Lancet (1974) II, 128–131.
12. Whittaker, J. A., Lilleyman, J. S., Jacobs, A., Balfour, I: Immunotherapy with intravenous B.C.G. Lancet (1973) II, 1454.

Androgens and Long-Term Complete Remission in Acute Granulopoietic Leukemias

D. Hollard, R. Berthier, and J. J. Sotto

At the present time, androgens are the only drug accepted as being efficient on hematopoiesis insufficiency. This has been clearly demonstrated, especially in bone marrow aplasia [7, 21]. Therefore, we have been using androgens as an adjuvant therapy for 7 years, expecting to improve the myeloid behavior and the tolerance to chemotherapy. Thus, among a series of 22 patients having achieved complete remission after low dose induction and maintenance therapy, six are still alive more than 3 years after they entered complete remission. And nine patients are definitely expected to achieve the same result.

Long-term remission in acute granulopoietic leukemia (AGL) is very rare, especially after a maintenance therapy with 6-mercaptopurine (6-MP) and methotrexate [1, 3]. Therefore, we think the androgens therapy is undoubtedly the reason why almost 50% of our patients are still alive more than 4 years after the onset of AGL. This study stopped in July, 1975. Presently, we are waiting for the results of a cooperative therapeutic trial in which androgenotherapy is being used in a randomized study.

This paper is devoted to the study of our first group of patients and to convincing other research workers to apply the same therapeutic method.

Another aim of this paper is to discuss the mode of efficiency of androgens. A great deal of experimental results are now available, leading us to believe that the leukemic cells or the hematopoietic process during AGL are still regulated by physiologic processes. Bone marrow cultures in AGL have demonstrated that leukemic cells are able to grow by stimulating factors in vitro. On the other hand, it is believed that androgens, which act on normal stem cells in Go, or resting cells [5] are able to act on "leukemic stem cells" both in vitro and in vivo.

Methods

The main characteristics of our group of patients have been given previously [11, 20].

1. Study of Patients Entering This Trial

a. Table 1 shows the main results for the group of patients. All the patients were submitted to the same induction and maintenance therapy. Briefly, the induction phase of the therapeutic program utilized rubidomycine, vincristine, and prednisone. The doses varied according to the age. The maintenance therapy consisted in the alternance of 6-MP and methotrexate with a reduction every 3 months, as in the above-mentioned papers.

The androgenotherapy consisted in stanozolol (α-derivate of androstane with pyrazol ring) at *low dosage* (0,15 mg/kg/day) for an indefinite period of time.

b. The criteria for classification of the AGL were the generally accepted ones.

Acute myeloblastic leukemia was diagnosed if Auer's bodies were present or according to positivity of peroxydase, Sudan black, and myeloperoxydase reactions.

Acute promyelocytic leukemia was diagnosed if granulations were very dense and covered the nucleus.

D. Hollard, R. Berthier, and J. J. Sotto

Table 1. Patients in complete remission for more than 12 months: main hematologic data at diagnosis and present status

	Marrow		Peripheral blood							Age (years)	Sex	Results		Present status
	Blasts %	Bone marrow cellularity	R.B.C.	Hb	Retic.	Neut.	Plat.	Blasts %	Cytol. type			C.R. duration (months)	Survival duration	
1 MER	87	+++	3,0	10,60	8 000	108	30 000	/	MBl	26	M	77	78	Alive[a]
2 LAB	90	+++	2,8	8,90	/	3 000	20 000	90	MBl	41	F	67	69	Alive[a]
3 BRA	96	+++	1,8	6	2 000	2 100	10 000	97,7	MBl	26	F	68	70	Dead[a]
4 DUP	66	+++	4,1	9,50	200 000	1 400	<10 000	87,5	MBl	6	M	36	70	Dead
5 FER	60	+	2,5	9	42 000	2 500	40 000	35	MBl	22	F	70	72	Alive[a]
6 BAU	80	+++	4,8	14,8	/	1 798	180 000	73	MBl	44	M	54	60	Alive[b]
7 ROD	75	++	1,6	5,9	82 000	1 250	<10 000	19	PMo	18	F	55	59	Alive[b]
8 THI	95	++	1,7	5	/	150	45 000	/	MBl	54	F	18	20	Dead[a]
9 DUJ	80	++	2,5	8,6	800	110	63 000	16	MBl	3	M	39	40	Alive[a]
10 FIC	100	+++	1,8	5,4	42 000	1 320	<10 000	77,5	MBl	6	F	23	20	Alive
11 VIL	100	+++	2,8	8,4	4 000	3 700	40 000	96	MBl	9	M	28	29	Alive
12 MIL	95	+++	2,3	7,8	35 000	1 100	230 000	21	MBl	50	F	13	15	Alive

PMo: Promyelocytic
a : off the treatment
b : Relapse
MBl: Myeloblastic

Myelomonocytic leukemia was diagnosed if a specific reaction was positive (naphtol acetate).

c. Table 2 shows the number of patients according to the cytologic classification.

Complete remission was accepted according to the usual criteria: less than 5% of blast cells in bone marrow, a normal count of red cells, polymorphonuclei and platelets in the peripheral blood reflecting a normal hematopoiesis in the bone marrow.

Table 2. Results according to cytologic type

	Myeloblastic AL	Myelomonocytic AL	Promyelocytic AL	Total
Complete remission	17	4	1	22
Failures	23	0	2	25
Total	40	4	3	47

2. Hematologic Data at Onset

The hematologic data for the nine patients still alive and maintaining complete remission were reviewed. In each case, as shown in Table 1, there was a large infiltration of the bone marrow and blood by the leukemic cells and a usual cytopenia.

3. In Vitro Analysis

The in vitro bone marrow and blood cell culture technique was used according to the original technique of PIKE and ROBINSON [18]. All the patients in complete remission were studied and the normality of the clusters and colonies counted on the 10th day constituted even greater supporting evidence for the normality of hematopoiesis.

In another way, the "density cut technique" according to MOORE et al. [16] was used to separate "low-density leukemic cells" from high-density cells. Since this technique is based on a buoyant density separation, we know that a normal light-heavy cell rate is another means of following up the level of leukemic cells. Unfortunately, not all the patients were investigated at the onset by this technique. Nevertheless, this procedure was used to follow up some patients in partial remission, and we believe the normality of the low-density cell population provides a good method for confirming complete remission.

Some patients were studied by the "thymidine suicide" technique of ISCOVE et al. [12] as modified by GREENBERG and SCHRIER [9]. We know this technique is an assay for cells in the S phase and has a range of 35–45% in normal bone marrow.

Results

The actuarial curves were calculated according to the usual procedure.

Out of the 46 patients who were investigated and treated, 22 achieved a complete remission. They are investigated at least every 3 months. The actuarial curves of survival and duration of complete remission were calculated as usual.

1. Hematologic and Clinical Data at Diagnosis

In order to avoid an unintentional selection of patients with a "good prognosis," all the blood and bone marrow smears were reviewed. Because this study was finished a year ago, this group is the same as the one already published [11, 22]. Briefly, to restate the main points (Table 1):

a. All patients with less than 60% of blast cells in the nucleated cells counted in the bone marrow were discarded from the study. In every case, there were more than 1000 blasts/mm³ in the peripheral blood. The bone marrow insufficiency was always well-marked (platelet counts were of less than 30,000/ml) except in one case where there was, at diagnosis, a blast infiltration in the peripheral blood of 190,000/mm³.

b. The results according to age, sex, and cytologic type are shown in Tables 2, 3, and 4. In spite of the low number of patients, a normal distribution is evident, especially for the young patients and the promyelocytic types [2] of AGL. The relationship between the number of the complete remission and the age is also normal, with a worse prognosis for adults.

Table 3. Results according to sex

	Males	Females	Total
Complete remission	12	10	22
Failures	14	11	25
Total	26	21	47

Table 4. Results according to age

	15 years	15–40 years	40–60 years	Total
Complete remission	7	8	7	22
Failures	0	5	20	25
Total	7	13	27	47

2. Results for Patients in Complete Remission

If we consider the slope of the actuarial curves (Fig. 1), some important factors emerge:

a. The low number of patients who relapsed during the 1st year is the main result: only six patients relapsed during this period of observation. In two cases (patients ROD and DUP), it was possible to put them in complete remission again. Comparing the slope of the curve with other results, it is possible to accept that this rate of continuous complete remission is much lower than the other one with the same drug regiment [19]. It is the reason why the number of patients who died during the first 3 months after we started the treatment is lower than that of other therapeutic results—we will discuss that later on.

b. Among the five patients who died during the first 3 years, only four relapsed. Two patients died in complete remission, three patients died because of relapse—they were only in partial remission after an initial stage in complete remission.

c. Two patients died in complete remission.

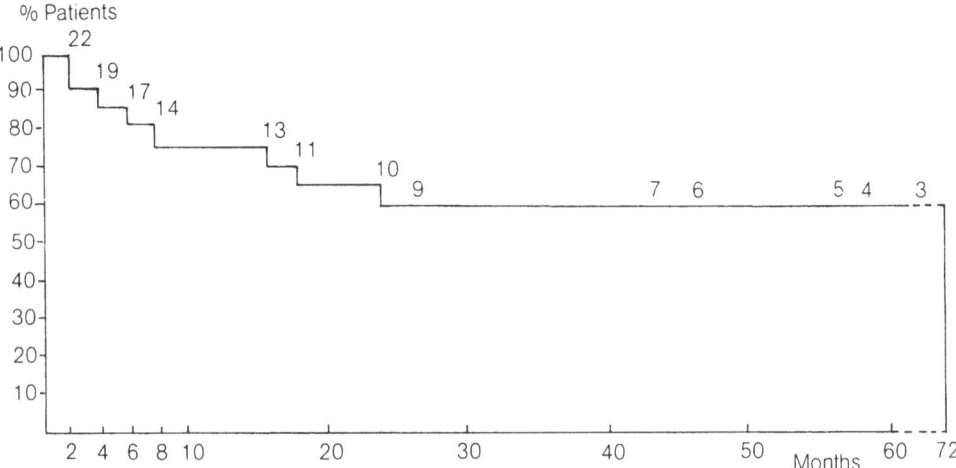

Fig. 1. Acturial survival curve (July 1976)

In one case, a surgical fault was directly the cause of death: surgical excision of a superficial abcess. This death was due to a massive loss of blood considered as normal in a "leukemic patient." The patient was admitted dying to our department.

In the other case (THT), the death was secondary to hepatic disease considered to be toxic. The postmortem examination confirmed the complete remission and a hepatic necrosis, perhaps secondary to the androgenotherapy or another infectious hepatitis.

d. One patient relapsed after a lengthy complete remission (70 months). The treatment had been discontinued because of the side effects of the androgens in women and because of the long-term complete remission.

e. For the other patients, still alive 2 years after they entered complete remission, the main feature is indeed the maintenance of a steady state.

Seven patients have remained in complete remission for more than 2 years, five for more than 4 years.

Two of them are now off the treatment after 5 years of maintenance therapy.

During this entire period, we were unable to discover any leukemic cells in the bone marrow. In one case (BAU), 4 years after the beginning of complete remission, a central nervous relapse with myeloblasts in the cerebrospinal fluid without any bone marrow relapse was detected.

3. In Vitro Study

The agar culture of marrow and blood was used to investigate all the patients in complete remission.

Figs. 2 and 3 show the results for 18 cases of AGL. Unfortunately, the cases studied before 1973 were not submitted to that investigation. Nevertheless, we can verify the behavior of the bone marrow and the blood of every patient in complete remission. According to others [14], the normality is confirmed, either by the colony and cluster formation [15] or by the rate of low-density cells [16] after a simple buoyant density separation according to the density cut technique of Moore et al. [16].

However, for two patients, the in vitro culture failed to confirm complete remission.

In the first (FER), although the blood peripheral cell count and marrow smears were

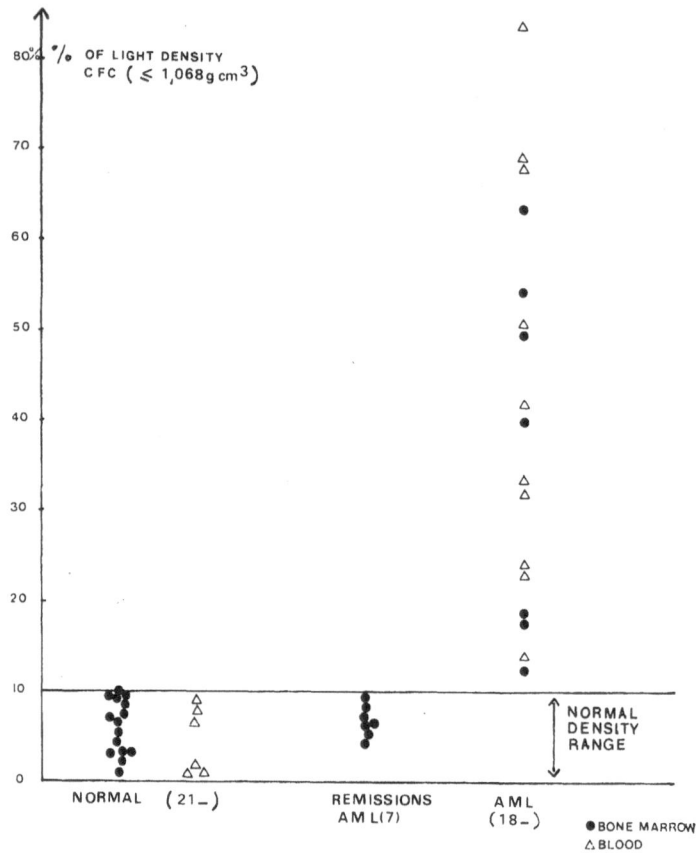

Fig. 2. Density cut distribution of CFC in marrow and blood cells of normal subjects and A.M.L. patients in remission and at diagnosis

entirely normal, the number of colonies was low [8] as was the incidence of clusters, but the rate of low-density cells was normal. This patient was off treatment (STA had been stopped for 6 months). Three months after the cessation of androgenotherapy, the behavior of bone marrow cells in culture is again normal.

In this second case (BAU), suffering from a partial relapse (CNS), the leukemic cells from a sample of the spinal fluid failed to grow. Moreover, the number of colonies and clusters in the agar culture system was lower than normal.

Discussion

In spite of the lack of randomized studies, the unusual number of patients in long-term complete remission in this series encourages us to attempt an experimental study on the mechanism of action in leukemic hematopoiesis and "leukemic cells differentiation." Therefore, we would like to discuss some practical and theoretical view points.

It is evident that our group of patients was selected neither for each prognostic factor nor for

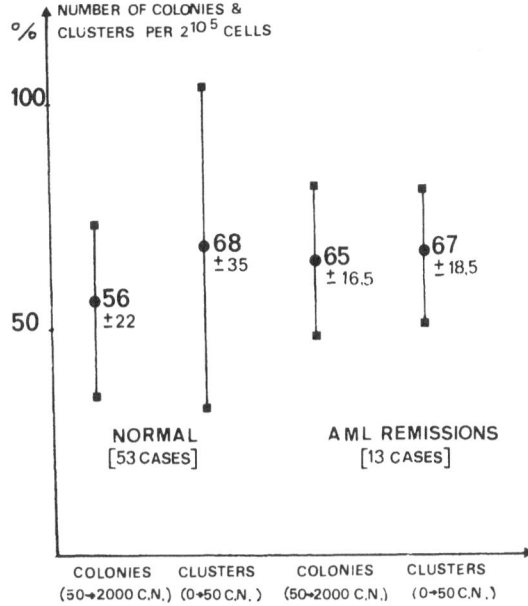

Fig. 3. Incidence of clusters and colonies per 2^{10^5} marrow cells in normal subjects and A.M.L. patients in remission (agar culture tests of PIKE and ROBINSON)

the probable diagnosis. Above all, it is not possible to suspect any slow or subacute leukemic progress (i.e., "smouldering" or oligoblastic leukemia). Moreover, it is well-known that these processes are poorly sensitive to androgenotherapy as well as to chemotherapy. In one case, the in vitro procedure seemed to show a particular feature with regard to the evolution of leukemic cells during androgenotherapy in a smouldering leukemia treated by 6-MP and methotrexate.

Other points for discussion:

1. The Low Doses of Androgens

In aplastic bone marrow insufficiency, it is well-known that only high doses (more than 1 mg/kg/day) are efficient. For this reason, we have to discuss high-dose androgenotherapy. First of all, we can confirm the reality of androgenotherapy. The side effects, especially the virilization of female patients, were well-marked. These side effects hindered a few patients from continuing the treatment. In one case (THI), it was possible to suspect androgenotherapy as a cause of fatal hepatic necrosis.

Nevertheless, we are wondering about this low-dose procedure. In a preceding paper [10], we reported on a study in which we began to try high doses on elderly patients during the first 3 months of treatment. Therefore, it is possible to obtain some other results in a phase of induction therapy. As a result of this discussion, we have come to two conclusions.

a. Androgenotherapy seems efficient at low doses and only in maintenance therapy associated with 6-MP and methotrexate.

b. Androgenotherapy can be efficient at high doses for the achievement of complete remission.

2. Possible Mechanism of Action of Androgenotherapy

Experimental results are now available to confirm the action of androgens on hematopoiesis
[8]. The in vivo study of Byron [4] demonstrated that androgens act on resting stem cells (or
in differentiated or cell-forming units (CFUs). The decrease in CFUs and the increase of
cells killed by the thymidine suicide procedure of hydroxyurea allow us to conclude that
androgens put cells into the S phase and sensitize them to cell cycle dependent drugs. Tfm
mice [6] which are genetically deprived of androgen-binding receptors on erythrogenic
precursors are nevertheless able to respond to androgen-producing granulopoietic stem
cells.

The in vitro studies of Rosenblum and Carbone [19] led them to believe in the existence of
a dose-response relationship in the production of CFUs in vitro. Nevertheless, it is
hazardous to extend these results to the leukemic hematopoiesis, and we need further
studies to approach these fascinating questions.

However, some hypotheses can be put forward:

a. A direct effect of androgens in leukemic blast cells themselves is the boldest hypothesis.
In one case, not included in this study, the in vitro growth pattern and the density
characteristics of high-density cells clearly showed some progressive modifications. The
patient was in partial remission; the results will be published elsewhere.

b. The possibility of androgen acting as a "recruitment drug" is offered. This could be the
explanation for good results with a usually poorly active chemotherapy [17].

c. The third hypothesis is probably the best. The stimulation of normal hematopoiesis by
androgens inhibits the growth of leukemic clones. We know that normal CFUs reduce the
growth of leukemic cells and vice-versa.

In any case, it would be of very great interest to confirm and to verify whether our results
are consistent with the view that leukemic cells are still regulated by normal factors of
growth and/or differentiation [13].

References

1. Bernard, J., Jacquillat, C., Weill, M., Gemon Auclerc, M. F.: Long term survivals (L.T.S.)
   in acute leukemias. In: The 16th International Congress of Hematology. (Abstract S-56-1) Main
   Topics and Symposia, Kyoto, 1976, p. 175.
2. Bernard, J., Weill, M., Boiron, M., Jacquillat, C., Flandrin, G., Gemon Auclerc, M. F.:
   Acute promyelocytic leukemia: results of treatment by daunorubidomycin. Blood 41, 489–496
   (1973).
3. Burchenal, J. H.: Long term survivors of acute leukemia. In: The 16th International Congress
   of Hematology. (Abstract S-56-3) Main Topics and Symposia, Kyoto, 1976, p. 176.
4. Byron, J. W.: Effect of steroids on the cycling of haemopoietic stem cells. Nature 228, 1204 (1970).
5. Byron, J. W.: Comparison of the action of ^{3}H-thymidine and hydroxyurea on testosterone-
   treated haemopoietic stem cells. Blood 40, 198–203 (1972).
6. Byron, J. W.: Application of the Tf$_m$ mutant mouse to the study of the haematopoietic action of
   androgens. In: IVth Annual Conference. (Abstract). International Society for Experimental
   Hematology, Trojer Croatia, Yougoslavia, 1975, p. 37.
7. Gardner, F. H., Pringle, J. C.: Androgens and erythropoiesis. Arch. intern. Med. 107, 846–862
   (1961).
8. Gorshein, D., Hait, W. N., Besa, E. C., Jepson, J. H. Gardner, F. H.: Rapid stem cell
   differentiation induced by 19-nortestosterone decanoate. Brit. J. Haemat. 26, 215–225 (1974).
9. Greenberg, P. L., Schrier, S. L.: Granulopoiesis in neutropenic disorders. Blood 41, 753–769
   (1973).
10. Hollard, D., Schaerer, R., Sotto, J. J.: The place of the androgenotherapy in acute leukemia
    treatment. In: Proceedings of International Meeting on Therapy of Acute Leukemias, Rome, 1973.
    Mandelli, R., Amadori, S., Mariani, G., (eds.). Rome: Centro Minerva Medica, 1975, pp. 527–536.

11. HOLLARD, D., SOTTO, J. J., BACHELOT, C., MICHALLET, M., RIBAUD, P., SCHAERER, R., WAGUET, J-C.: Essai d'androgénothérapie dans le traitement des leucémies aiguës non lymphoblastiques. Nouv. Presse méd. 5, 1289–1293 (1976).
12. ISCOVE, N. N., SENN, J. S., TILL, J. E., McCULLOCH, E. A.: Colony formation by normal and leukemic marrow cells in culture—effect of conditioned medium from human leukocytes. Blood 37, 1–5 (1971).
13. McCULLOCH, E. A., TILL, J. E.: Leukemia considered as defective differentiation complementary in vivo and culture methods applied to the clinical problem. In: The Nature of Leukemia. Vincent, P.C. (ed.). Sydney: W. C. Blight, 1972, p. 119.
14. METCALF, D., MOORE, M. A. S.: Haemopoietic cells. Amsterdam-London: North Holland, 1971.
15. MOORE, M. A. S.: In vitro studies in the myeloid leukaemias. In: Advances in Acute Leukaemia. Cleton, F. J. Crowther, D., Malpas, D. (eds.). Amsterdam-Oxford: North Holland-New York: American Elsevier, 1974, pp. 161–218.
16. MOORE, M. A. S., WILLIAMS, N., METCALF, D.: In vitro colony formation by normal and leukemic human hematopoietic cells: characterization of the colony forming cells. J. nat. Cancer Inst. 50, 603–623 (1973).
17. PAVLOVSKY, S., PENALVER, J., EPPINGER-HELFT, M., SACKMANN MURIEL, F., BERGNA, L., ARGIMIRO, S., VILASECA, G., PAVLOVSKY, A. A., PAVLOVSKY, A.: Induction and maintenance of remission in acute leukemia. Cancer 31, 272–278 (1973).
18. PIKE, B. L., ROBINSON, W. A.: Human bone marrow colony growth in agar gel. J. cell. Physiol. 76, 77–84 (1970).
19. ROSENBLUM, A. L., CARBONE, P. P.: Androgenic hormones and human granulopoiesis in vitro. Blood 43, 351–356 (1974).
20. SOTTO, J. J., HOLLARD, D., SCHAERER, R., BENSA, J. C., SEIGNEURIN, D.: Androgènes et rémissions prolongées dans les leucémies aiguës non lymphoblastiques: résultats d'un traitement systématique par le stanozolol associé à la chimiothérapie. Nouv. Rev. fr. Hémat. 15, 57–72 (1975).
21. ZITTOUN, R., BERNADOU, A., BLANC, C. M., BILSKI-PASQUIER, G., BOUSSER, J.: La méténolone dans le traitement des insuffisances médullaires. Presse méd. 76, 445–449 (1968).

Treatment by Radiophosphorus Versus Busulfan in Polycythemia Vera: A Randomized Trial (E.O.R.T.C.'s*) "Leukemias and Hematosarcomas" Group

CHAIRMAN: H. O. KLEIN; COUNCILLOR: G. MATHÉ; SECRETARY: M. HAYAT

Participating members of the group:
Amsterdam: J. F. CLETON; Anvers: M. PEETERMANS; Barcelona: C. FERRAN; Bologna: M. BACCARANI, S. TURA; Bordeaux: B. HOERNI, S. HOERNI-SIMON; Brussels: C. CAUCHIE, Y. KENIS, J. MICHELS, J. P. NAETS, P. STRYCKMANS, H. TAGNON; Cologne: R. GROSS, W. HIRSCHMANN, H. O. KLEIN; Dublin: J. B. HEALY; La Haye: H. KERKHOFS, C. H. W. LEEKSMA; Leiden: F. ELKERBOUT; Liège: J. M. ANDRIEN, P. CONINX, J. HUGUES; Lyon: D. FIERE, L. REVOL; Mayence: J. FISHER; Nijmegen: C. HAANEN, M. C. DALE; Paris: A. BERNADOU, G. BILSKI-PASQUIER, G. M. BLANC, J. BOUSSER, J. DEBRAY, M. KRULIK, R. ZITTOUN; Reims: A. CATTAN; Rotterdam: W. F. STENFERT-KROESE; Rouen: H. PIGUET; Villejuif: J. L. AMIEL, M. HAYAT, G. MATHÉ, P. POUILLART, L. SCHWARZENBERG, F. DE VASSAL

Polycythemia vera is a relatively rare disease with an average annual incidence rate of from 0.6–1.6/100,000 population. The mean age of onset is 55–60 years, and there is an increasing annual incidence rate with advancing age. Males fall more often ill than females (approximately 2:1; [2, 13, 18]). The mean survival time of untreated patients is only about 18 months [2].

Generally, the disease is considered a myeloproliferative syndrome [1] or a myelodysplastic disease [2] which involves, in addition to erythropoiesis, granulopoiesis as well as thrombopoiesis. The pathogenesis of the disease is still unknown although there seems to be evidence that an intrinsic cell defect at the stem cell level might be responsible for extensively uncontrolled proliferation of bone marrow cells [2, 3]. Therefore, only symptomatic therapeutic measures such as phlebotomy and treatment with radioactive phosphorus as well as cytostatic agents are available to date.

Concerning phlebotomy, earlier studies revealed that ^{32}P treatment and myelosuppressive agents may yield better results [ref. in 2], although in 1971 SILVERSTEIN and LANIER [18] showed no significant differences—however, their series was small.

In so-called phase II studies, it could be shown that ^{32}P and cytostatic agents induce long-lasting remissions and prolong survival considerably [4, 5, 9, 16, 17, 19]. Unfortunately, both treatment procedures are said to also induce high rates of side effects, especially acute leukemia and myelofibrosis [8, 14, 15]. There is a lack of randomized trials comparing both treatments.

In 1967, our group started a phase III trial trying to close the gap of knowledge. The aim of the study was to assess the effects of both treatment methods on (1) the remission duration, (2) the length of survival, and (3) the frequency and types of complications occurring in patients with polycythemia vera, especially the incidence of acute leukemia, so-called "spent" polycythemia, and myelofibrosis.

---

* European Organisation for Research on the Treatment of Cancer.

Materials and Methods

Since 1967, 251 patients—never treated before by one of the two treatment methods—were included in this trial and allocated to ^{32}P or busulfan treatment at random. However, 26 out of the 251 patients were eliminated from the trial because of lack of news.

Diagnosis of polycythemia vera was based on erythrocytosis with elevated red blood cell mass and on signs of panmyelosis in the bone marrow. Patients with secondary erythrocytosis were excluded. Table 1 shows the mean age and the distribution of males and females as well as the hematologic parameters for patients of both treatment groups. There are statistically significantly more females in the busulfan group than in the ^{32}P group.

Treatment was performed by radiophosphorus as well as by busulfan. Radiophosphorus was administered intraveneously (dosage 0.5–1.0 mCi/10 kg body weight). Busulfan was given orally in a dosage of 4–6 mg/day till hypoplasia of the bone marrow and normalization of the red cell mass was observed. In Table 2 are listed the different initial doses of radiophosphorus (mean dose 5.9 mCi) and the different doses of busulfan necessary to induce first complete remission (mean total dose 310.6 mg). In each group phlebotomy was used as a means to correct red cell mass—the hematocrit count should be maintained between 42 and 47%. The rate of phlebotomy was equal in both groups (Table 2).

Results and Discussion

Results of this randomized cooperative trial are shown in Table 3. Of the patients treated by busulfan, 59% are still in their first complete remission compared to only 34% in the

Table 1. Comparison of the two groups prior to any treatment

Therapeutic group		^{32}P	Busulfan	Statistical significance
		% or mean	% or mean	
Sex	Male	58%	44%	p = 0.05
	Female	42%	56%	
Age		60 ± 2 years	60 ± 2 years	NS
Erythrocytes × 10⁶		7.18 ± 0,2	7.13 ± 0,2	NS
Hemoglobin		20.4	19	NS
Reticulocytes × 10⁴		10.2 ± 3	9.4 ± 2	NS
Polynuclears × 10²		72 ± 6	71 ± 6	NS
Mononuclears × 10²		20 ± 2	20 ± 2	NS
Thrombocytes × 10⁴		42.5 ± 10	42 ± 5	NS
Blood volume		90.5 ml/kg	90.3 ml/kg	NS
Red cell mass		60 ml/kg	61 ml/kg	NS
Plasma volume		41 ml/kg	43 ml/kg	NS
Blood viscosity		8.5	8	NS

Hematologic parameters in patients with polycythemia vera.

Table 2. Polycythemia vera (doses of ^{32}p and Busulfan)

^{32}p		Busulfan		
First doses	Number of patients	Total doses		Number of patients
			dose < 80 mg	11
3.0 mCi < dose < 4.5 mCi	7	80	dose < 160 mg	17
4.5 mCi < dose < 6.0 mCi	42	160	dose < 410 mg	60
dose < 6.0 mCi	58	410	dose < 700 mg	30

Mean dose of ^{32}p at the first administration: 5.9 mCi; mean total dose of busulfan for first remission induction 310.6 mg.

Therapeutic group	^{32}p		Busulfan	
	Number of patients	%	Number of patients	%
With phlebotomy	27	25	21	18
Without phlebotomy	80	75	97	82

Rate of phlebotomy in patients with polycythemia vera. Results are not significant statistically.

Table 3. Polycythemia vera remissions and relapses after nine years of follow-up

Therapeutic groups	^{32}p		Busulfan	
	Number of patients	%	Number of patients	%
Patients in first complete remission	36	34	70	59
Relapses	71	66	48	41

Differences are statistically significant $p = 0,001$

Survival and death after nine years of follow-up

Therapeutic groups	^{32}p		Busulfan	
	Number of patients	%	Number of patients	%
Alive	93	87%	110	93%
Deceased	14	13%	8	7%

Results after treatment of polycythemia vera by radiophosphorus or busulfan.

radiophosphorus group. The result is statistically significant. However, the survival rates in both groups are not statistically different.

The duration of first complete remission and the actuarial curve of survival are demonstrated in Figure 1. Of the busulfan treated patients, 50% display a remission duration of about 4 years, which is in good agreement with data in the literature [20]. On the other hand, remission duration for 50% of our radiophosphorus treated patients is only about 2½ years. In a recent review of ^{32}P treatment in polycythemia vera, similar data were recorded [7].

Many reports deal with hematologic complications after radiophosphorus treatment, especially for acute myeloid leukemia and myelofibrosis [ref. in 8]. Table 4 shows causes of death in our patients with polycythemia vera. At present, there is no case due to acute leukemia and only one case with myelofibrosis. Vascular complications caused death for the most part in both groups of treatment, as is also stated in the literature [ref. in 2].

A further interesting observation was made by our group when remission duration was plotted according to sex. Females do better than male patients (Fig. 2).

In summary, despite the present short observation time of about 6–9 years, it was thought worthwhile to present these data, which display the partly statistically significantly better

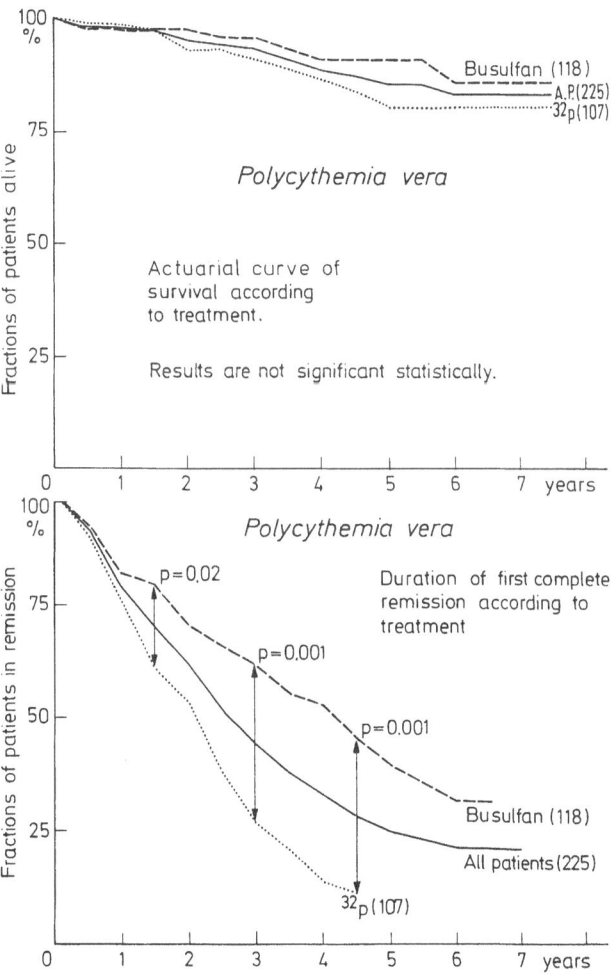

Fig. 1

Table 4. Causes of death in patients with polycythemia vera

Causes	^{32}p	Busulfan
Relapses	2	1
Vascular complications	9	5
Myelofibrosis	1	1
Other causes	1 (infection)	1 (gangrene)
Unknown causes	1	0

results of busulfan treatment compared with ^{32}P with regard to remission duration, death rate, and incidence of vascular complications. Furthermore, the statistically better results in females compared with males were also of particular interest for there were already indications in the literature pointing out this fact [6, further ref. in 8].

A high incidence rate of acute leukemia following radiophosphorus therapy is well-known from the studies of MODAN [14, 15], TUBIANA and co-workers [19], and LAWRENCE et al [10]. It averages 10–20% in most published series, but at least two large series have been reported in which no cases of leukemia occurred, and in some small series, leukemia represented more than 50% of the total number of deaths [ref. in 8]. According to MODAN and LILIENFELD [14], the incidence rate increases with the dose of ^{32}P; with 3–12 mCi, the incidence rate was 0–4%; with 15–35 mCi, it was 12–22%; and with 50–75 mCi, it was 28%. This was confirmed by TUBIANA et al. [19]. However, it is not clear from all the studies whether polycythemia vera per se already bears a high risk for developing leukemia. LANDAW [8] reported a compilation of more than 50 cases of acute leukemia developing in patients with polycythemia vera treated only by phlebotomy or chemotherapy. TUBIANA et al. [19] and MODAN and LILIENFELD [14] found that a biological factor—a high initial white cell count and a large palpable spleen [19] or the number of immature white cells in

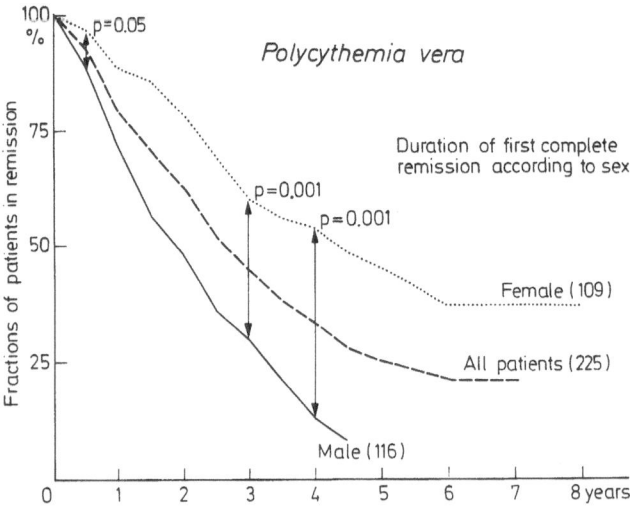

Fig. 2

the blood prior to therapy [14]—is of importance for the occurrence of leukemia. TUBIANA and co-workers [19] stated that these patients also needed a higher dose of ^{32}P to enter remission than patients who did not show these clinical symptoms. The authors suggested that these biological factors plus high doses of ^{32}P are responsible for the early appearance of leukemia and other hematologic complications in their patients. To date, in our trial, no patient with acute leukemia has been observed. This might be due to the relatively short observation time of 6–8 years. However, LEDLIE [11] and also TUBIANA et al. [19] showed that in patients under radiophosphorus therapy, leukemia may already appear 1½–4 years after the onset of treatment.

A further follow-up of our patients will demonstrate whether some cases have yet to develop acute leukemia and also whether a statistically significant difference of survival between the two groups of treatment will appear. The latter seems unlikely because there are already several phase II trials showing no real difference in survival time [4, 5, 9, 16, 17, 19]. Later on, our results may also be compared with findings of the Polycythemia Vera Study Group which is conducting a trial proving the therapeutic effect of ^{32}P and chemotherapy as well as phlebotomy [12].

References

1. DAMESHEK, W.: Some speculations on the myeloproliferative syndromes. Blood 6, 372 (1951).
2. GILBERT, H. S.: Definition, clinical features and diagnosis of polycythemia vera. Clin. Haematol. 4, 263 (1975).
3. GURNEY, C. W.: Mechanisms underlying the polycythemias. In: Regulation of Hematopoiesis. Red Cell Production. Gordon, A. S. (ed.). New York: Appleton Century Crofts, Educational Division, Meredith Corporation, 1970, Vol I, p. 611.
4. HALNAN, K. E., RUSSELL, M. H.: Polycythemia vera. Comparison of survival and causes of death in patients managed with and without radiotherapy. Lancet (1965) II, 760.
5. HARMAN, J. B., LEDLIE, E. M.: Survival of polycythemia vera patients treated with radioactive phosphorus. Brit. Med. J. 2, 146 (1967).
6. HENNING, K., FRANKE, W. J., STRIETZEL, M.: Eigene Erfahrungen in der Radiophosphorbehandlung bei Polycythaemia vera. Zschr. ges. inn. Med. 20, 14 (1965).
7. HÖR, G., PABST, H. W.: Radiophosphortherapie der Polycythaemia vera. Revue therapeutique 30, 789 (1973).
8. LANDAW, ST. A.: Acute leukemia in polycythemia vera. Sem. Hematol. 13, 33 (1976).
9. LAWRENCE, J. H.: Polycythemia. Physiology, diagnosis, and treatment. New York: Grune and Stratton, 1955.
10. LAWRENCE, J. H., WINDELL, H. S., DONALD, W. G.: Leukemia in polycythemia vera. Ann. intern. Med. 70, 763 (1969).
11. LEDLIE, E. M.: The incidence of leukemia in patients with polycythemia vera treated by ^{32}P. Clin. Radiol. 11, 130 (1960).
12. LOEB, V.: Treatment of polycythemia vera. Clin. Haematol. 4, 441 (1975).
13. MODAN, B.: An epidemiological study of polycythemia vera. Blood 26, 657 (1965).
14. MODAN, B., LILIENFELD, A. N.: Polycythemia vera and leukemia: role of radiation. Treatment study of 1222 patients. Medicine 44, 305 (1965).
15. MODAN, B.: Inter-relationship between polycythemia vera, leukemia, and myeloid metaplasia. Clin. Haematol. 4, 427 (1975).
16. OSGOOD, E. E.: Polycythemia vera: age relationship and survival. Blood 26, 243 (1965).
17. PERKINS, J., ISRAELS, M. C. G., WILKINSON, J. F.: Polycythemia vera: clinical studies on a series of 127 patients managed without radiation therapy. Quart. J. Med. 33, 499 (1964).
18. SILVERSTEIN, M. N., LARNIER, A. P.: Polycythemia vera, 1935–1969: an epidemiologic survey in Rochester, Minnesota. Mayo Clinic Proceedings 46, 771 (1971).
19. TUBIANA, M. R., FLAMANT, ATTIE, E., HAYAT, M.: A study of hematological complications occurring in patients with polycythemia vera treated with ^{32}P. (Based on a series of 296 patients). Blood 32, 536 (1968).
20. URASINSKI, J., MYSIK, M.: Die Therapie der Polycythaemia vera mit Busulfan (Myleran^R). Bericht über die Behandlungsergebnisse von 40 Kranken. Folia haemat. (Leipzig) 94, 360 (1970).

The Strategy of Treatment of Hodgkin's Disease*

B. Hœrni, J. Chauvergne, and C. Lagarde

The treatment of Hodgkin's disease has greatly evolved during the last decade. It has actually reached a degree of maturity which can lead to a general consensus on the main points [1, 6, 7, 8, 9].

Methods of Treatment

First, we will do a quick revision of the available therapeutic methods and of their main characteristics. It is particularly important to separate them into two groups.

Localized methods, radiotherapy and surgery, are very active but limited as they can only be applied to a part of the body.

Generalized methods, chemotherapy and immunotherapy, are a little less active but capable of acting on the totality of the organism and on neoplasic cells no matter where they may be. Let us emphasize that this therapeutic arsenal is important and very efficacious, one of the most efficacious in all oncology. Therefore, the main problem for the treatment of Hodgkin's disease, as well as for some other cancers, is no longer to do the maximum, but rather to do the minimum while assuring the same high chance of cure.

Following the works of Gilbert, Peters, and Kaplan, in particular, *radiotherapy* has constituted the main treatment of Hodgkin's disease until these last years.

It is capable of sterilizing areas to which it is applied at relatively weak doses of about 40 gray in 4 weeks. This allows the extension of the field by covering adjacent lymph node areas in order to prevent further relapses, which have a preference for these same areas; but, the necessity of this field extension can be debated if one associates a chemotherapy which can also sterilize the tumoral microfoci. We will come back to this point later on.

The inconveniences of this type of treatment are firstly the limitation of application. Thus, it necessitates a precise staging topography for the localization of the tumoral foci to be irradiated. Technical progress has now greatly reduced the local complications such as myelitis and pericarditis which should no longer be seen nowadays. The oncogenic risk persists as with all radiotherapy, minimal perhaps, but not negligible, especially for Hodgkin's patients who are often young.

Surgery can be of interest for the lymph nodes or for the spleen. The lymph node biopsy is necessary for diagnostic purposes, but the surgical dissection sometimes proposed in the attempt at tumoral reduction has almost no interest.

Splenectomy is more interesting. A moderate splenic involvement can be sterilized just as well by radiotherapy or, in our opinion, even better by chemotherapy, but we think that for a large splenomegaly, splenectomy offers the best eradication of spleen foci. The infectious risk seems to be limited and due to Hodgkin's disease, as well as to the absence of the spleen. On the other hand, one presently insists on the abdominal complications provoked by radiotherapy after a prior laparotomy.

Chemotherapy has the great advantage of being a general treatment able to reach Hodgkin's tumoral foci, no matter where they may be in the organism.

---

* Communication to the 1976 Villejuif-Paris Immuno-Oncology Week.

Single drug chemotherapy is no longer employed. Many protocols of combinations exist, such as MOPP, (Mustard, oncovin, procarbazine, prednisone) and others more recently proposed. These combinations are very active and have proved their capacity in sterilizing tumoral foci, if they are small enough [2]. Let us note that the uncured patients, among those treated by chemotherapy alone, had presented relapses in the areas which initially had large tumoral formations—so-called icebergs—too large to be sterilized by chemotherapy alone and consequently needing a complementary localized radiotherapy.

The inconvenience of this treatment is that if often brings about masculine sterility and, as radiotherapy, increases the hazards of a second cancer.

Lastly, *immunotherapy* can have a certain effectiveness. The results we have obtained with BCG in a randomized study including all malignant lymphomas but with a majority of Hodgkin's disease are significantly in favor of the utilization of BCG in weekly cutaneous scarifications [4].

Strategy of Treatment

After having reviewed the methods of treatment, we will now take a look at the optimal way of combining them. It is practical to distinguish the apparently localized forms, corresponding to clinical stages I, II, and IIIa for which a local treatment, thus radiotherapy, is the most important, from the generalized forms, corresponding to clinical stages IIIb and IV, for which a general treatment, thus chemotherapy, is the most important.

For *stages I and II*, irradiation alone gives long-term survival in 40–50% of cases, or properly speaking cures, as indicated by almost all published series. Consequently, these results indicate that half of the clinical stages I and II forms are actually generalized or at least more extensive. This observation has led to divergent viewpoints. Radiologists, like KAPLAN, claiming that the relapses were often abdominal, have proposed a systematic laparotomy to detect abdominal microfoci and consequently to irradiate them. On the other hand, oncologists, claiming that the relapses were also often generalized, prefer to combine a generalized chemotherapy associated with radiotherapy. This is the case in our group in Bordeaux.

Fig. 1 shows the actuarial curves of remissions for clinical stages I and II in the past decade in the Fondation Bergonié [5]. With radiotherapy alone, the plateau is established at about 50% beyond 5 years. With an association of a combined chemotherapy prior to radiotherapy, the initial complete remission rate is significantly higher. Secondly, the plateau is established higher and sooner, mainly if there is a consolidating chemotherapy of about 15 days following the radiotherapy. These results are obtained without laparotomy, spleen irradiation, maintenance chemotherapy.

Fig. 2 indicates our present protocol of treatment for clinical stages I and II, using a chemotherapy combination as previously described [1].

Therapeutic trials of ROSENBERG and KAPLAN [10] show that the association of chemo-plus radiotherapy appears useful even for patients who have had a laparotomy and extended irradiation.

Summing up, for stages I and II and probably IIIa, we can say that laparotomy is useless if one systematically combines a vigorous chemotherapy, as clearly indicated by the preliminary results of the H_2 trial of E.O.R.T.C. [3].

Secondly, one should try to lighten the treatment in order to reduce the therapeutic complications:

1. Can we withhold chemotherapy from certain forms with excellent prognosis which relapse in only 10–20% of cases just after radiotherapy alone, keeping in mind the

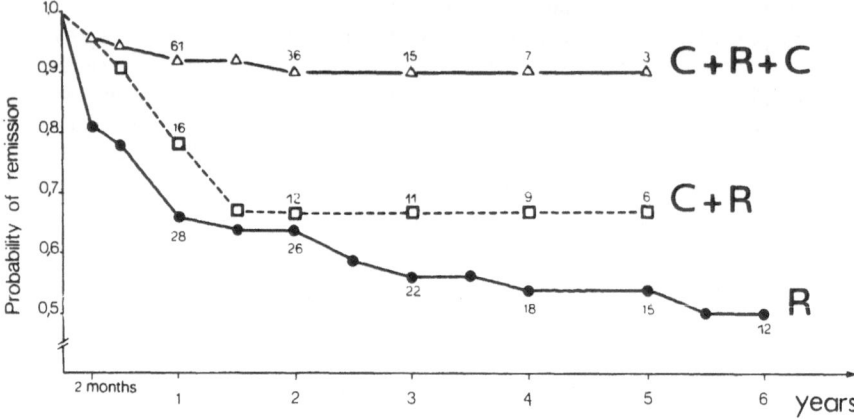

Fig. 1. Actuarial complete remission curves for clinical stages I and II treated by radiotherapy alone (R), chemo + radiotherapy (C + R) or chemo + radio + chemotherapy (C + R + C), Fondation Bergonié, 1965–1974

possibility of secondarily curing these patients after their relapse with the present available chemotherapy?

2. Can we reduce the size of the radiotherapy fields by calling upon chemotherapy to sterilize the microscopic lymph node foci?

To answer these two questions randomized studies are needed.

For *diseases obviously generalized* corresponding to clinical stages IIIb and IV, general chemotherapy is the main treatment. It should be completed by an irradiation of icebergs. Furthermore, we can propose an immunotherapy trial.

Finally, the majority of Hodgkin's diseases have localized macroscopic components, more or less extended, and a generalized dissemination, usually infraclinical, inconstant but more frequent than one believed in the past. These two components both need treatment: (1) on the one hand, a general chemotherapy more or less vigorous, according to the possibility or the certitude of the generalization and according to its importance and (2) on the other hand, a radiotherapy, which until now has been the surest way to sterilize the tumoral sites visualized by clinical and radiologic assessment.

In conclusion, 80% of patients with Hodgkin's disease can and should be cured by the present methods of treatment. Therapeutic studies should be oriented to clarify the optimal equilibrium between chemotherapy and radiotherapy.

The remaining 20% of patients constitute the failures: (1) one-quarter (5%) present a primary resistance to treatment and perhaps the pathologists will be able to identify them,

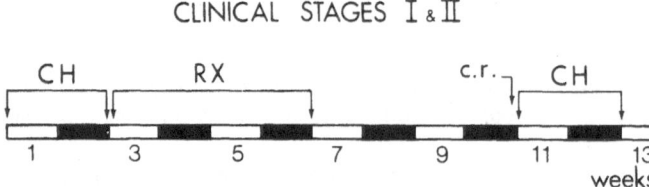

Fig. 2. Therapeutic schedule for treatment of Hodgkin's disease, clinical stages I and II (c.r. = complete remission)

(2) one-quarter are aged patients who cannot tolerate the optimal treatment, they incite us to look not for more efficacious treatments but rather more tolerable treatments, (3) one-quarter have enormous tumoral masses and are beyond any possible curative therapy, only an early diagnosis can eliminate this problem, and (4) lastly, one-quarter of the failures are actually unexplainable.

So there has been dramatic progress in the treatment of Hodgkin's disease but there is still a lot of work to be accomplished.

Summary

The treatment of Hodgkin's disease necessitates, in most cases, an association of radio-therapy for the macroscopic tumoral masses and chemotherapy for the cells generalized in the organism. Whenever a systematic chemotherapy is associated with radiotherapy, a precise staging topography with laparotomy is useless. The current therapeutic trials should seek methods to lighten these treatments by determining the best equilibrium between the two principal methods and by specifying the eventual place of immunotherapy. The present possibility of curing more than three-fourths of Hodgkin's patients incites us to look for means of reducing the treatment and its inconveniences for the curable forms, and search for more active or tolerable treatments for the uncurable forms.

References

1. CHAUVERGNE, J., HŒRNI, B., HŒRNI-SIMON, G., DURAND, M., LAGARDE, C.: Chimiothérapie de la maladie de Hodgkin associant procarbazine, vinblastine, cyclophosphamide et methyl-prednisolone. Analyse d'une série de 124 cures. Z. Krebsforsch, *80*, 179–188 (1973).
2. DE VITA, V. T., SERPICK, A. A., CARBONE, P. P.: Combination chemotherapy in the treatment of advanced Hodgkin's disease. Ann. intem. Med. *73*, 881–895 (1970).
3. E.O.R.T.C. Radiochemotherapy Group: Splenectomy vs splenic irradiation. Annual plenary meeting of the E.O.R.T.C., June 24, 1976
4. HŒRNI, B., CHAUVERGNE, J., HŒRNI-SIMON, G., DURAND, M., LAGARDE, C.: The utility of BCG in the immunotherapy of malignant lymphomas. Results of a controlled trial. Cancer Immunol. Immunother. (1977) (in press).
5. HŒRNI, B., CHAUVERGNE, J., TOUCHARD, J., MEUGÉ, C., HŒRNI-SIMON, G., DURAND, M., BRUNET, R., LAGARDE, C.: Résultats du traitement de la maladie de Hodgkin. Stades cliniques I et II, Fondation Bergonié, 1965–1975. IIème Congrès français d'Hématologie, Le Touquet, 25 mai 1976.
6. LAGARDE, C., CHAUVERGNE, J., HŒRNI, B.: La maladie de Hodgkin. Paris: Masson et Cie, 1971.
7. LAGARDE, C., CHAUVERGNE, J., HŒRNI, B.: Les lymphomes malins. Paris: Masson, 1975.
8. LAGARDE, C., CHAUVERGNE, J., TOUCHARD, J., DURAND, M., HŒRNI-SIMON, G., BRUNET, R.: Traitement des stades cliniques I et II de maladie de Hodgkin. Résultats obtenus chez 100 malades par l'association à la radiothérapie d'un ou deux cycles de chimiothérapie. Acta Haemat. *55*, 257–264 (1976).
9. MATHÉ, G., TUBIANA, M.: The natural history, diagnosis and treatment of Hodgkin's disease. Series hæmat. *6*, 5–269 (1973).
10. ROSENBERG, S. A., KAPLAN, H. S.: The management of stages I, II and III of Hodgkin's disease with combined radiotherapy and chemotherapy. Cancer, Philad. *35*, 55–63 (1975).

2. Solid tumors

Limb Preservation in Osteogenic Sarcoma: A Preliminary Report*

N. JAFFE, H. WATTS, E. FREI, D. TRAGGIS, G. VAWTER, and K. FELLOWS

Introduction

Optimum treatment for osteogenic sarcoma involves a rapid definitive attack upon the primary tumor and systemic treatment to destroy pulmonary metastases [2, 4, 5, 6, 10, 11, 13, 14, 16]. Traditionally, the first objective is attempted by amputation, although radiation therapy has also been employed [1]. The latter, however, has not met with universal approval since osteogenic sarcoma is generally considered a radioresistant tumor, and retention of an uninhibited source of metastases is contrary to sound principles of cancer management. Not infrequently, tumor growth after irradiation required amputation for palliation [9].

The advances achieved with chemotherapy in osteogenic sarcoma during the past 5 years prompted a reconsideration of alternative modes of therapy for ablation of the primary tumor. We were attracted to the concept of intensive preoperative treatment with chemotherapy followed by local en bloc resection and insertion of an internal prosthesis. Such treatment could exert an effect concurrently against the primary tumor and systemic micrometastases. This communication will present our preliminary results.

Eligibility for Entry into Trial

1. Attainment of Complete or Nearly Complete Physical Growth for Patients With Lesions of the Lower Extremities

This was recommended to avoid a short stature or gait problems which could follow normal growth of the uninvolved limb. It was recognized that some patients who had not attained full growth could subsequently undergo epiphysiodesis of the uninvolved limb at a later stage if needed. However, until the results of this experimental approach have been evaluated, we have avoided making such plans.

2. The Lesion was Considered Safely Resectable

The major artery did not show tumor encasement on the angiogram although gradual displacement of the vessels by tumor was not considered a contraindication.

* Supported in part by a research grant (CA06516) from the National Cancer Institute and by a grant (RR-05526) from the Division of Research Facilities and Resources, National Institutes of Health.

3. Absence of Metastases

Although the presence of metastases need not necessarily obviate an en bloc resection, it was elected to re-evaluate recommendations for this procedure after observing the response of metastases to chemotherapy. A complete or partial response might be a reasonable incentive to proceed with limb preservation.

4. Awareness of Risks

Patients and parents were to be fully appraised that the procedure was of an investigational nature and that limb ablation might be required at any stage because of failure or other complications occurring during the treatment program.

Patients (Table 1)

Eight patients were entered into the program from January, 1974 to September, 1976. Their ages ranged 13–18 years. Three had primary lesions of the distal femur, three of the proximal and one of the middle tibia, and one of the upper humerus. No patient had roentgenographically visible pulmonary or bone metastases at the initiation of treatment. All had measurable soft tissue involvement of variable degree.

All patients were subjected to a full physical examination, pulmonary tomograms, angiographic studies of the tumor, radionucleotide bone scans and anthropometric radiographs, and measurements of the affected limb for manufacture of a suitable endoprosthesis. The results were correlated, and the feasibility of performing a local en bloc resection was determined. An affirmative decision was followed by definitive entry into the program.

Procedure

The limb preservation program comprised four basic components:
1. Weekly courses of vincristine, high-dose methotrexate, and citrovorum factor (VCR-MTX-CF)
2. Intra-arterial adriamycin (ADR)
3. Local en bloc resection
4. Insertion of an internal prosthesis

1. Weekly VCR-MTX-CF (Fig. 1)

This involves the administration of VCR, 2 mg/m^2 (maximum 2 mg) $\frac{1}{2}$ hour before initiation of a 6-hour infusion of intravenous MTX. The first, second, and subsequent doses of MTX are 3, 6, and 7.5 g/m^2, respectively. Two hours after the completion of MTX, CF (CF "rescue") is administered at 15 mg q3h i.v. for the first 24 hours and 15 mg q6h p.o. for the subsequent 48 hours. The first p.o. dose commences 3 hours after the last i.v. dose. Prerequesites for treatment include a normal hemogram, creatinine clearance, liver

N. Jaffe, H. Watts, E. Frei, D. Traggis, G. Vawter, K. Fellows

Table 1

Patient	Age	Site of primary	VCR-MTX-CF courses	ADR	Clinical response	Angiographic response	% Viable tumor	Pulmonary metastases (Mths)	Follow-up (Mths)	Comments
W.B.	18	Proximal humerus	4	Yes	+	+	<10		20	
K.F.	13	Proximal tibia	4	Yes	+	Mixed[a]	<10	Yes (13)	14	Adr. slough. Amputation
C.G.	16	Proximal tibia	8		+	+	20		9	Ulcer over prosthesis
C.S.	17	Proximal tibia	8		−	−	90	Yes (6)	10	Small wound dehiscence
J.C.	15	Middle tibia	6		+	No change[b]	10–20		8	Dislocation, distal end of prosthesis
M.M.	16	Distal femur	8		+	Mixed[a]	60	Yes (5)	6	Sepsis
L.W.	18	Distal femur	8	Yes	+	Mixed[a]	50		6	
M.N.	16	Distal femur	2	Yes	−	Mixed[a]	50		2	Amputation because of possible escape

+ = Distinct improvement.

− = No improvement, possible deterioration.

[a] Regression of tumor neovascularity in some areas and increase or persistence of neovascularity elsewhere.

[b] Hypovascular tumor. No change in tumor size pre- and postangiography.

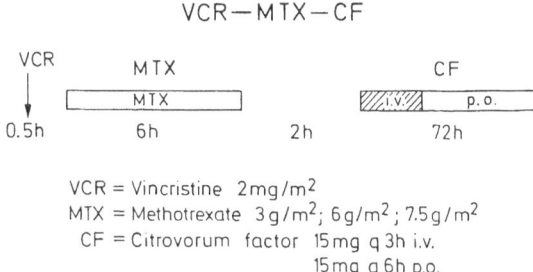

Fig. 1. High-dose MTX program. VCR, 2 mg/m² (maximum 2 mg) is administered ½ hour before the initiation of a 6-hour infusion of MTX. The first, second, and subsequent doses of MTX are 3 gm/m², 6 gm/m², and 7.5 gm/m², respectively. Two hours after completion of the MTX infusion, CF is initiated. Courses are administered at weekly intervals for 4–8 weeks

function tests, adequate hydration, and absence of toxicity attributable to VCR and MTX. Throughout the period of treatment, weekly chest radiographs and clinical and radiographic examinations of the primary lesion are obtained. Any evidence of "escape" or growth of the primary lesion is followed by immediate amputation.

In the initial study, four weekly doses of VCR-MTX-CF were administered [7]. Subsequently, after the safety of the procedure was determined and since, in several instances, a suitable endoprosthesis had not been manufactured after 4 weeks, the number of courses was extended to eight. Following the last VCR-MTX-CF course, a repeat angiographic study was performed.

2. Intra-Arterial ADR

In three patients, intra-arterial ADR was administered by Harvard pump. One received 45 mg/m² by 6-hour infusion with the first angiographic study. The second received 70 mg/m² over 6 hours and the third 75 mg/m² over 72 hours, with the second angiographic studies, respectively.

3. Local En Bloc Resection

This operation was performed 10–14 days after the last administration of chemotherapy, provided the hemogram was normal and no complications had developed. Each tumor was resected with wide margins. Seven cm of bone proximal to femoral lesions or distal tibial or humoral lesions were removed—the limit of the tumor estimated by bone scan. The entire knee joint, including the patella, all ligaments, and suprapatellar arch, was removed in each lower extremity tumor. Femoral lesions included the proximal tibia just proximal to the infrapatellar ligament. Tibial lesions included sufficient distal femur to be just proximal to the suprapatellar arch. Active extension of the knee was made possible by transferring the hamstring muscles anteriorly.

4. Internal Prostheses

A variety of prostheses were used. Knee joints were modified Guepan knees with solid segments designed to replace the resected bone. These prostheses took approximately 8 weeks for individual manufacture. The Guepan knee was chosen because it is intrinsically stable in extension. One tibial tumor in an obese boy (125 kg) was replaced with resected intramedullary Kuntscher rods plus steel mesh and cement. The humoral lesion was resected together with the scapula and shoulder joint; the humerus was stabilized with a Buchholz shoulder prosthesis modified to give adequate length for the resected bone and the glenoid component was cemented into the residual clavicle. Other graphs were not used because our experience with chemotherapy shows that graphs of any sort are extremely slow to heal.

Patients were treated with intravenous antibiotics during the operation and more recently postoperatively for 1 week. Oral antibiotics were prescribed thereafter for variable periods of time until complete healing and the absence of infection were demonstrated. The limbs were immobilized for 2–3 weeks and gradually allowed motion. Full weight bearing was permitted as soon as the patients could stand comfortably, usually at 5–7 days. Adjuvant chemotherapy with VCR-MTX-CF and ADR [6] was initiated 3 weeks after the operation.

Results (Table 1)

In six of the eight patients, subjective and objective improvement was noted on clinical and radiographic examination. The clinical responses were characterized by complete or nearly complete disappearance of pain, reduction in tumor size, improved mobility, and reduction in local temperature within 2–3 weeks. In C.S., the tumor remained stationary and only slight reduction in pain was noted. In M.N., a new subcutaneous nodule developed adjacent to the primary tumor approximately 3 weeks after initiation of treatment. No patient developed pulmonary metastases during the period of intensive chemotherapy.

Angiographic evidence of response generally comprised reduction or disappearance of tumor neovascularity, although other changes were also noted. This was demonstrable on the resected specimens and is presented as estimates of viable tumor seen on pathologic examination. An example of the response obtained in W.B. with osteogenic sarcoma of the humerus is outlined in Figures 2a and 2b and the corresponding histologic features are outlined in Figures 3a and 3b. A more intensive correlation of the angiographic studies and pathologic results is in preparation.

The patients who received 75 mg/m^2 of ADR by intra-arterial infusion with the second angiographic study developed an area of brawny induration and erythema approximately 5 cm below the tip of the catheter 24 hours after initiation of the infusion. Examination with a Wood's lamp failed to reveal evidence of fluorescence and the intra-arterial infusion was maintained. However, 2 weeks later, sloughing of the indurated area occurred; local resection was not considered possible and an amputation was performed. Intra-arterial ADR in the other patients proceeded without untoward effect. Amputation was also performed in the patient who developed a subcutaneous nodule during the preoperative chemotherapy phase.

Of the six patients who underwent prosthetic limb replacement, one developed a staphylococcal infection approximately 3 months postoperatively. This was treated successfully by debridement and antibiotics, leaving the prosthesis in place. One patient developed a wound slough at the site of the previous biopsy which had been performed elsewhere transversely to the long axis of the leg and resulted in a cross-shaped closure. A third patient developed an ulcer over the prosthesis requiring a cross leg pedicle flap for closure, and a fourth developed displacement of the distal end of his tibial prosthesis which was recemented. Despite these complications, the potential for retention of a useful functioning

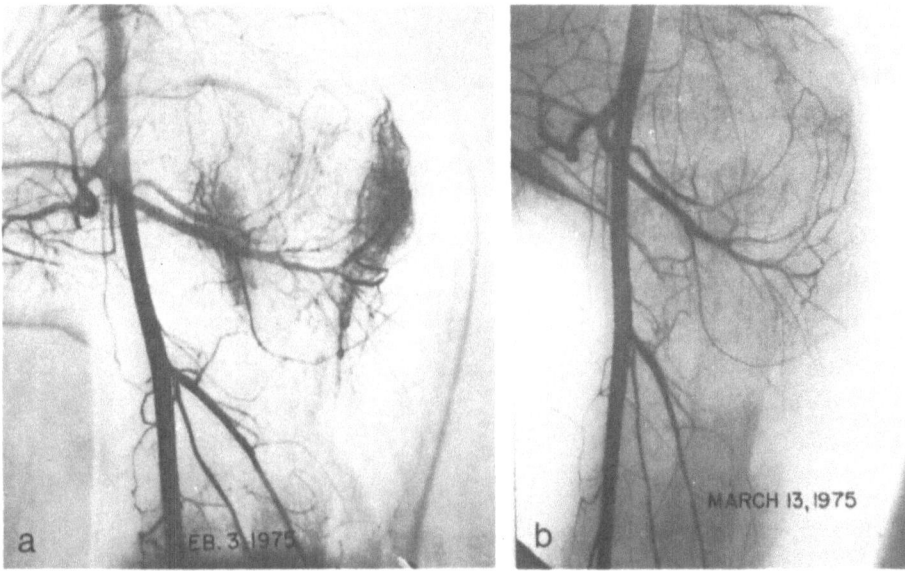

Fig. 2a and b. (a) Selective axillary artery injection demonstrating enlarged normal arterial branches supplying a hypervascular densely staining circumferential tumor of the humoral head. Soft tissue and joint extension of the tumor is moderate; (b) Repeat selective axillary artery injection (postchemotherapy) demonstrating absence of tumor neovascularity and staining with diminished soft tissue involvement. The decreased tumor vascularity is also reflected in the decreased size of the normal arteries supplying the region of the humoral head

limb remains in each patient. An example of the function achieved in the upper limb of the patient who underwent a local en bloc resection is illustrated in Figure 4. Full function of the elbow, forearm, and hand has been achieved with stability at the shoulder.

During the subsequent periods of adjuvant chemotherapy, three patients, including one who underwent amputation, developed isolated pulmonary metastases at 6, 6, and 12 months, respectively. In the amputated patient, the metastasis has been removed and the other patients are undergoing multidisciplinary treatment with similar intent [8].

Discussion

Local en bloc resection as primary definitive treatment is not a new therapeutic concept. It has been successfully employed in patients with benign and less aggressive malignant tumors where the potential for local recurrence and dissemination is minimal. The approach, however, has not been advocated for osteogenic sarcoma. Rather, optimum treatment for such patients is considered to be immediate ablation to remove the source of metastases (and death). This concept has been bolstered by a body of opinion advocating disarticulation for extremity lesions rather than transmedullary amputation because of an increased potential for local recurrence from residual microscopic disease or undetected "skip" lesions [3]. However, such complications have not been encountered in over 30 patients undergoing transmedullary amputation who received chemotherapy in our clinics. These

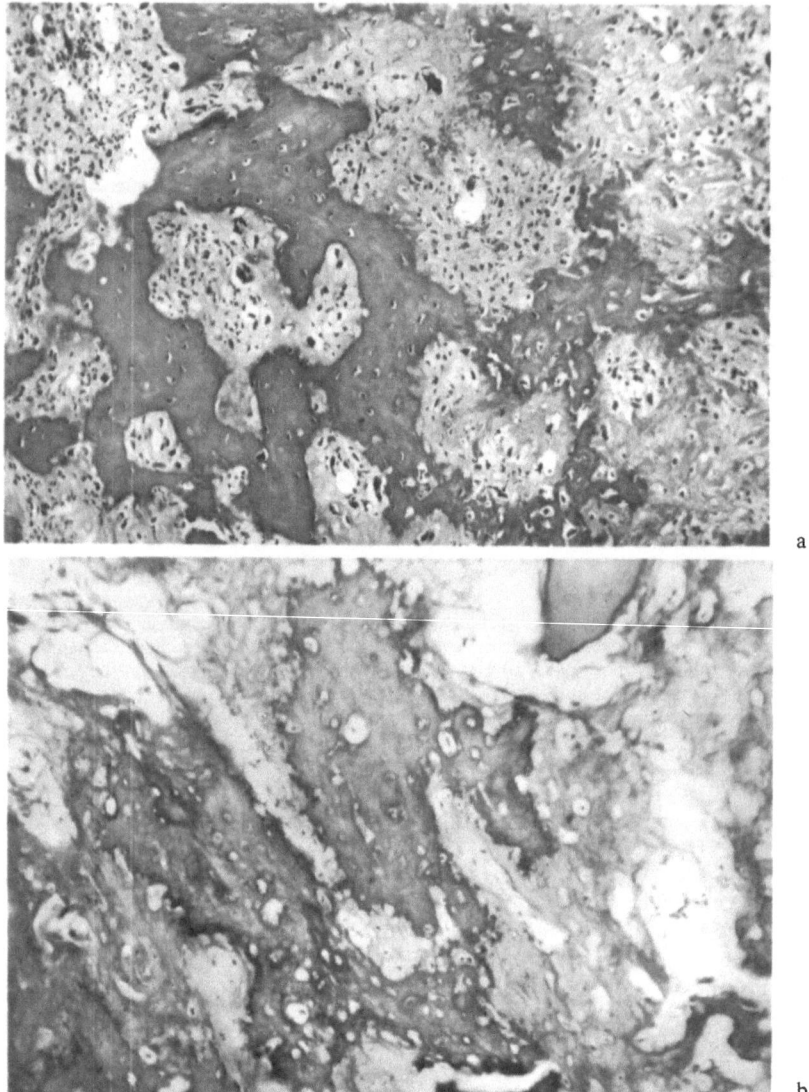

a

b

Fig. 3a and b. (a) Intramedullary tumor. Biopsy specimen showing moderate cellular and pleomorphic sclerosing osteogenic sarcoma; (b) Neoplastic bone and stroma are virtually devoid of cells. Residual nuclei are pyknotic and small. A few fibroblastic cells lie in the interstices of the tumor

procedures were performed a minimum of 7 cm above the highest level of reactivity seen on bone scan [15].

Encouraged by these results and also by a report by ROSEN et al. [12] demonstrating the feasibility of local en bloc resection, we embarked upon a program of limb preservation in selected cases. Support for the investigation was further obtained by reviewing experiences at the Sidney Farber Cancer Institute and Children's Hospital Medical Center where substantial destruction of overt metastases in the lungs and bones had been noted on clinical and pathologic examination in a number of patients. The preliminary observations in at

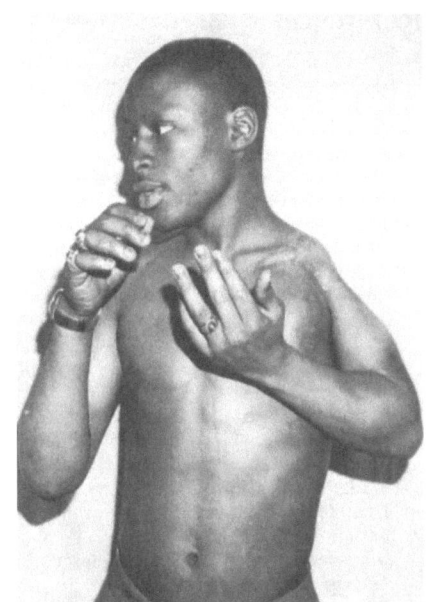

Fig. 4. Appearance of patient several weeks
after the operation demonstrating function of
left upper limb

least four of these patients are in accord with these experiences (percentage of viable tumor 20% or less).

Effective preoperative chemotherapy can markedly decrease the viability of the tumor and prevent growth of a primary lesion, thereby improving the potential for success. However, this experience should not be utilized as a mechanism to render inoperable tumors operable. The program must still be considered experimental until its potential is demonstrated by further follow-up. We consider patients candidates for limb preservation if the primary tumor appears locally resectable ab initio and administer chemotherapy to improve the prospects for total tumor eradication. Bone replacement should also not be considered a substitute for amputation which carries the potential for immediate cure.

Retention of viable tumor as an unhibited source of metastases may be advanced as an argument against the limb preservation program. However, in six of the eight cases, high-dose MTX was shown to be variably effective against the primary tumor by clinical, pathologic, and radiographic parameters. Aggressive, systemic treatment during the preoperative phase also constitutes a powerful attack against pulmonary micrometastases, and it appears unlikely that such metastases will seed or become firmly established during this period. Notwithstanding, any evidence of escape or failure of control by chemotherapy should be followed by immediate amputation as was performed in one patient.

Intra-arterial ADR may have been responsible for some degree of tumor destruction in two patients. This procedure, however, is not without risk. Erythema and subsequent necrosis of the tissues in one of the patients necessitated an amputation. This therapeutic approach is consequently undergoing review and cannot be recommended with confidence until more information is accumulated. Further, limb preservation must still be considered an investigational procedure and should be undertaken only in specialized centers.

References

1. CADE, S.: Osteogenic sarcoma: a study based on 133 patients. J. R. Coll. Surg. Edinb. *1*, 79–111 (1955).
2. CORTES, E. P., HOLLAND, J. F., WANG, J. J., SINKS, L. F., BLOM, J., SENN, H., BANK, A., GLIDEWELL, O.: Amputation and adriamycin in primary osteosarcoma. N. Engl. J. Med. *291*, 998–1000 (1974).
3. ENNEKING, W. F., KAGAN, A.: The implications of "skip" metastases in osteosarcoma. Clin, Orthop. and Related Res. *111*, 33–41 (1975).
4. JAFFE, N.: Recent advances in the chemotherapy of metastatic osteogenic sarcoma. Cancer *30*, 1627–1631 (1972).
5. JAFFE, N., FREI, E., III, TRAGGIS, D., BISHOP, Y.: Adjuvant methotrexate-citrovorum factor treatment of osteogenic sarcoma. N. Engl. J. Med. *291*, 994–997 (1974).
6. JAFFE, N.: The potential for an improved prognosis with chemotherapy in osteogenic sarcoma. Clin. Orthop. *113*, 111–118 (1975).
7. JAFFE, N., FREI, E., III, TRAGGIS, D., WATTS, H.: Weekly high-dose methotrexate-citrovorum factor in osteogenic sarcoma: pre-surgical treatment of primary tumor and of overt pulmonary metastases. Cancer *39*, 45–50 (1977).
8. JAFFE, N., TRAGGIS, D., CASSADY, J. R., FILLER, R. M., WATTS, H., FREI, E., III: Multidisciplinary treatment for macrometastatic osteogenic sarcoma. Brit. Med. J. *2*, 1039–1041 (1976).
9. JENKIN, R. D. T., ALLT, W. E. C., FITZPATRICK, P. J.: Osteosarcoma. An assessment of management with particular reference to primary irradiation and selective delayed amputation. Cancer *30*, 393–400 (1972).
10. PRATT, C. B., HUSTU, H. O., SHANKS, E. C.: Cyclic multiple drug adjuvant chemotherapy for osteogenic sarcoma. Proc. AACR/ASCO, Abstract No. 76 (1974).
11. ROSEN, G., TAN, C., SANMANEECHAI, A., BEATTIE, E. J., JR., MARCOVE, R., MURPHY, M. L.: The rationale for multiple drug chemotherapy in the treatment of osteogenic sarcoma. Cancer *35*, 936–945 (1975).
12. ROSEN, G., MURPHY, M. L., HUVOS, A. G., GUTIERREZ, M., MARCOVE, R. C.: Chemotherapy, en bloc resection, and prosthetic bone replacement in the treatment of osteogenic sarcoma. Cancer *37*, 1–11 (1976).
13. SUTOW, W. W., GEHAN, E. A., VIETTI, T. J., FRIAS, A. E., DYMENT, P. G.: Multidrug chemotherapy in primary treatment of osteosarcoma. J. Bone Jt. Surg. *58-A*, 629–633 (1976).
14. SUTOW, W. W., SULLIVAN, M. P., FERNBACH, D. J., CANGIR, A., GEORGE, S. L.: Adjuvant chemotherapy in primary treatment of osteogenic sarcoma. A Southwest Oncology Group Study. Cancer *36*, 1598–1602 (1975).
15. WATTS, H., JAFFE, N.: (Unpublished data).
16. WILBUR, J. R., ETCUBANAS, E., LONG, T., GLATSTEIN, E., LEAVITT, T.: 4 drug therapy and irradiation in primary and metastatic osteogenic sarcoma. Proc. AACR/ASCO, Abstract No. 816 (1974).

Breast Cancer: Changing Strategy for Treatment

P. CARBONE

The concept that breast cancer presents as localized tumor and disseminates only late in its clinical course has been challenged in the last few years. The traditional application of surgery or surgery plus radtiotherapy has resulted in essentially no change in the overall prognosis or survival over the last 40 years [14]. Moreover, the major operations, even the superradical and the segmental resection used for treating breast cancer, were devised almost 80 years ago. Improvements in survival have not occurred by refinements in the application of these various localized treatments. More recently, there has been the advocation of less surgery with a possibility of substituting radiotherapy to treat the primary tumor with results rather comparable to the more radical surgical procedures [19].

The question about the optimal primary treatment of breast cancer can be looked at as problems in surgical technique or in terms of biological questions. Clinical trials have demonstrated that less surgery, i.e., a simple mastectomy, may be equivalent to a radical mastectomy [1]. Radiation therapy added to a radical mastectomy does not increase the chances of cure [7]. Studies have attempted to look at less surgical procedures such as the segmental mastectomy or even excisional biopsy and radiation therapy. These studies have clearly shown that the kind of surgery or the use of surgery plus radiotherapy does not significantly add to the overall survival of patients with localized breast cancer. The major determining factor, whether the patient has recurrent, disseminated disease, is the presence of lymph node involvement. Removal of these lymph nodes per se does not improve the survival of patients with breast cancer. The clear-cut implication of these studies indicates that the biological behavior of most breast cancer is not one of a localized disease but rather that, in a significant portion of patients, the disease is already disseminated by the time the patient comes to the surgeon. Results indicate that those patients with histologically negative nodes have a 75% chance of having disease-free survival for 10 years. For patients with positive lymph nodes, only 25% are alive without recurrence after 10 years [9].

Knowledge about the cell kinetics and growth rates of cancer indicate that a tumor about 1 cm in size contains a billion tumor cells. Thus, if one has a doubling time of roughly 30–60 days, one can postulate that the cancer has been in the patient anywhere from 2–4 years. The tumors have had many opportunities to shed into the circulation and establish distant metastases. The local lymph nodes are not efficient mechanical traps for cancer cells. The local control of cancer with surgery or surgery plus radiotherapy can be achieved by a variety of methods. However, the cure or control of occult metastases requires systemic treatment. The number and size of these tumor deposits will eventually determine the curability.

In the management of micrometastases, the principles of systemic treatment have been evaluated in a variety of experimental systems by SCHABEL [13], STOFFI et al. [16], and BOGDEN et al. [2]. In general, cancer chemotherapeutic drugs kill by first order kinetics. This implies that each dose of drug kills a proportion of the tumor cells rather than an absolute number [20]. Thus, one must continue treatment until the probability exists that all the cancer cells are either killed or decreased in number so that the normal host immune system can take care of the few remaining cells. The sensitivity of the tumor cells to drugs is related to their growth kinetics. Removal of the gross tumor has been shown to increase the growth fraction and shorten the average cell cycle time [15]. The response of the gross clinical tumor may not predict the sensitivity of the micrometastases to the chemotherapeutic drugs. In general, the micrometastases are more vulnerable to chemotherapy.

Systemic approaches to human breast cancer include chemotherapy, both hormonal and cytotoxic, and immunotherapy. A variety of many neoplastic drugs, both alone and in combination, have a high degree of effectiveness in controlling or decreasing tumor size in patients with advanced disease. Combinations have been shown to produce higher response rates than single agents [4]. To develop the most effective systemic treatment for combining with effective local treatment, several important principles are worth reviewing.

First, in attempting to answer the question about which drugs to use, one has to consider questions such as safety, tolerance by the patient, and acceptability by both the physician and the patient. Response rates to a variety of single agents, adriamycin (ADR), methotrexate (MTX), cyclophosphamide (CPM), L-phenylalanine mustard (L-PAM), vincristine (VCR), and 5-fluorouracil (FU) ranges from 18–37% [5]. Combinations of these drugs produce responses in up to 80% of patients. However, in patients with advanced breast cancer, rarely are complete remissions achieved or does the duration of the response persist for more than a few months. Survival is rarely prolonged more than 12–24 months. In the design of chemotherapeutic trials for patients with what appears to be clinically resectable localized breast cancer, one must consider seriously the acceptability of the treatment regimen by the patient and the surgeon. The regimen must avoid severe side effects and must have some demonstration of effectiveness in patients with advanced disease. In the design of the original L-PAM studies by the NSABP (National Surgical Adjuvant Breast Group) and the Eastern Cooperative Oncology Group, L-PAM was chosen since it could be given orally and had minimal side effects except bone marrow toxicity [8]. Likewise, a three-drug regimen which did not include prednisone and VCR was also a likely choice for a second trial done by BONADONNA and the Milan Cancer Institute [3]. This had been previously shown to be more effective than L-PAM in achieving response in patients with advanced breast cancer by an Eastern Group trial [17].

In the experimental systems, there is little relationship between activity against the advanced clinically obvious tumor and the effectiveness of the same regimen in the adjuvant or micrometastatic state. Thus, one does not need the highly curative regimens against advanced disease to see an effect in patients with early disease. This lack of correlation between activity in advanced disease and the adjuvant situation is extremely important. As mentioned in a study reported by the Eastern Cooperative Oncology Group using L-PAM, response was first seen in 19% of patients using a single agent as compared to 53% with CMF [17]. Both of these regimens have been shown to cause significant delay in recurrences in patients in the adjuvant situation when used following a radical mastectomy in patients with N+ disease. Since neither of these regimens were curative in the advanced situation, the effect seen in the adjuvant situation clearly supports the experimental data. The data of BONADONNA and his colleagues would indicate that CMF is a highly effective postoperative regimen in patients with N+ disease [3]. Likewise, L-PAM in the subset of patients who are premenopausal also produced a significant decrease in recurrence rate [8].

While endocrine therapy has been a major therapeutic tool in the management of breast cancer, its use in the adjuvant situation has had equivocal results. Prophylactic castration has not been shown to prolong survival [11]. More recently, DAO and his colleagues have suggested that radical mastectomy combined with adrenalectomy can delay recurrences significantly in patients with node-positive disease following radical mastectomy [6]. There are several trials underway which are attempting to combine chemotherapy with hormone therapy in patients with advanced disease [5]. It may help to show how endocrine therapy can be used in the adjuvant situation. Most likely, it will occur in patients who are ER+ and who will be treated with chemotherapy and hormone therapy. The simple addition of hormones and chemotherapy may not necessarily be additive. While estrogens can stimulate the hormonal-dependent breast cancer cells to undergo DNA synthesis, the removal of estrogenic stimulation, such as with an oophorectomy or hypophysectomy, may result in a decrease in DNA synthesis and therefore competition with cell cycle specific chemotherapeutic agents. Moreover, if there are two populations of cells, both ER+ and ER−, a hypothesis which has not yet been proven, the strategy employed in developing combined hormonal and cytotoxic chemotherapy may be different.

Immunotherapy has had a major effect on the treatment of cancer patients including stage III breast cancer [12]. In general, these effects have been most notable when combined with chemotherapy. There are several studies now in adjuvant breast cancer combining immunotherapy with chemotherapy which may prove to show this same sort of effect in patients in the combined modality mode [5]. In patients with advanced breast cancer, one study has demonstrated that there is a prolongation of remission, although not an improved response rate using immunotherapy combined with chemotherapy [10].

The changing approaches to breast cancer require use of multiple, well-designed clinical trials to obtain the necessary information to the most obvious questions. I believe the questions that need to be answered are the following:

1. What is the best treatment, producing the best results, with the least toxicity, that can be combined with surgery to improve the disease-free survival as well as the overall survival?
2. What is the best immunotherapy that can be added to chemotherapy to improve the overall survival?
3. How can endocrine therapy be added to chemotherapy to produce significant additive or synergistic effects?
4. What is the optimal duration of treatment for combined modality approaches?
5. What factors can be used to identify those patients who have histologically negative nodes and yet are bound to fail so that they can be treated with adjuvant chemotherapy? Likewise, can treatment be spared those patients who are lymph node-positive and who will not have a recurrence following effective surgical primary treatment?

The answer to some of these questions may require specific tumor cell markers that correlate with the clinical course of the patient. Several of the studies to date have indicated that carcinoembryonic antigen and other products of tumor cells may be helpful as markers of active disease [20]. As yet, we do not have a completely reliable marker such as the paraproteins in myeloma or human chorionic gonadotrophin in choriocarcinoma that can identify high risk patients and also help select the duration and intensity of treatment. The answers to these questions can only be obtained by using well-designed clinical trials.

References

1. ATKINS, H., HAYWARD, J. L., KLUGMAN, D. J., WAYTE, A. B.: Treatment of breast cancer: a report after ten years of a clinical trial. Brit. Med. J. 20, 423 (1972).
2. BOGDEN, A. E., ESBER, H. J., TAYLOR, D. J., GRAY, J. H.: Comparative study on the effects of surgery, chemotherapy and immunotherapy, alone and in combination, on metastases of the 13762 mammary adenocarcinoma. Cancer Res. 34, 1627–1631 (1974).
3. BONADONNA, G., BRUSAMOLINO, E., VALAGUSSA, P., ROSSI, A., BRUGNATELLI, L., BRAMBILLA, C., DELENA, M., TANCINI, G., BAJETTA, E., MUSUMECI, R., VERONESI, V.: Combination chemotherapy as an adjuvant treatment in operable breast cancer. N. Engl. J. Med. 294, 405–410 (1976).
4. BRODER, L., TORMEY, D. C.: Combination chemotherapy of carcinoma of the breast: a review. Cancer Treatment Reviews 1, 183–203 (1974).
5. CARBONE, P. P.: The role of chemotherapy in treatment for breast cancer. In: Cancer Chemotherapy—Fundamental Concepts and Recent Advances Year Book. Chicago: Medical Publishers, Inc., 1975, pp. 311–322.
6. DAO, T. L., NEMOTO, T., CHAMBERLAIN, A., BROSS, I.: Adrenalectomy with radical mastectomy in the treatment of high risk breast cancer. Cancer 35, 474–482 (1975).
7. FISHER, B., SLACK, N. H., CAVANAUGH, P. J., GARDNER, B., RAVDIN, R. G. (and Cooperating Investigators): Postoperative radiotherapy in the treatment of breast cancer: results of the NSABP clinical trial. Annals of Surg. 172, 711 (1970).

8. FISHER, B., CARBONE, P. P., ECONOMOU, S. G., FRELICK, R., GLASS, A., LERNER, H., REDMOND, C., ZELEN, M., KATRYCH, D. L., WOLMARK, N., BAND, P., FISHER, E. R.: L-phenylalanine mustard (L-PAM) in the management of primary breast cancer: a report of early findings. N. Engl. J. Med. 292, 117–122 (1975).
9. FISHER, B., SLACK, N., KATRYCH, D., WOLMARK, N.: Ten year follow-up of breast cancer patients in a cooperative clinical trial evaluating surgical adjuvant chemotherapy. Surg. Gynecol. Obstet. 140, 528–534 (1975).
10. GUTTERMAN, J. V., MAGLIVIT, M. A., BURGESS, M. A., CARDENAS, J. O., BLUMENSCHEIN, G. R., GOTTLIEB, J. A., McBRIDE, K. B., McCREDIE, K. B., BODEY, G. P., RODRIGUEZ, V., FREIREICH, E. J., HIRSH, E. M.: Immunotherapy of breast cancer, malignant melanoma, and acute leukemia with BCG; prolongation of disease free interval and survival. Cancer Immunol. and Immunotherapy 1, 99–107 (1976).
11. RAVDIN, R. G., LEWISON, E. F. SLACK, N. H., DAO, T. L., GARDNER, B., STATE, D., FISHER, B.: Results of a clinical trial concerning the worth of prophylactic oophorectomy for breast cancer. Surg. Gyn. & Obst. 131, 1055–1064 (1970).
12. ROJAS, A. F., MICKIEWICZ, E., FEIERSTEIN, J. N., GLAIT, H., OLIVARI, A. J.: Levamisole in advanced human breast cancer. Lancet (1976) I, 211–215.
13. SCHABEL, F. M., Jr.: The use of tumor growth kinetics in planning "curative" chemotherapy of advanced solid tumors. Cancer Res. 29, 2384–2389 (1969).
14. SILVERBERG, E., HOLLEB, A. I.: Major trends in cancer: 25 year survey. Cancer 25, 2–7 (1975).
15. SIMPSON-HERREN, L., GRISWOLD, D. P.: Studies on the kinetics of growth and regression of 7,12-dimethylbenz(α)anthracene induced mammary adenocarcinoma in Sprague-Dawley rats. Cancer Res. 30, 813–818 (1970).
16. STOLFI, R. L., MARTIN, D. S., FUGMANN, R. A.: Spontaneous murine mammary adenocarcinoma: model system for evaluation of combined methods of therapy. Cancer Chemo. Reps. 55, 239–249 (1971).
17. TAYLOR, S. G., CANELLOS, G. P., BAND, P., POCOCK, S.: Combination chemotherapy for advanced breast cancer: randomized comparison with single drug therapy. Proc. Amer. Soc. Clin. Oncol. 15, 175 (1974).
18. TORMEY, D. C., WAALKES, T. P., AHMANN, D., GEHRKE, C. W., ZUMWALT, R. W., SNYDER, J., HANSEN, H.: Biological markers in breast cancer. I. Incidence of abnormalities of CEA, HCG, three polyamines and three minor nucleosides. Cancer 35, 1095–1100 (1975).
19. WEICHSELBAUM, R. R., MARCK, A. HELLMAN, S.: Role of postoperative irradiation in carcinoma of the breast. Cancer 37, 2682–2690 (1976).
20. WILCOX, W. S.: The last surviving cancer cell: the chances of killing it. Cancer Chemo. Reps. 50, 541–542 (1966).

Radiotherapy in the Therapeutic Strategy to Breast Cancer

J. STJERNSWÄRD

There is a great uncertainty regarding the optimal therapeutic strategy for breast cancer, not only in regard to the traditional role of surgery and radiotherapy, but also the optimal effect of cytotoxic chemotherapy treatment designs with a minimal toxicity, the optimal adjuvant hormone therapy, and the possibility of immunotherapy. The role of radiotherapy in a combined modality approach to breast cancer needs reevaluation, trying to explore the optimal effectiveness of each treatment method: surgery, radiotherapy, chemotherapy, and hormonotherapy, perhaps also immunotherapy. Much remains to be understood about how these treatment modalities work in synergism or in antagonism with each other and their optimal timing and combination so as not to over or undertreat the patient. The old hierarchic approach of using the above treatment modalities sequentially should be forgotten and replaced by an active search and identification of high risk groups with occult widespread disease at the time of diagnosis, offering these women systemic therapies. In addition, local therapies should be combined and explored wisely so as to achieve minimal morbidity and an optimal effect of systemic therapies, allowing an identification of patients with high risk for disseminated disease. There is no doubt, however, that the search for systemic adjuvant therapies that may be curative is a sound therapeutic principle in a disease that presently is disseminated in most cases at the time of diagnosis.

Radiotherapy like surgery is a localized form of therapy but in contrast to surgery, it has a systemic effect which may positively or negatively influence the effect of later systemic therapies.

As a general rule, however, it could be said that when doubt exists as to which local therapy to apply in the present clinical routine, it appears possible to state that there is no great difference in survival with any of the available localized forms of treatment. The simplest, easiest method with the least morbidity and to which the doctor is accustomed can, therefore, be used without great objection.

However, based on the present knowledge of the biology of breast cancer disease, certain important points can be underlined in regard to the role of radiotherapy.

Radiotherapy Before or After Surgery?

A great deal of evidence argues in favor of a combined surgery and radiotherapy approach, therapeutically and for achieving best local cosmesis. The failure of radiotherapy to cure bulky, extensive carcinomas and the failure of surgery to cure occult tumor spread warrants a combined approach.

The use of radiotherapy depends very much on the size of the primary tumor as well as on the stage of disease. Its use will be analyzed according to stages:

1. Stage I and Minimal Cancers

With early diagnosis, e.g., by mammography, local radiotherapy of the breast without surgery may be envisaged, offering women the possibility of saving their breast. Surgery may, in certain cases, even be completely unnecessary at this stage of disease. Encouraging results, mainly from France [1, 3, 4, 17, 18, 20] indicate that irradiation alone plus later surgery produces the same results as maximal mutilating surgery [4]. By exploring advances in radiobiology, it will hopefully be possible to neutralize very small tumors by irradiation alone and leave women with an acceptable "normal breast" after therapy. Surgery in the form of axillary tail dissection, however, still seems advisable to enable identification of the small percentage of women with a lymph node spread in spite of a small tumor and to offer these patients systemic therapies, especially if they are premenopausal. Axillary dissection seems to be sufficient for identifying this group of patients [10]. Surgery of the primary tumors, even if it is less than 1 cm, may be judged desirable in university clinics that are searching for a way via primary pathology of identifying the small group of patients that will develop direct hematogenous spread.

2. Stage II of Breast Cancer Disease

a) The Role of Preoperative Irradiation
The biological rationale for preoperative irradiation in this stage of disease is highly questionable for four reasons:
No survival benefits from preoperative irradiation of patients in stage II. These patients have a high probability of occult dissemination of the disease at the time of irradiation and can thus, with a clinical, localized, easily resectable lesion, not logically be expected to benefit from preoperative irradiation. Easily resectable tumors and patients with micrometastases have been pointed out as a group biologically and therapeutically unsuitable for pre-operative irradiation [18].
Lymph node status lost. This is the most important criterion for selecting high risk patients. It is highly desirable in stage II disease to identify high risk patients by the lymph node status.
Spread at time of operation probably not main factor for metastases. The old concept of spread of tumor cells at time of operation and increased later incidence of metastases does not seem to hold true. It is partially denied by the data, indicating that more than 50% of the metastases seem to have occurred before surgery [31], as well as by the investigation of venous tumors spread at the time of operation, with no correlation to survival [22].
Overtreatment. This is a practical and not to be neglected argument against preoperative irradiation in stage II disease. A very large number of patients are unnecessarily irradiated. There is, thus, little rationale for preoperative irradiation in stage II disease as pointed out earlier [18]. Nonetheless, a trial has been undertaken [24], and it will be interesting to see whether the biological and logical objections raised against the rationale or preoperative irradiation in operable breast cancer will be confirmed.

b) Routine Post-operative Irradiation
I will stress the word routine. Most probably there is a subgroup of patients, e.g., with internal quadrant tumors and outer axillary lymph node positive for tumor cells, that may benefit. This assumption is based on the logic from the results of extended local interventions, studied in a large randomized surgical trial [14], where the above subgroup of patients (13%) were shown to have a significant increase in survival after extended radical mastectomy as compared to radical mastectomy only. Whether there will be an increased survival benefit to such a subgroup after postoperative irradiation remains to be demonstrated in a controlled clinical trial.
There are points for and against the routine use of postoperative irradiation:
In favor of its use is the *decrease in frequency of local regional recurrences* which has been convincingly demonstrated. Approximatively 10–15% decrease in local regional recur-rences was achieved by postoperative radiotherapy in the randomized trials [29]. This is a

more realistic figure than the more exaggerated figures repeatedly quoted from a center highly sophisticated in radiotherapy but basing its figures on nonrandomized patient material [9].

Against the routine use of postoperative radiotherapy are:

Overtreatment. Less than 10% have local regional disease without also having simultaneous, or shortly following, distant metastases [29]. We are thus "overtreating" at least 90% of the patients. In the patients where recurrence occurs, a recent study demonstrates that close to 70% are completely controlled by modern radiotherapy [6].

Increased morbidity. There is a local increased morbidity, e.g. apical lung fibrosis, skin fibrosis, impaired shoulder movement, arm lymphoedema, vascular, cardiac, and pulmonary changes, and a long-lasting lymphopenia which are enhanced by adding routine postoperative radiotherapy. More worrying are data indicating that mortality may also be increased. Without any selection, all available randomized trials have been analyzed for this question. After the first report, showing in the first five available trials an increased mortality of 1–10% in the groups where postoperative radiotherapy was added [27] and an even higher increased or earlier mortality in certain subgroups such as premenopausal women, an updated analysis shows [29, 30] that out of ten randomized trials, eight estimate survival at 4 or 5 years. Seven out of these eight trials show an increased mortality rate in the group that is irradiated. This is in itself significant. Six out of these eight trials also include node negative patients, and in two of the eight trials, adjuvant castration was carried out in all premenopausal women. The observed decreased survival after adding postoperative radiotherapy is revealed in spite of the fact that, in most trials, 5 years postoperative has been arbitrary used as the time of assessment and that most of the trials include lymph node negative patients, a group with low risk for microdissemination and thus risk of earlier appearance of micrometastases, if now irradiation-induced immunosuppression is one of the many possible mechanisms that may be relevant. Results from most animal model systems suggest that irradiation of breast cancer or of the breast host results in an increase of distant metastases [for review see 28]. How far in vivo models of experimental medicine are valid for human medicine is a recurring question [15].

Cost-benefit ratio. Although this is a neglected aspect of cancer therapy, the cost-benefit ratio can, due to the increasing costs for medical care, not be neglected. Routine postoperative radiotherapy is convincingly shown not to increase survival, and it is highly questionable if the marginal effect on local-regional recurrence warrants its routine use, especially in premenopausal women where the more logical systemic therapies, e.g., multiple drug chemotherapy, seem to have their best effect on soft tissue disease rather than on visceral and bone metastases [2].

Unknown interactions with systemic therapies. Data indicate that the irradiation-induced immunosupression may diminish the effect of given systemic therapies such as chemotherapy, hormonotherapy, and perhaps also immunotherapy as will be discussed below. However, by the same mechanism causing an accelerated earlier appearance of diatant metastases, it may be theoretically possible that a positive effect may also be achieved by an augmented sensitivity to chemotherapy.

In conclusion, in stage II disease, surgery remains the primary localized form of therapy, and radiotherapy probably only plays a role in a very small subgroup of patients not yet identified in a trial.

3. Stage III—Radiotherapy and/or Surgery

Radiotherapy has here a clear therapeutic role in tumors limited to the breast in order to make them operable and postoperatively, also in stages that "should not have been operated" and where there is known residual local disease. An improved local therapeutic ratio ought to result from exploring advancements in radiobiology, using radiosensitizers, high energy particle radiation, and hyperthermia in connection with chemotherapy/ radiotherapy. With increasingly more efficient systemic therapies, local tumor control in stage III will hopefully lead to increased survival.

4. Stage IV

The local role of surgery here is limited mainly to toilet mastectomy. The palliative effect of radiotherapy is well-established.

Radiotherapy and Systemic Therapies

The interaction of radiotherapy with systemic therapies such as chemotherapy, hormono-therapy, and immunotherapy needs clarification, and much remains to be understood about how the different treatment modalities interact positively or negatively with each other and how to optimally time them and in what combinations.

It has been stated [8] that "the radical procedure (surgery) actually makes irradiation less effective because the vascular supply is disturbed resulting in some hypoxice of the tissue of the chest wall." We know that radiotherapy causes vascular endothelial changes. With the same logic, it has to be excluded that radiotherapy will not have a negative effect on the tumor-inhibiting properties of chemotherapy given later.

Not only locally in the area of the primary tumor, but also distantly, there are interactions of which one should be aware. In spite of radiotherapy being a localized form of therapy, it has systemic effects, e.g., a long-lasting lymphopenia [25]. Change in white blood cells and trombocytes induced by radiotherapy may not allow a full dose of aggressive chemotherapy [23]. Another negative interaction that has to be definitely excluded is the indication that the response to given hormonotherapy in patients with low lymphocyte values after irradiation will be diminished [16]. In patients treated with estrogens and androgens, the successful responders were found to have significantly higher pretreatment peripheral lymphocytic counts than the intermediate responders and failures [11, 12, 13]. Animal data exist showing that suppression of host immunity by previous irradiation [5] decreases the therapeutic effect of both cyclophosphamide and melphalan against a mouse mammary carcinoma [21]. The clinical interaction of local radiotherapy with active immunotherapy is unknown. Irradiation-induced immunologic change [22] is only one of many possible mechanisms to explain the observed earlier appearance of distant metastases after adding postoperative irradiation to operable breast cancer patients. With the increased use of systemic adjuvant therapies, the interaction of radiotherapy with these is an important clinical area that needs clarification.

Irradiation as a Systemic Form of Therapy

Agents that kill cells in all phases of cell cycle, regardless of the proliferative state, especially cells in the Go phase, would be desirable in the therapy of breast cancer. Irradiation has this ability. There is, thus, a logic for adjuvant total body irradiation. The biological rationale and the possibility of applying total body irradiation in breast cancer patients has been investigated and data exist on the experience of hundreds of patients [7]. A single exposure to doses in the range of 500–1000 rad to half of the body, repeated at monthly intervals to the other half of the body, has indeed achieved positive palliative effect in patients with symptomatic advanced disease. Evidence suggests that a single dose of 300 rad has a cell lethality of 90%, but at 800 rad it is 99.5%. Thus, if a cancer has a doubling time of 3 months, a remission of approximately 30 months is anticipated, and for longer doubling times such as 6 months, a remission of 5 years. The acute radiation syndrome was never severe and never a major clinical problem. Using the half-body technique with doses of 500 rad as an adjuvant in breast cancers with poor prognosis was speculation on the part of the investigators [7].

Whether total half-body/total body irradiation of identifiably very high risk operable stage II breast cancers is worth a clinical trial is open to discussion. If it were to be considered, radiotherapy might here enter a new area, from being a localized therapy to offering systemic adjuvant therapy. With the risk of secondary tumors, especially in the lymphatic system after irradiation, such a trial may, however, be questionable, even if it were to be technically feasible. The severity of the prognosis has to be balanced against the risks as well as the possibility of efficient therapy through other systemic therapies.

Conclusion

Table 1 tries to summarize the optimal strategy and interaction of radiotherapy with other forms of therapy in the treatment of breast cancer.

Based on present knowledge and latest advances in treatment of breast cancer, Table 2 tries to identify some pertinent and relevent therapeutic questions in relation to radiotherapy that could be investigated.

Table 1. Combination of therapies in breast cancer: role of radiotherapy

Stage	Surgery	Radiotherapy	Systemic therapies
I	+	+ (curative)	$-$ [a]
II	+	?/+ (curative in a subgroup to be identified)	$-N_{(-)}$ $+N_{(+)}$ [b]
III	±	+ (palliative)	+
IV	−	+ (palliative)	+

[a] The 25% with direct hematogenous spread not yet identifiable.
[b] Half-body/total body irradiation to very high risk groups may be discussed.

Table 2. Present advances and questions of priority in relation to radiotherapy and breast cancer

Stage I:	Earlier diagnosis: Irradiation of breast—saving breast
Stage II:	Systemic therapies—survival improved (?) Stop routine postop RT—resource allocation Identify subgroup(s) for RT with survival benefit Interaction with systemic therapies? Possibility of systemic RT?

Table 2 (continued)

Stage III: Innovation to be applied:
             Improved local therapeutic ratio by: radiosensitizers
                                                  particle radiation
                                                  hyperthermia?
                                                  chemotherapy
             Improved survival by added systemic treatment?
             Optimal timing—interaction of RT/systemic therapies

Stage IV: Improved palliation
             Optimal schedules
             Half/total body RT

References

1. AMALRIC, R., CLEMENT, F., SANTAMARIA, F., AYME, Y., BRANDONE, H., CLERC, S., POLLET, J. F., D'ESTIENNE Y D'ORUES, J. F., SPITALIER, J. M.: Radiothérapie curative à expérance conservatrice des cancers du sein operables. 403 cas de 5 ans. Bulletin du Cancer 63, 239–248 (1976).
2. BRODER, L. E., TORMEY, D. C.: Combination chemotherapy of carcinoma of the breast. Cancer Treatment Reviews 1, 183–203 (1974).
3. CALLE, R., PILLERON, J. P., SCHLIENGER, P.: Thérapeutiques "à visée conservatrice" des épithéliomas mammaires. Bulletin du Cancer 60, 217–231 (1973).
4. CALLE, R.: The role of radiation therapy in the loco-regional treatment of breast cancer. In: Breast Cancer: A Multidiscipliniary Approach, Recent Results in Cancer Research. Berlin-Heidelberg-New York: Springer-Verlag, 1976, Vol. LVII, pp. 164–175.
5. CASTRO, J. E.: Orchidectomy and the immune response. I. Effect of orchidectomy on lymphoid tissue of mice. Proc. R. Soc. Lond. (Biol) 185, 425–436 (1974).
6. CHU, F. C., LIN, F. J., KIM, J. H., HUH, S. H., GARMATICS, C. J.: Locally recurrent carcinoma of the breast. Cancer 37, 2677–2681 (1976).
7. FITZPATRICK, P. J., RIDER, W. D.: Half body radiotherapy. Int. J. Radiation Oncology Biol. Phys. 1, 197–207 (1976).
8. FLETCHER, G. H., MONTAGUE, E., NELSON, A. J.: Combination of conservative surgery and irradiation for cancer of the breast. Amer. J. Roentg. 162, 216–222 (1976).
9. FLETCHER, G. H.: Reflections on breast cancer. Int. J. Radiation Oncology Biol. Phys. 1, 759–779 (1976).
10. FORREST, A. P. M., ROBERTS, M. M., CANT, E., SHIVAS, A. A.: Simple mastectomy and pectoral node biopsy. Brit. J. Surg. 63, 569–575 (1976).
11. FRANK, C. R., WILLIAMS, Y.: Prognosis value of peripheral lymphocyte count in hormone therapy of advanced breast cancer. Brit. J. Cancer 34, 641–644 (1976).
12. HOLT, J. E., LEE, Y. T.: Peripheral lymphocyte counts and results of therapeutic castration for advanced mammary cancer. Ann. Surg., 175, 403–408, 1972.
13. HOGE, A. F., HARTSACK, J. M., KOLLMORGEN, G. M., SHILLING, J. A.: Endocrine and immunological studies in breast cancer. Amer. J. Surg. 126, 722–727 (1973).
14. LA COUR, J., BUCALOSSI, V., CACERS, E., JACOBELLI, G., KOSZAROWSKI, T., LE, M., RUMEAU-ROUQUETTE, C., VERONESI, U.: Radical mastectomy versus radical mastectomy plus internal dissection. Five year results of an international cooperative study. Cancer 37, 206–214 (1976).
15. MATHÉ, G.: How far are in vivo models of experimental medicine valid for human medicine. Biomedicine 24, 225–226 (1976).
16. MEYER, K. K.: Radiation-induced lymphocyte-immune deficiency. A factor in the increased visceral metastases and decreased hormone responsiveness of breast cancer. Arch. Surg. 101, 114–121 (1970).
17. PAPILLON, J., MONTBARBON, J. H., INGELS, J.: Le traitement conservateur du cancer du sein par l'association tumorectomie + radiation. J. Belge Radiol. (10) 55, 129–137 (1972).
18. PEREZ, C. A.: Pre-operative irradiation and the treatment of cancer. Front. Rad. Therapy Onc. 5, 1–7 (1970).
19. PIERQUIN, B.: Les techniques d'irradiation exclusive des cancers du sein. J. Radiol. Electrol. 56, 443–445 (1975).
20. PIERQUIN, B., CHASSAGNE, D., COX, J. D.: Toward consistent local control of certain malignant tumors. Endoradiotherapy with Iridium 192. Radiology 99, 661–667 (1971).

21. RADOV, L. A., HASKILL, J. S., KAN, J. H.: Host immune potentiation of drug responses to a murine mammary adenocarcinoma. Int. J. Cancer *17*, 773–779 (1976).
22. SALSBURY, A. J.: The significance of circulating cancer cells. Cancer Treatment Review *2*, 55–72 (1975).
23. SAMUEL, M. L., LANZOTTI, V. J., HOLOYE, P. Y., BOYLE, L. E., SMITH, T. L., JOHNSON, D. E.: Combination chemotherapy in germinal cell tumors. Cancer Treatment Review. Hellman, K., Carter, S. K. (eds.). *3*, 185–204 (1976).
24. DE SCHRYVER, A.: The Stockholm breast cancer trial: preliminary report of a randomized study concerning the value of pre-operative radiotherapy in operable disease. Int. J. Oncology Biol. Phys. *1*, 601–609 (1976).
25. STJERNSWÄRD, J.: Immunological changes after radiotherapy for mammary carcinoma. Ann. Ins. Pasteur *122*, 883–894 (1972).
26. STJERNSWÄRD, J., JONDAL, M., VANKY, F., WIGZELL, H., SEALY, R.: Lymphopenia and change in distribution of human B and T lymphocytes in peripheral blood induced by irradiation for mammary carcinoma. Lancet (1972) I, 1352–1356,
27. STJERNSWÄRD, J.: Decreased survival correlated to local irradiation in "early" operable breast cancer. Lancet (1974) II, 1285–1286.
28. STJERNSWÄRD, J.: Radiotherapy, host immunity and cancer spread. In: Secondary Spread in Breast Cancer. News Aspects of Breast Cancer. Stoll, B. (ed.). London: Heinemann Med. Books Ltd., 1977, Vol. III, pp. 139–167.
29. STJERNSWÄRD, J.: Adjuvant radiotherapy trials in breast cancer: a report to the profession. Washington, 1976. Cancer *39*, 2846–2867 (1977).
30. STJERNSWÄRD, J.: Can survival be decreased by post-operative irradiation. In: Current Concepts in Cancer—Up Dated Breast Cancer. Int. J. of Radiation Oncology, 1977 (in press).
31. TUBIANA, M., CHAUVEL, P., RENAUD, A., MALAISE, E. P.: Vitesse de croissance et histoire naturelle du cancer du sein. Bull. du Cancer *62*, 341–358 (1975).

Adjuvant Combination Chemotherapy in Primary Mammary Carcinoma: The CMF Program

A. Rossi, G. Bonadonna, P. Valagussa, and U. Veronesi

Introduction

The contemporary revolution in the field of cancer treatment involves primarily a multidisciplinary approach for diseases at high risk of early relapse. This applies particularly to those solid tumors which present clinically in a local-regional stage but whose natural history indicates that a considerable fraction of patients had undetected distant micro-metastases at the time of optimal surgery and/or radiotherapy. The plateau reached by local treatments in the cure of various neoplastic diseases has recently stimulated new conceptual and operational attitudes [5].

Due to its incidence as well as to its responsiveness to diverse therapeutic modalities, breast cancer appears to be probably the most important single tumor on which to test the validity of new treatment strategies. In fact, no dramatic progress has been reported in the disease-free survival of this neoplasm over the past 30 years despite different forms of local treatment [6]. The different figures reported in the literature are practically always related to the overall survival rate and not specifically to the disease-free survival. It is well-known that, besides selection of patients for surgery, the overall survival can also be influenced by effective secondary treatments (endocrine manipulations, chemotherapy) as well as by the course of the disease related to metastatic pattern. Furthermore, when the disease has invaded the ipsilateral axillary nodes, the percent of patients free of disease 10 years after radical mastectomy falls from 76% (N−) to 24% (N+) [8]. This simply indicates that, all other prognostic factors being equal, the presence (and the number) of histologically positive axillary lymph nodes represents for clinical purposes the single most useful prognostic sign.

Since resectable breast cancer with positive axillary nodes behaves in about three-fourths of patients as a systemic disease, a systemic treatment is required in combination with the local modality to improve the disease-free period and, hopefully, the disease-free survival. In recent years, chemotherapy, especially with cyclic multiple drug regimens, has proved to be effective in the control of different forms of metastatic neoplasms, including breast cancer. In particular, patients with disseminated mammary carcinoma achieving complete or good partial remission with combination chemotherapy have shown an improved median survival compared with those with no regression or a minimal response [3]. A number of pioneering studies carried out in experimental animal systems [9, 11, 12] have provided interesting and useful guidelines for applying chemotherapy and immunochemotherapy in human neoplasms and in breast cancer in particular [10]. The initial clinical results with prolonged adjuvant single agent (melphalan) and combination (CMF) chemotherapy [1, 7] have indicated that both the concepts and findings derived from animal models were to a large extent therapeutically predictive for human breast cancer.

The scope of this paper is to update our results with adjuvant CMF, a combination evaluated in advanced breast cancer by ECOG [13] as a modification from a quadruple regimen originally designed by the NCI group [4].

Patients and Methods

The details of the study were recently described elsewhere [1]. Briefly, from June 1, 1973 to September 11, 1975, all female patients who underwent radical (Halsted or extended) mastectomy at the Instituto Nazionale Tumori, Milan for potentially curable mammary carcinoma and who were proved to have histologically positive axillary lymph nodes were considered eligible for the prospective randomized study. Extended radical mastectomy was performed in patients with either primary tumors larger than 7 cm in diameter or with disease located in the medial quadrants.

The most important protocol requirements were as follows: (1) primary tumor classified as T_1, T_2, T_{3a}—N_0, N_{1a-b} (TNM international classification 1974), (2) negative chest x-ray, skeletal survey, and liver scan, (3) adequate bone marrow reserve and renal function tests within normal limits, and (4) geographic accessibility for frequent follow-up observation. The conditions for ineligibility included age over 75 years, pregnancy or lactation, previous treatment for current neoplasm, previous or concomitant neoplasms, and high surgical risk patients having nonmalignant systemic disease.

After stratification according to age ($\leqslant 49$ or 50–75 years), number of involved axillary nodes (1–3 or $\geqslant 4$), and type of radical mastectomy (Halsted or extended), patients were randomly allocated to receive either no further therapy or 12 cycles of CMF as outlined in Table 1. CMF was started 2–4 weeks after surgery. Besides physical examination, follow-up studies included chest x-ray and blood chemistry every 3 months and bone survey and liver scan every 6 months. Bone and brain scans as well as peritoneoscopy with multiple liver biopsies were done only in patients in whom it was suspected that the treatment had failed. Whenever technically feasible, the presence of relapse was confirmed by biopsy.

Table 2 shows the number of patients randomized and evaluable in both treatment groups. Off-protocol patients were included in the analysis only for the period from mastectomy to the evidence of second primary neoplasm or to death secondary to cerebrovascular accident, respectively. The characteristics of evaluable patients are summarized in Table 3. The treatment groups are comparable in terms of stratification parameters, type of mastectomy, T extent, and histologic subgroup. At the time of present analysis, 124 of 207 patients (60%) have completed 12 cycles of CMF. In particular, 99 of 124 (79.8%) have been followed for a minimum of 3 months and for a median of 10 months from completion of chemotherapy. In 27 of 207 patients (13%), chemotherapy was administered with some protocol deviations. In particular, in 21 of 207 (10%), CMF was discontinued before the 12th cycle because the patients refused to complete the combination chemotherapy, while in six patients (3%), the administration of CMF was temporarily interrupted for a period of 2–3 months for reasons other than toxicity.

Table 1. CMF Combination (one cycle)

Drugs	Route	mg/m²	Days of treatment ①2 3 4 5 6 7⑧9 10 11 12 13 14 15⟶28
Cyclophosphamide	p.o.	100	⟶
Methotrexate	i.v.	40 [a]	↑ ↑ Rest Period
Fluorouracil	i.v.	600 [b]	↑ ↑

In patients older than 65 years: [a] 30 mg/m²; [b] 400 mg/m².
During treatment a dose attenuation schedule is carried out in the presence of myelosuppression as detected by blood counts on days 1 and 8 [1].

Table 2. Patient population

Total	Control	CMF
Randomized	181	210
Not evaluable	2	3
Intercurrent death[a]	1	1
Protocol violation	1	2
Evaluable	179	207
Off-protocol		
2nd primary tumor[b]	2	—
Death in absence of relapse[c]	—	2

[a] Cardiovascular disease within 2 months from mastectomy.
[b] Cervical ca. (in situ), malignant melanoma.
[c] Cerebrovascular accident.

Table 3. Characteristics of evaluable patients

	Control	CMF
Total	179	207
Nodes: 1–3	126	140
≥ 4	53 (29.6%)	67 (32.3%)
Age: ≤ 49 years	74	95
≥ 50 years	105	112
median	52 (29–75)	51 (26–73)
Menopause: pre	82	95
post	97	112
Mastectomy: radical	131	148
extended	48 (26.8%)	59 (28.5%)
Stage: T_1	22	18
T_2	136 (75.9%)	153 (73.9%)
T_3	21	36
Histology: ductal	158 (88.2%)	180 (86.9%)
lobular	15	21
other	6	6

Results

Treatment Failure

Table 4 presents the treatment failures observed as of April 1, 1976. The minimum period of observation was 6 months, the maximum 34 months. The overall recurrence rate was 29.6% for the group treated only with mastectomy compared with 12% for that treated with surgery plus CMF. As reported by Fisher et al. [7] and in our previous publication [1], the highest relapse rate was observed in patients with four or more involved axillary nodes. Our results indicate that CMF was effective in reducing the relapse rate irrespective of the menopausal status or the size and location of the primary tumor. At the present time, 14

Table 4. Observed treatment failures (data are as of April 1, 1976)

	Control		CMF	
	No.	%	No.	%
Total with recurrence	53	29.6	25	12.0
Nodes: 1–3	28	22.2	14	10.0
≥ 4	25	47.1	11	16.4
Age: ≤ 49	23	31.1	11	11.5
≥ 50	30	28.5	14	12.5
Menopause: pre	26	31.7	8	8.4
post	27	27.8	17	15.1
Mastectomy: radical	34	25.9	18	12.1
extended	19	39.5	7	11.8

Table 5. Observed treatment failures in relation to the number of histologically involved axillary lymph nodes

	Control		CMF	
	No.	%	No.	%
1	17/70	24.2	5/63	7.9
2	3/34	8.8	6/50	12.0
3	8/22	36.3	3/27	11.1
4	5/17	29.4	3/16	18.7
5–6	8/15	53.3	3/11	27.2
≥ 7	12/21	57.1	5/40	12.5

control patients and six treated with CMF have already died of progressive disease. However, the difference is not statistically significant. Table 5 shows the comparative relapse rate related to the number of positive axillary nodes. The advantage in favor of CMF appears evident even in the presence of one involved lymph node.

The comparative relapse rate during the first 30 months from the beginning of the study is graphically illustrated in Figure 1 according to the direct method. For risk patients at 30 months after mastectomy, the failure rate was 52% for the control group and 10% for the CMF group. At present, of the total number of control patients in relapse, 39.6% (21 of 53) relapsed after the 12th month after mastectomy. An almost identical finding (10 of 25 or 40%) was observed in the CMF group. It should be pointed out, however, that four of ten patients had received chemotherapy with protocol deviations. Figures 2 and 3 present the same type of analysis related to different numbers of involved axillary nodes. In the group with one to three involved lymph nodes, 44.4% of the control patients have relapsed at 30 months after mastectomy compared with 5.5% of those given CMF. In the group with four or more involved nodes, five of seven risk controls at 30 months showed treatment failure whereas the two CMF risk patients for the same period of time are presently free of disease. The comparative analysis of the curves resulted in a significant level of $p = 0.0001$ for the whole series; a similar calculation for patients with one to three involved nodes gave $p = 0.03$, while for patients with four or more involved nodes, the level of p was $= 0.001$.

A. Rossi, G. Bonadonna, P. Valagussa, and U. Veronesi

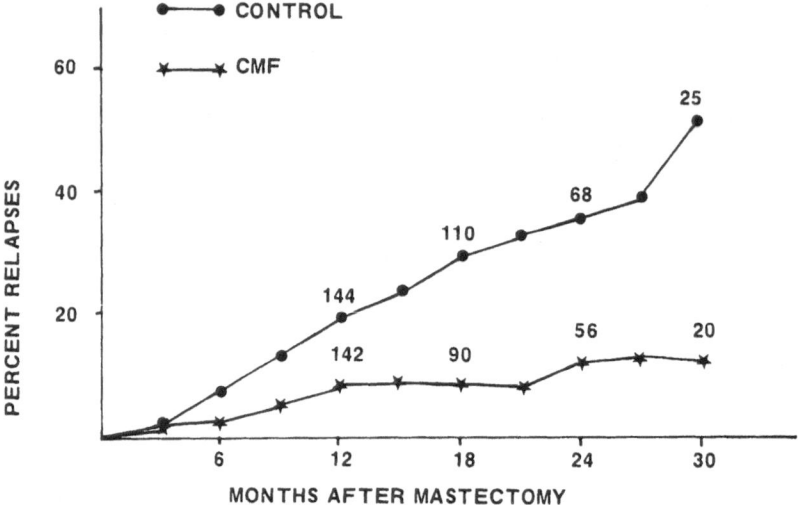

Fig. 1. Treatment failure rates in all evaluable patients

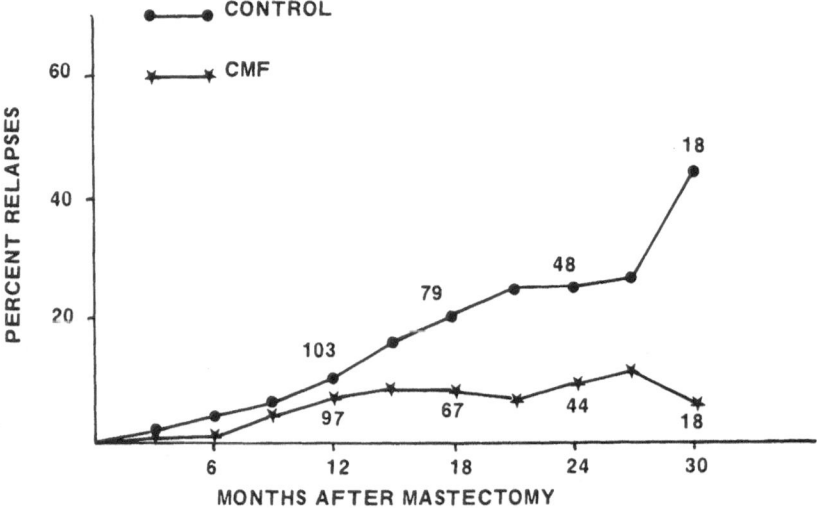

Fig. 2. Treatment failure rates in patients with one to three positive axillary nodes

Table 6 illustrates the sites of initial treatment failure. The pattern of relapse appears somewhat similar in the two groups. In fact, the clinical evidence of disease occurred preferentially in distant sites and particularly in the skeleton. The incidence of relapses at different sites was lower in the CMF group in relation to the lower relapse rate of patients given chemotherapy compared with those treated only with surgery. However, the difference in terms of multiple site involvement is particularly striking (p = 0.005). As far as local-regional recurrences is concerned, it should be added that six of 18 patients with limited initial treatment failure showed subsequent dissemination of disease within a short

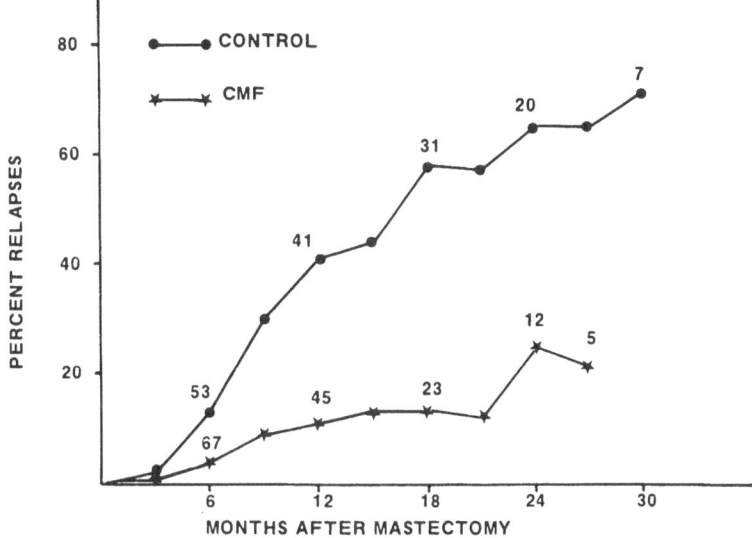

Fig. 3. Treatment failure rates in patients with four or more positive axillary nodes

Table 6. Site of initial relapse

	Control (179 patients)		CMF (207 patients)	
	No.	%	No.	%
Local-regional[a]	13	7.3	5	2.4
Distant (± local-regional)	38	21.2	18	8.7
bone	18	10.0	10	4.8
viscera	5	2.8	6	2.9
soft tissues	2	1.1	1	0.5
multiple sites	13	7.3	1	0.5
Second breast primary	2	1.1	2	0.9

[a] Chest wall and/or ipsilateral supraclavicular region.

period of time after the first documented relapse. Second breast primary tumors were detected in a total of four patients as a single sign of treatment failure. Contralateral breast cancer was also observed in two other control patients in association with multiple recurrences.

Toxicity

The side effects observed during treatment with CMF are summarized in Table 7. Reversible myelosuppression was a rather common finding and the most frequent dose-limiting factor. The incidence of severe leukopenia and thrombocytopenia was limited and in no instance was it complicated by infections or episodes of bleeding. Nausea, vomiting, loss of hair, and amenorrhea were at times psychologically disturbing side effects. However,

Table 7. Toxic manifestations

	No.	%
Leukopenia:[a]		
3999–2500	148	71
< 2500	12	6
Thrombocytopenia[b]		
129,000–75,000	125	60
< 75,000	36	17
Oral mucositis	49	19
Conjunctivitis	55	27
Loss of hair	126	61
Cystitis	63	30
Amenorrhea	69/95	72
No toxicity	4	2

[a] Leukocytes/mm^3
[b] Platelets/mm^3

it should be emphasized that nausea and vomiting were generally limited to the day of drug administration, and the loss of hair was cosmetically irrelevant in the large majority of patients. So far, amenorrhea was reversible in 22% of patients.

Fig. 4 shows the percent of the optimal doses administered during the 12 cycles of CMF. It appears evident that treatment did not produce cumulative toxicity. The average total dose of cyclophosphamide is slightly lower than that of methotrexate and fluorouracil either because its administration was temporarily discontinued in the presence of chemical cystitis or because few patients arbitrarily interrupted the oral treatment for a limited number of days because of prolonged nausea.

Comment

The results of this updated analysis substantially confirm the data reported in previous publications [1, 2]. Adjuvant treatment with full or nearly full doses of CMF is definitely effective in reducing the incidence of early relapses after radical surgery irrespective of the number of positive axillary lymph nodes and of the menopausal status. The short-term toxicity appears consistently acceptable. The long-term therapeutic efficacy of CMF remains, at present, unknown since the median follow-up period of this series is still limited. Therefore, all considerations concerning effects on survival and "cure" as well as implications about reduced extent of surgery and late side effects of systemic treatment are, on the basis of present findings, premature. Time remains an essential ingredient to provide and to evaluate clinical results.

On the other hand, present data once more provide unquestionable evidence that operable breast cancer with involved axillary nodes behaves as a systemic disease in a large fraction of patients. Therefore, a vigorous and prolonged systemic treatment is indicated to affect the growth of widespread micrometastases. Although the ultimate therapeutic value of adjuvant chemotherapy in breast cancer cannot yet be fully defined, it is hard to deny that

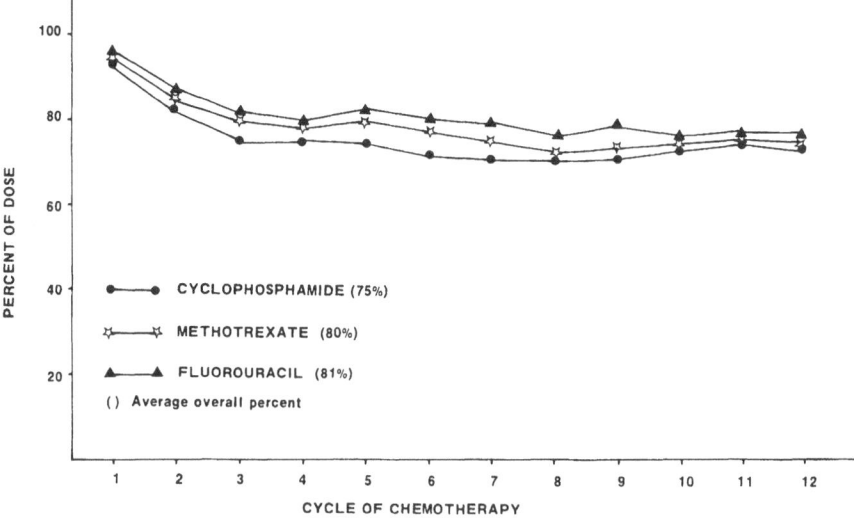

Fig. 4. Percent of the optimal doses administered during the 12 cycles of CMF

the consistent preliminary results of the two largest contemporary studies [1, 7] have already made a remarkable impact on the new concept of curative treatment for primary breast cancer at high risk of early relapse.

Now that the concept of interdisciplinary treatment for primary breast cancer is being gradually accepted by clinical oncologists as well as by general surgeons, it is essential for future progress to design new treatment modalities for any given stage of the disease on the basis only of sound results provided by controlled studies. Systemic treatment will certainly be improved through future studies where new combinations and new treatment schedules will be carefully evaluated. To limit the clinical use of effective adjuvant treatments for high risk groups to research institutions appears neither possible nor useful. However, physicians should be aware that the indiscriminate use of unproven local and systemic treatment modalities could be hazardous.

Acknowledgements

The work reported herein was partially supported by Contract NO1-CM-33714 with DCT, NCI, NIH.

References

1. BONADONNA, G., BRUSAMOLINO, E., VALAGUSSA, P., ROSSI, A., BRUGNATELLI, L., BRAMBILLA, C., DE LENA, M., TANCINI, G., BAJETTA, E., MUSUMECI, R., VERONESI, U.: Combination chemotherapy as an adjuvant treatment in operable breast cancer. N. Engl. J. Med. *294*, 405–410 (1976).

2. BONADONNA, G., VALAGUSSA, P., VERONESI, U.: Results of ongoing clinical trials with adjuvant chemotherapy in operable breast cancer. In: Breast Cancer: Trends in Research and Treatment. Heuson, J. C., Mattheiem, W. H., Rozencweig, M. (eds.). New York: Raven Press, 1976, p. 239.
3. BRODER, L. E., TORMEY, D. C.: Combination chemotherapy of carcinoma of the breast. Cancer Treat. Rev. *1*, 183–203 (1974).
4. CANELLOS, G. P., DE VITA, V. T., GOLD, G. L., CHABNER, B. A., SCHEIN, P. S., YOUNG, R. C.: Cyclical combination chemotherapy for advanced breast carcinoma. Brit. Med. J. *1*, 218–220 (1974).
5. CARTER, S. K., SOPER, W. T.: Integration of chemotherapy into combined modality treatment of solid tumors. I. The overall strategy. Cancer Treat. Rev. *1*, 1–13 (1974).
6. CUTLER S. J., MYERS, M. H., GREEN, S. B.: Trends in survival rates of patients with cancer. N. Engl. J. Med. *293*, 122–124 (1975).
7. FISHER, B., CARBONE, P., ECONOMOU, S. G., FRELICK, R., GLASS, A., LERNER, H., EDMOND, C., ZELEN, M., BAND, P., KATRYCH, D. L., WOLLMARK, N., FISHER, E. R. (and other co-operating investigators): 1-phenylalanine mustard (L-PAM) in the management of primary breast cancer. A report of early findings. N. Engl. J. Med. *292*, 117–122 (1975).
8. FISHER, B., SLACK, N., KATRYCH, D., WOLLMARK, N.: Ten year follow-up results of patients with carcinoma of the breast in a cooperative clinical trial evaluating surgical adjuvant chemotherapy. Surg. Gynecol. Obstet. *140*, 528–534 (1975).
9. MARTIN, D. S., FUGMANN, R., STOLFI, R., HAYWORTH, P. E.: Rationale of combined modality therapy for cancer. Cancer Chemother. Rep. *4*, 13–24 (1974).
10. MARTIN, D. S., FUGMANN, R. A., STOLFI, R. L., HAYWORTH, P. E.: Solid tumor animal model therapeutically predictive for human breast cancer. Cancer Chemother. Rep. *5*, 89–109 (1975).
11. MARTIN, D. S., HAYWORTH, P. E., FUGMANN, R. A.: Enhanced cures of spontaneous murine mammary tumors with surgery, combination chemotherapy, and immunotherapy. Cancer Res. *30*, 709–716 (1970).
12. SCHABEL, F. M.: Concepts for systemic treatment of micrometastases. Cancer *35*, 15–24 (1975).
13. TAYLOR, S. G., III, CANELLOS, G. P., BAND, P., POCOCK, S.: Combination chemotherapy for advanced breast cancer. Randomized comparison with single agent therapy. Proc. Am. Soc. Clin. Oncol. *15*, 175 (1974).

Chemo Immunotherapy of Advanced Breast Cancer With BCG*

G. N. Hortobagyi, J. U. Gutterman, G. R. Blumenschein, A. Buzdar,
M. A. Burgess, S. P. Richman, C. K. Tashima, M. Schwarz, and E. M.
Hersh

Introduction

Breast cancer continues to be the leading cause of cancer death among females [5, 7]. With
the development of combination chemotherapy programs, utilizing a variety of active drugs
with different modalities of action and toxicity, an encouraging increase in remission rates
among patients with advanced disease has been achieved [3, 4, 13]. The introduction of
adriamycin in various combination programs has produced remission rates of 50–70%
[11, 13].
Despite this encouraging trend in remission rates, the duration of these responses has been
short with a median of 5–10 months. The overall median survival with most of these
combination chemotherapy programs has improved to approximately 10–15 months.
The importance of host defense mechanisms in the control of breast cancer and other
tumors has become increasingly evident [1, 2]. As a result, immunotherapy is becoming
increasingly important in the therapeutic strategy of the cancer patient [16]. We recently
demonstrated that immunotherapy with BCG prolonged chemotherapy-induced remissions
and survival of patients with disseminated melanoma [15] and acute myelogenous leukemia
[14]. After we successfully worked out the use of intermittent chemotherapy with
immunotherapy, we explored the question of whether BCG immunotherapy could (1)
increase remission rates, (2) prolong remission duration, and (3) prolong overall survival of
patients with metastatic breast cancer who were receiving combination chemotherapy.
Thus, a program of chemoimmunotherapy for disseminated breast cancer was initiated,
combining BCG with our previous best combination chemotherapy regimen of 5-
fluorouracil (5-FU), adriamycin (ADR), and cyclophosphamide (CPM). Our preliminary
reports have been published elsewhere [13], and we report now on an extension of the
results for 105 patients.

Materials and Methods

Since March, 1974, 105 evaluable patients with disseminated breast cancer have been
treated with chemoimmunotherapy consisting of 5-FU (500 mg/m2 i.v. on days 1 and 8 of
each course), ADR (50 mg/m2 i.v. on day 1), and CPM (500 mg/m2 i.v. on day 1).
Lyophilized Tice or Pasteur strain BCG at a dose of 6×10^8 viable units was given by

* This work has been supported by Contract NO1-CB-33888 and Grants 05831 and 11520 from the
National Cancer Institute, Bethesda, Maryland 20014. Dr. Gutterman is the recipient of a Career
Development Award (CA 71007-02) from the National Cancer Institute, Bethesda, Maryland 20014.

scarification, rotating all four proximal extremities as previously described on days 9, 13, and 17 of each course [17]. Courses of chemoimmunotherapy were repeated every 21 days if hematologic recovery permitted. Dose escalation or de-escalation was performed in order to maintain the lowest granulocyte count, between 1000 and 2000 per mm^3, and the lowest platelet count, above 50,000. Documented infection and/or hemorrhage required a dose reduction of 25% regardless of changes in the blood count.

The results of this series were compared with those obtained in a comparable group of 44 patients treated with the same chemotherapy (FAC) immediately prior to the study, between August, 1973, and March, 1974 [13].

Sixty-four patients were entered on the FAC chemotherapy study. Six patients were inevaluable since two died before the first course of therapy was completed (early death) and four patients had major protocol violations with totally inadequate doses of chemotherapy. Fifty-eight patients were eligible for evaluation of the response rate, which was 79% (see below). Only 44 were evaluable for remission duration and survival since 14 of the patients were given BCG after they achieved remissions. Thus, 44 patients were treated with FAC chemotherapy for the entire duration of therapy and serve as the chemotherapy control group.

One hundred and twenty-eight patients were entered on the FAC-BCG treatment program. Twenty-three (18%) were excluded from evaluation for the following reasons: nine of them received either no BCG or an inadequate dose schedule of BCG, five patients were lost to follow-up after their first course of chemotherapy, six patients had major chemotherapy-related protocol deviations, and three patients died before day 14 (early death) of the first course of treatment.

The total dose of ADR was limited to 550 mg/m2 in the first 44 patients and subsequently to 450 mg/m2 in order to prevent ADR-related cardiotoxicity. At the time ADR was stopped, maintenance therapy consisted of the CMF regimen: CPM, 500 mg/m2 p.o. on day 2, methotrexate (MTX), 30 mg/m2 i.m. on days 1 and 8, and 5-FU, 500 mg/m2 p.o. on days 1 and 8. In the chemoimmunotherapy group, BCG was continued on days 9, 13, and 17 of each 21-day maintenance course.

Criteria for eligibility for the FAC-BCG studies were as follows: evidence of progressive metastatic breast cancer with clearly measurable tumor, either by physical examination, radiologic or radioisotopic criteria. Patients with overt congestive heart failure were not eligible for this trial. Although prior chemotherapy did not exclude the patients from entering the FAC or FAC-BCG program, evidence of progression with prior CPM, ADR, or 5-FU precluded their inclusion in the treatment programs.

The criteria of response to treatment were as follows: complete remission was defined as the complete disappearance of all objective and subjective evidence of disease, including complete recalcification of bone lesions; partial remission was interpreted as a 50% or greater reduction in the product of the diameter of measurable lesions, including partial recalcification of bone metastases. Patients with less than 50% reduction or less than 25% increase in tumor size for a minimum period of 2 months were considered to have stable disease. Progression or relapse were defined as more than 25% increase in existing tumor masses or the appearance of any new lesions.

Remission duration was determined from the date of achieving remission until the day of progression or relapse. Survival was measured from the start of treatment to the date of death or last follow-up examination.

The statistical methods used included the method of KAPLAN and MEIER for calculating and plotting remission and survival curves [20] and a generalized Wilcoxon test with a one-tailed analysis for testing the difference between remission and survival curves [10].

Results

Pretreatment characteristics of evaluable patients in both groups are shown on Table 1. Factors known to alter the prognosis of these patients were similar in both groups. Distribution of metastatic sites was comparable among the two groups of patients (Table 2). Thirty-two patients of 44 (73%) treated with FAC and 78 of 105 (75%) treated with FAC-BCG achieved a partial or complete remission (Table 3). The proportion of partial and complete remissions was similar among both groups. The response according to metastatic sites was also similar in both treatment groups (Table 4). The median time to partial and complete remission was 2–3 months, respectively. The age, menopausal status, disease-free interval, and response to prior hormonal manipulation did not influence the response to chemotherapy.

Table 1. Chemoimmunotherapy of advanced breast cancer: population characteristics

	FAC	FAC-BCG
No. of patients	44	105
Age (range)	51 (29–67)	53 (25–72)
Premenopausal	31%	23%
Postmenopausal	69%	77%
Prior hormonal therapy	79%	65%
Prior chemotherapy	7%	14%
Disease-free interval (months)	15 (0–104)	16 (0–140)

Table 2. Chemoimmunotherapy of advanced breast cancer: distribution of metastatic sites

	FAC	FAC-BCG
Soft tissue	44%	33%
Lymph nodes	32%	28%
Bone	66%	61%
Lung	55%	33%
Pleura	16%	24%
Liver	20%	22%

Table 3. Chemoimmunotherapy of advanced breast cancer: response rates

	FAC	FAC-BCG
Total no. patients	44	105
CR	6 (14%)	20 (19%)
PR	26 (59%)	58 (55.2%)
Stable	12 (27%)	21 (20%)
Progression	—	6 (6%)

CR: complete remission; PR: partial remission.

G. N. Hortobagyi et al.

Table 4. Chemoimmunotherapy of advanced breast cancer:
response by sites

	FAC	FAC-BCG
Breast and soft tissue	(83%)	(80%)
Lymph nodes	(100%)	(86%)
Bone	(41%)	(67%)
Lung	(66%)	(69%)
Pleura	(63%)	(76%)
Liver	(58%)	(61%)

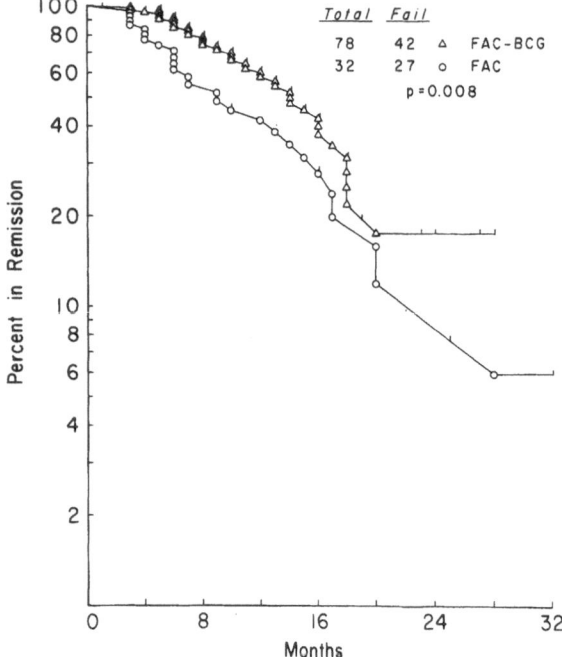

Fig 1. Chemoimmunotherapy of stage IV breast cancer duration of remission

The duration of remission is shown in Fig. 1. Twenty-seven of 32 patients in the FAC group have relapsed with a median duration of 9 months. Forty-two of the 78 patients on FAC-BCG have relapsed with a median duration of 14 months. These differences are statistically significant, p = .008. The median duration of remission for FAC complete responders was 9 months and 14 months for the FAC-BCG complete responders. This was not statistically significant, p = 0.2. Four of 26 partial responders on the FAC program are still in remission with a median of 9 months. In contrast, 26 of 58 patients achieving partial remission on the FAC-BCG group are still in remission with a median duration of 14 months, p = .07. The duration of stability was identical for both groups.

The most important effect of chemoimmunotherapy was prolongation of survival. Shown in Fig. 2 is the survival of the responding patients. Eleven of 32 patients in the FAC group who achieved remission are still alive with a median survival of 16 months. Fifty-one of 78 patients on FAC-BCG are still alive with a median survival of 22.5 months. These differences are statistically significantly, p = .004.

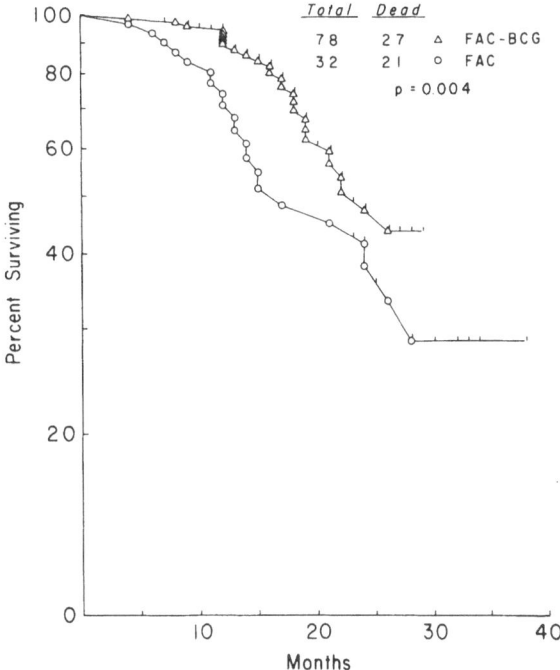

Fig. 2. Chemoimmunotherapy of stage IV breast cancer survival of responders

At this point, survival of stable patients is superior for FAC-BCG (median = 13.5 months) compared to FAC (median = 12 months). These differences are not significant.

The survival for all patients treated with an adequate trial is shown in Fig. 3. Thirty-one of the 44 FAC-BCG patients have died with a median survival of 14.8 months. Forty-five of 105 patients on FAC-BCG have died with a median survival of 20.7 months. These differences are statistically significant, p = .02.

After progression, most of the patients in both studies were treated with second line chemotherapeutic agents such as MTX, vincristine (VCR), mitomycin-C, Baker's antifol, ifosphamide, and occasional hormonal manipulation. A comparative analysis of the response to secondary modalities of treatment between the two groups did not suggest any significant differences in responses after the first relapse.

Toxicity

Treatment in both groups was well-tolerated. Although nausea, vomiting, and alopecia occurred in virtually all patients, the dose-limiting toxicity was myelosuppression. Granulocytopenia was very predictable. The lowest granulocyte count was usually encountered between days 12–18 of each course. The recovery was prompt and the majority of patients were able to start their courses of treatment every 21 days. Thrombocytopenia was rarely measured and was of little clinical significance. Myelosuppression was slightly cumulative, proven by the fact that by the sixth course, 50% of the patients were able to tolerate only 80% of the calculated dose.

Infectious episodes associated with granulocytopenia occurred in a small fraction of the

G. N. Hortobagyi et al.

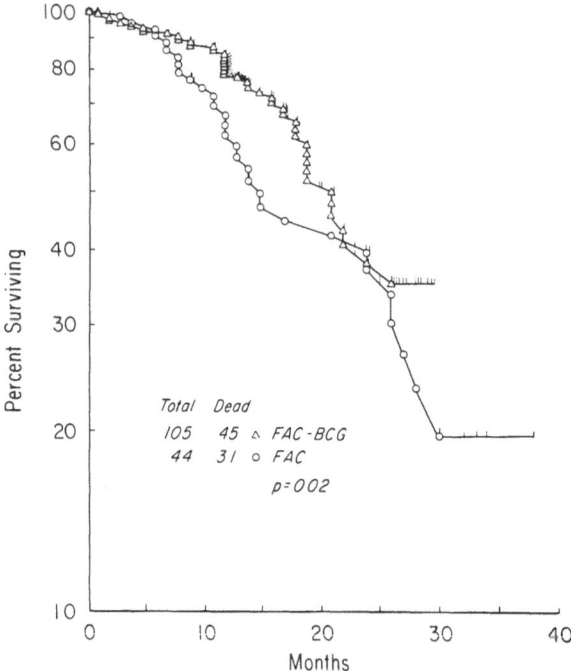

Fig. 3. Chemoimmunotherapy of stage IV breast cancer survival all patients

patients in both groups, but none of these patients died as a consequence of an infectious episode. Immunotherapy did not seem to influence the degree of myelosuppression or the incidence of infectious complications.

Side effects related to BCG were mild and consisted mainly of local soreness and itching, a low grade fever and an ill-defined influenza-like syndrome for 12–24 hours following most scarifications. Although a generalized rash (with a histologic picture of a hypersensitivity vasculitis) was observed in three patients, no disseminated BCG disease occurred and tuberculostatic chemotherapy was not required.

Congestive heart failure, presumably secondary to ADR-related cardiomyopathy was observed in five patients of the FAC group and four patients of the FAC-BCG group. In all cases, digitalis and diuretic treatment achieved symptomatic control. None of the patients died as a direct consequence of the cardiotoxic effects of ADR.

Discussion

This study suggests that the prognosis of patients with advanced breast cancer treated with cyclic combination chemotherapy has been improved by the addition of immunotherapy. Remission rates have not been influenced by BCG immunotherapy; however, durations of remissions have been highly significantly prolonged with FAC-CMF-BCG compared to the chemotherapy control group. However, only 20% of the patients are projected to remain in remission at 20 months even with chemoimmunotherapy.

The most important therapeutic effect of BCG immunotherapy in the current study was the increase of survival among the responders. Thus, less than half the patients who achieved remission with FAC chemotherapy survived 18 months (median = 15 months). In contrast, a projected 75% of the patients achieving remission with FAC-BCG will survive longer than 18 months. Thus, the .75 percentile is already 18 months. It is important to point out that the data from our FAC control group treated just prior to the FAC-BCG trial are nearly identical to those reported by JONES and co-workers with a similar chemotherapy combination [19] (ADR plus cytoxan = AC). The survival of patients in partial remission (FAC = 15 months, AC = 17 months) and overall survival (median = 15 months for both studies) are identical. The allocation of 14 patients onto FAC-CMF-BCG therapy from the original 58 patients treated with FAC does not appear to have influenced the control group and thus serves as a suitable historical control.

The results, if confirmed, extend the principles established in other chemoimmunotherapy trials with BCG where remission rates were not significantly increased (except for tumor size regional to BCG scarification), but remission durations and particularly survival were significantly increased compared to chemotherapy alone [15]. Similar results have been reported previously when C. parvum was added to chemotherapy in breast cancer [18]. It is hoped that this preliminary report will stimulate additional trials of chemoimmunotherapy in advanced breast cancer.

Despite the encouraging results with BCG, improved modalities of immunotherapy and combination chemotherapy are needed to increase the remission rates in visceral regions as well as to shift the partial remissions to complete remissions. Other immunologic approaches have suggested benefits in breast cancer [22, 23].

Finally, since adjuvant chemotherapy has prolonged the disease-free interval and survival in breast cancer patients with histologic evidence of spread to regional lymph nodes [4, 9] and adjuvant immunotherapy has been beneficial in colorectal cancer [21] and malignant melanoma [8, 17], programs of combination chemotherapy and immunotherapy should be designed for patients with suspected residual microscopic disease after surgery.

Results with FAC-BCG as a postoperative adjuvant therapy for breast cancer patients with positive nodes show a highly significant prolongation of disease-free interval and survival compared to historical surgical controls (BUZDAR, A., GUTTERMAN, J., BLUMENSCHEIN, G., HORTOBAGYI, G., et al.: Proc. Amer. Soc. Clin. Oncology submitted, 1977).

References

1. BLACK, M. M., KERPE, S., SPEER, F. D.: Lymph node structure in patients with cancer of the breast. Amer. J. Pathol. 29, 505–521 (1953).
2. BLOOM, H. J., RICHARDSON, W. W., FIELD, J. R.: Host resistance and survival in carcinoma of the breast: a study of 104 cases of medullar carcinoma in a series of 1,411 cases of breast cancer followed for 20 years. Brit. Med. J. 3, 181–188 (1970).
3. BLUMENSCHEIN, G. R., CARDENAS, J. O., FREIREICH, E. J., GOTTLIEB, J. A.: FAC chemotherapy for breast cancer. Amer. Soc. Clin. Oncol. (Abstract No. 839) 15, 193 (1974).
4. BONADONNA, G., BRUSAMALINO, E., VALAGUSSA, P., ROSSI, A., BRUGNATELLI, L., BRAMBILLA, C., DE LENA, M., TANCINI, G., BAJETTA, E., MUSUMECI, T., VERNOESI, U.: Combination chemotherapy as an adjuvant treatment in operable breast cancer. New Engl. J. Med. 294–   (1976).
5. American Cancer Society, Inc.: Cancer facts and figures. New York, 1975.
6. CANELLOS, G. P., DEVITA, V. T., GOLD, G. L., CHABNER, B. A., SCHEIN, P. S., YOUNG, R. C.: Cyclical combination chemotherapy for advanced breast carcinoma. Brit. Med. J. 1, 218–220 (1974).
7. CUTLER, S. J.: Classification of extent of disease in breast cancer. Seminars in Oncology 1, 91–96 (1974).
8. EILBER, F. R., MORTON, D. L., HOLMES, E. C., SPARKS, F. C., RAMMING, K. P.: Immunotherapy with BCG in treatment of regional-lymph-node metastases from malignant melanoma. New Engl. J. Med. 294, 237–240 (1976).

9. FISHER, B., CARBONE, P., ECONOMOU, S. G., FRELICK, R., GLASS, A., LEINER, H., REDMOND, C., ZELEN, M., BAND, P., KATRYCH, D., WOLMARK, N., FISHER, E. R.: 1-phenylalanine mustard (L-PAM) in the management of primary breast cancer. A report of early findings. New Engl. J. Med. 292, 117–122 (1975).

10. GEHAN, E. A.: A generalized Wilcoxan test for comparing arbitrarily singly-censored samples. Biometrika 52, 203–223 (1965).

11. GOTTLIEB, J. A., BLUMENSCHEIN, G. R., GUTTERMAN, J. U., FREIREICH, E. J., CARDENAS, J. O.: Adriamycin in the treatment of breast cancer. Adriamycin Review IV, 249–256 (1975).

12. GREENSPAN, E. M.: Combination cytoxic chemotherapy in advanced disseminated breast carcinoma. J. Mt. Sinai Hosp. 33, 1–27 (1966).

13. GUTTERMAN, J. U., CARDENAS, J. O., BLUMENSCHEIN, G. R., HORTOBAGYI, G., BURGESS, M. A., LIVINGSTON, R. B., MAVLIGIT, G. M., GOTTLIEB, J. A., FREIREICH, E. J., HERSH, E. M.: Chemoimmunotherapy of advanced breast cancer: prolongation of remission and survival with BCG. Brit. Med. J. 2, 1222–1225 (1976).

14. GUTTERMAN, J. U., HERSH, E. M., RODRIGUEZ, V., McCREDIE, K. B., MAVLIGIT, G., REED, R., BURGESS, M. A., SMITH, T., GEHAN, E., BODEY, G. P., Sr., FREIREICH, E. J.: Prolongation of remission in myeloblastic leukemia with BCG. Lancet (1974) II, 1405–1409.

15. GUTTERMAN, J. U., MAVLIGIT, G., GOTTLIEB, J. A., BURGESS, M. A., McBRIDE, C. E., EINHORN, L., FREIREICH, E. J., HERSH, E. M.: Chemoimmunotherapy of disseminated malignant melanoma with DTIC and BCG. New Engl. J. Med. 391, 592–597 (1974).

16. GUTTERMAN, J. U., MAVLIGIT, G. M., HERSH, E. M.: Chemoimmunotherapy of human solid tumors. Medical Clinics of North America 60, 441–462 (1976).

17. GUTTERMAN, J. U., MAVLIGIT, G., McBRIDE, C., FREI, E. III., FREIREICH, E. J., HERSH, E. M.: Active immunotherapy with BCG for recurrent malignant melanoma. Lancet (1973) I, 1208–1212.

18. ISRAEL, L., EDELSTEIN, R.: Non-specific immunostimulation with C. parvum in human cancer. In: Immunologic Aspects of Neoplasia, 26th Symposium. Baltimore, Maryland: William and Wilkins, 1976.

19. JONES, S. E., DURIE, B. G., SALMON, S. E.: Combination chemoimmunotherapy with adriamycin and cyclophosphamide for advanced breast cancer. Cancer 36, 90–97 (1975).

20. KAPLAN, E. L., MEIER, P.: Non-parametric estimation from incomplete observations. J. Amer. Stat. Assoc. 53, 457–481 (1958).

21. MAVLIGIT, G. M., GUTTERMAN, J. U., BURGESS, M. A., KHANKHANKIAN, M., SEIBERT, B. B., SPEER, J. F., JUBERT, A. V., MARTIN, R. C., McBRIDE, C. M., COPELAND, E. M., GEHAN, E. A., HERSH, E. M.: Prolongation of post operative disease free interval and survival in human colorectal cancer by bacillus calmette guerin (BCG) or BCG plus 5-fluorouracil. Lancet (1976) I, 871–875.

22. OETTGEN, H. F., OLD, L. J., FARROW, J. H., VALENTINE, F. T., LAWRENCE, H. S., THOMAS, L.: Effects of dialyzable transfer factor in patients with breast cancer. Proc. Natl. Acad. Sci. 71, 2319–2323 (1974).

23. ROJAS, A. F., MICKIEWICZ, E., FEIRSTEIN, J. N., GLAIT, H., OLIVARI, A. J.: Levamisole in advanced human breast cancer. Lancet (1976) I, 211–215.

Trial of BCG Immunotherapy in the Treatment of Resectable Squamous Cell Carcinoma of the Bronchus (Stages I and II)

P. POUILLART, G. MATHÉ, T. PALANGIE, L. SCHWARZENBERG, P. HUGUENIN, P. MORIN, H. GAUTIER, and A. BARON

Introduction

Squamous cell carcinoma of the lung ranks as one of the most prevalent and lethal of all malignancies. Though bronchogenic carcinoma responds to both chemotherapy [10] and radiotherapy, the survival of lung cancer patients has not greatly increased, and cure is anticipated only when complete surgical resection is possible; under actual therapeutical conditions, no more than 7.5–10% of patients with squamous cell carcinoma of the lung can be cured, and chemotherapy systematically applied after surgery has been demonstrated as ineffective [1, 11].

The goal of the present work was to study the role of BCG applied in patients after surgical resection of squamous cell carcinoma of the lung.

Patients and Method

Thirty-nine patients operated on for squamous cell carcinoma of the bronchus took part in this trial, which began in October, 1973 (Table 1). Eighteen patients were selected at random for the group to be submitted to BCG application, and the other 21 patients received no further treatment after surgery. The distribution according to age and sex is shown in Table 1 and, in Table 2, distribution according to anatomical staging.

Table 1. Resectable squamous cell carcinoma of the bronchus: median age of the patients

	BCG	No treatment
Number of patients	18	21
Median age	58 (37–68)	59 (45–67)

Table 2. Resectable squamous cell carcinoma of the bronchus: distribution according to anatomical staging

	BCG	No treatment
Stage I	9	11
Stage II	9	10

Treatment

The 18 patients submitted to immunotherapy received weekly applications of Pasteur Institute BCG on a scarification 1 m long applied to the proximal extremity of each of the four limbs. The dose of live BCG applied was 75 mg once a week (living bacilli).

Surveillance of the Patients

The condition of the patients was followed in three ways: clinically, radiologically, and immunologically. The clinical examination of the patients was systematic: survey of the peripheral lymph node areas of the liver, of the neurologic state, and of the weight curve. Routine monthly radiologic examinations were associated with cine γ-encephalographic examinations every 3 months or at the time of the appearance of recent neurologic troubles. Pulmonary scintigraphic (197Hg) examinations were repeated every 4 months.

The immunologic surveillance of these patients was based on the regular study of delayed hypersensitivity skin reactions (DHS) of the secondary type, of the average number of circulating lymphocytes, and of the amount of serum LIF.

Finally, the average survival times of these patients were studied and presented actuarially.

Immunologic Surveillance

Six of the 18 patients in the group treated with BCG showed negative DHS reactions at the time of their entry into the trial. In all these patients, the skin tests for DHS became positive in the 3 months which followed the application of BCG. Three of them have since died and another is in relapse.

Seven of the 21 nontreated patients initially had negative DHS reactions, in three of them a spontaneous reversion to positive was noted in the 3 months following their entry into the trial. Five of these patients are now dead and another is in relapse.

Results

In the group treated with BCG, three patients died respectively at the 9th, 10th and 13th months, and two others relapsed at the 14th and 19th months but are still alive. In the nontreated group, eight patients died respectively at the 4th, 6th, 7th, 8th, 12th, 18th, and 35th months.

In the group treated with BCG, the three dead patients presented stage II of the disease, i.e., the histologic study of the part operated on showed a mediastinal ganglionic extension. In this group, a single patient in stage I has now relapsed at the 14th month (Fig. 1).

In the group left without treatment, three patients in stage I of the disease died and one is in relapse; five patients in stage II died and another is now in relapse.

Comparison of the actuarial curves of survival revealed a significant difference after the 18th month in favor of the group submitted to immunotherapy. In the group treated with BCG,

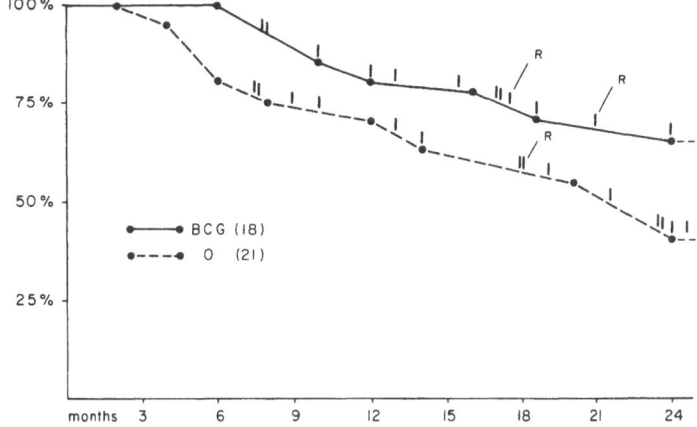

Fig. 1. Results of a controlled randomized trial of resectable bronchus carcinoma. Comparison of cumulative survival of patients submitted to BCG after operation and of patients receiving no postsurgery treatment. (Actuarial survival curve of 39 patients with squamous cell carcinoma of the bronchus (St. I, II) randomized trial: after surgical resection)

the chance of surviving for 2 years is 66% and only 38% in the nontreated group. This difference seems much more marked for the patients in stage I of the disease. Although the sample is small, the chance of surviving for 2 years for patients at this stage of the disease, and who have been submitted to treatment with BCG, is of the order of 90%, against 55% for the identical group of nontreated patients.

Discussion

Radical surgery remains the only effective means of treatment for patients with squamous cell carcinoma of the bronchus. However, the small percentage of patients apparently cured 5 years after satisfactory surgery encourages one to investigate complementary therapeutic means liable to improve results already obtained.

In this trial, we have studied, in 2 randomized groups of patients, the role of BCG applied systematically and regularly after surgery. The chance of surviving for 2 years is significantly higher for the treated patients than for the nontreated ones; but this difference is much more apparent if one considers only the patients in stage I of their illness.

The sample is too small for this difference to have anything but an indicative value, but it confirms once again the great efficacy of BCG in cases where the tumor mass has been reduced as much as possible [6].

The efficacy of immunotherapy after application of cyto-reducing treatment has already been shown [5, 7]. In addition, a correlation between prognosis and the state of delayed hypersensitivity reactions of the primary type [3, 8] or of the secondary type [4] has been shown in patients initially treated by surgery or secondarily treated by chemotherapy [9]. With regular administration of another systemic adjuvant of immunity (*Mycobacterium segmat*), DECROIX obtained a significantly greater chance of survival, in the order of nearly 3 years, for patients with operated bronchial cancers over the recorded groups of nontreated patients.

These results are confirmed in our study, which also indicates the differences in behavior of patients to DHS reactions ($-$), since in the two groups, in spite of a reversion of the skin tests to positive, either spontaneously or under BCG, the prognostic significance remains disappointing in midterm.

Finally, the patients in stage II of the disease do not seem to benefit notably from immunotherapy in the first 2 years.

This study is continuing along the same lines, but if the results are confirmed, the degree of significance of the differences becoming greater, then immunotherapy will be rapidly made part of the prescribed routine for the treatment of patients suffering from epidermal bronchial cancers.

Conclusion

Thirty-nine patients with squamous cell carcinoma of the bronchus were randomized into two groups after radical surgery. The first group of 18 patients received 75 mg of living BCG on a scratched area once a week; the second group of 21 patients received no further treatment. After 2 years, three patients of the group treated with BCG are dead and one is in relapse; eight patients of the control group are dead and two are in relapse.

In this study, the hope of survival for more than 2 years for patients with squamous cell carcinoma of the bronchus is 66% in the group of patients treated with BCG, and 38% in the control group. From these results, we can see the beneficial effect of BCG as a complementary treatment to surgery for patients with squamous cell carcinoma of the bronchus.

References

1. BRUNNER, K. W., MARHALER, T. H., MULLER, W.: Unfavorable effects of long term adjuvant chemotherapy with endoxan in radically operated bronchogenic carcinoma. Europ. J. Cancer 7, 285–288 (1971).
2. DECROIX, J.: Personal communication.
3. EILBER, F. R., MORTON, D. L.: Impaired immunologic reactivity and recurrence following cancer surgery. Cancer 25, 362, 367 (1970).
4. ISRAEL, L., MUGICA, J., CHA INIAN, P.: Prognosis of early bronchogenic carcinoma. Survival curves of 451 patients after resection of lung cancer in relation to the results of preoperative tuberculin skin tests. Biomedicine 19, 68–71 (1973).
5. MATHÉ, G., AMIEL, J. L., SCHWARZENBERG, L., CATTAN, A., SCHLUMBERGER, J. R., HAYAT, M., DE VASSAL, F.: Active immunotherapy for acute lymphoid leukemia. Lancet (1969) I, 697–699.
6. MATHÉ, G., POUILLART, P., LAPEYRAQUE, F.: Active immunotherapy of L1210 leukemia applied after the graft of tumor cell. Brit. J. Cancer 23, 814–816 (1969).
7. MATHÉ, G., POUILLART, P., SCHWARZENBERG, L., AMIEL, J. L., SCHNEIDER, M., HAYAT, M., DE VASSAL, F., JASMIN, C., ROSENFELD, C., WEINER, R., RAPPAPORT, H.: Attempt at immunotherapy of 100 acute lymphoid leukemia patients. Some factors influencing results. Nat. Cancer Inst. 35, 361–371 (1972).
8. MORTON, D. L., EILBER, F. R., MARMGREN, R. A., WOOD, W.: Immunological factors which influence response to immunotherapy in malignant melanoma. Surgery 68, 158–164 (1970).
9. POUILLART, P., BOTTO, G., GAUTIER, H., HUGUENIN, P., BARON, A., LAPARRE, C., HOANG THY, H. T., PARROT, R., MATHÉ, G.: Relation entre l'état immunitaire et la réponse à la chimiothérapie. Résultats chez 64 malades avec cancers bronchiques epidermoides inopérables. Nouv. Presse Med. 5, 1037–1042 (1976).

10. POUILLART, P., SCHWARZENBERG, L., AMIEL, J. L., MATHÉ, G., HUGUENIN, P., MORIN, P., BARON, A., LAPARRE, C., PARROT, C.: Combinaisons de drogues se potentialisant. 1. Application au traitement des cancers du sein. 2. Application au traitement des cancers des bronches. 3. Application au traitement des tumeurs primitives du système nerveux central. Nouv. Presse Med. *4*, 713–716 (1975).
11. SELAWRY, O. S., HANSEN, H. H.: Lung cancer in "cancer treatment." Holland, J., Frei, E., III (eds.). Philadelphia: Lea and Febiger, 1974.

Postoperative Nonspecific Immunotherapy in Primary Bronchogenic Carcinoma

V. Djurovic and G. Decroix

The results of surgery in primary bronchogenic carcinoma remain very poor.

The addition of some form of adjuvant therapy following surgery therefore appears necessary and even imperative.

In this regard, neither radiotherapy nor chemotherapy has proved its efficacy [1, 4, 8, 9, 11, 13, 19, 20].

We felt that adjuvant active nonspecific immunotherapy, by acting against "residual disease" might have some chance of preventing or delaying the appearance of metastases and improving postoperative survival [2].

The present therapeutic trial shows the survival rates observed 1 and 2 years after surgery.

The immunopotentiator we used is an original product prepared from a transformed strain of mycobacteria

The transformed strain was obtained by inoculating a mixture of a saprophytic mycobacterium: *M. smegmatis* ATCC 607, nonvirulent for mice and rapid-growing, and a virulent slow-growing bacillus: *M. tuberculosis* H37Rv, into the peritoneal cavity of mice. The amount of each type of bacilli in the mixture is evaluated according to their respective sensitivities to phagocytosis.

After 4 days of contact and modification of the two types of bacilli in peritoneal macrophages, a few sparse fast-growing bacilli survive and these can be isolated and cultured from peritoneal washings.

These bacilli differ from *M. smegmatis* by their virulence for mice, since they induce a 100% mortality rate in the animals 4 days after inoculation with an intentise bacilli survival (Fig. 1).

Thus, through phagocytosis by peritoneal macrophages, these rapid-growing saprophytic bacilli, *M. smegmatis*, have acquired one of the genetic charactéristics of *M. tuberculosis* H37Rv, namely virulence for mice.

This change of virulence has probably been obtained by absorption of *M. tuberculosis* H37Rv ADN through an increase of membrane permeability, allowing a coded figure, namely virulence, to integrate itself into their genetic material [5].

The immunopotentiator prepared from this new bacterial strain, killed by heating, was administered subcutaneously every 2 weeks or every month at four different sites beginning as soon as possible after surgery (15 days).

The dose and administration schedule were adapted to each individual patient depending on tumor extension, according to the TNM classification, the patient's immune status as assessed by responses to skin tests, and their reactions to the immunostimulus itself.

Tolerance to the product was satisfactory.

Between January, 1973 and May, 1976, 104 patients underwent surgery for primary bronchogenic carcinoma. Twenty-five of these patients were excluded from the trial for various reasons, and 79 were placed on postoperative immunotherapy.

At the present time, 54 of the patients who underwent surgery between January, 1973 and May, 1975 have been followed up postoperatively for 12–36 months. (Table 1).

A non randomized control group consisted of 71 patients who also underwent surgery between January, 1973 and May, 1975. (Table 2).

All operations were performed by the same surgical team, and all operative specimens were examined by the same pathologist.

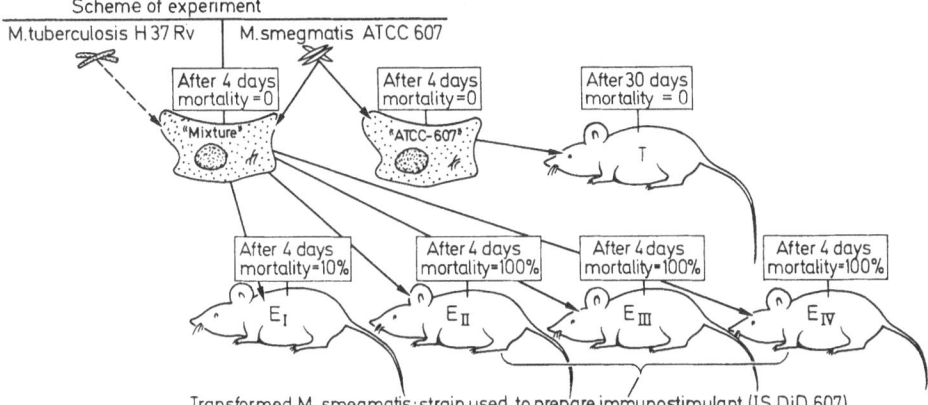

Fig. 1. Change of virulence of the saprophyte strain *M. smegmatis* ATCC 607 when mixed with *M. tuberculosis* H37Rv in mouse peritoneal cavity

$-\ -\ -\ =$ *M. tuberculosis* H37Rv = virulent.
$————— =$ *M. smegmatis* ATCC 607 = saprophytic and virulent transformed strains.
T: *M. smegmatis* ATCC 607 strain inoculated i.p. to mice designed as "ATCC 607," subsequently isolated from peritoneal washings and reinoculated to T group of mice.
E-I, E-II, E-III, E-IV: Four distinct colonies of a rapid-growing strain isolated from peritoneal washing 4 days after i.p. inoculation of mixture ATCC 607 and H37Rv, to mice designed as "mixture," and reinoculated into groups of mice E-I, E-II, E-III, E-IV

Table 1. Group of 54 patients on active nonspecific immunotherapy following resection (follow-up from 12–36 months after surgery)

Operation		Cell type			Total	%
		Oat cell 2%	Squamous cell 74%	Adenocarcinoma 24%		
Lobectomy		1	22	9	32	59.2
Pneumonectomy			18	4	22	40.8
TNM	No		18	7	25	46.2
	N+	1	22	26	29	53.8
Bronchial section involved			2	3	5	9.2

The treated group and the control group were comparable with regard to age, cell type, TNM classification, and the type of operation performed. (Table 3).
The main features of the 54 patients in the treated group are summarized in Table 1.
The control group has the same features (Table 2).
The postoperative survival rate is shown in Table 3.
The 1-year survival rate is 91% in the treated group and 60% in the control group. The 2-year survival rate is 80% in the treated group and 40% in the control group.

Table 2. Control group of 71 patients with primary bronchogenic carcinoma resected between January, 1973 and May, 1975 (no adjuvant immunotherapy) (same surgical team) (same pathologist)

Operation		Cell type			Total	%
		Oat cell 4%	Squamous cell 75%	Adenocarcinoma 21%		
Lobectomy		2	24	10	36	51
Pneumonectomy		1	29	5	35	49
TNM	No	0	27	9	36	51
	N+	3	26	6	35	49
Bronchial section involved		1		2	3	4

Table 3. Comparison of 1- and 2-year survival rates in patients on immunotherapy and untreated controls

Adjuvant	Lobectomy	Pneumonectomy	No	N+	1-year survival	2-year survival
Immunotherapy treated group	59%	41%	46%	54%	91%	80%
Non-treated control group	51%	49%	51%	49%	60%	40%

Table 4. Comparison of 1-year survival in the immunotherapy group, the untreated control group, and 21 surgical series taken from the literature

Authors	Year	Number of cases	Survival (%)
EISENBERG, VOSSCHULTE, BOUCOT, JONS, CHURCHILL, PAULSON (From 11)	1935 1957	5396	46
LONGEFAIT, BRANCADORO, BIGNALL, TALA, SABOUR, HUMBERT, SULZER, LAVAL, HERTZOG (From 11)	1947 1968	9614	58
HUET et al. [10], SHIELDS [20], POULET and BOUL [15], FRYJORDET and KLEVMARK [8], BROSS et al. [3], PRIOLLET [16]	1952 1972	5953	57
Control group	1973 1975	71	60
Immunotherapy group	1973 1975	54	91

Table 5. Overall 1-year mortality rates in resected bronchial carcinoma according to various authors: No N+ ratio (%)

Authors	Number of cases	No %	N+ %	1-year mortality (%)
Nohl [14]	211	52	48	42
Laval eta l. [12]	513	68	32	45
Edwards and Whitwell [7]	60	52	48	45
Renault [17]	356	55	45	40
Laval et al. [12]	951	68	32	42
Ribet [18]	120	75	25	40
Priollet [16]	263	50	50	40
Dubois and Vanderhoeft [6]	120	60	40	42
Control group	71	51	49	40
Immunotherapy group	54	46	54	9.2

Table 6. Study of responses to PPD skin tests in 54 patients with resected bronchogenic carcinoma treated by immunotherapy (follow-up from 12–36 months after surgery) (International standards)

Tumor histology	PPD Test 10 IP48 u (3 international u)			
	Before surgery		After surgery (6 months)	
	−	+	+	−
Oat cell	1		1	
Squamous cell	28	17	36	9
Adenocarcinoma	3	5	7	1
Total	32	22	44	10
%	59	41	81	19

The difference, according to the number of treated patients is statistically significant (p = 0,001).

Let us compare this 91% 1-year survival rate with the major survival series published in the literature. We have collected 1-year survival figures from 21 series all over the world totaling over 20,000 patients (Table 4).

In the best of cases, the 1-year survival rate did not exceed 60% as compared to 90% in our treated group.

The curve (Fig. 2) shows the results compared to those of the control group and those achieved in eight recent surgical series.

The 1-year survival rate in the treated group is 91% versus 60% in the other groups. And after 2 years, the survival rate is 80% in the treated group versus 40–45% in the other series. We have represented the present status of the actuarial survival curve up to 30 months (Fig. 3). The standard deviation increases as the number of patients with a sufficiently long follow-up become smaller and smaller. It can be seen, however, that the most pessimistic predictions still place the survival rate of treated patients above that of patients from available surgical series.

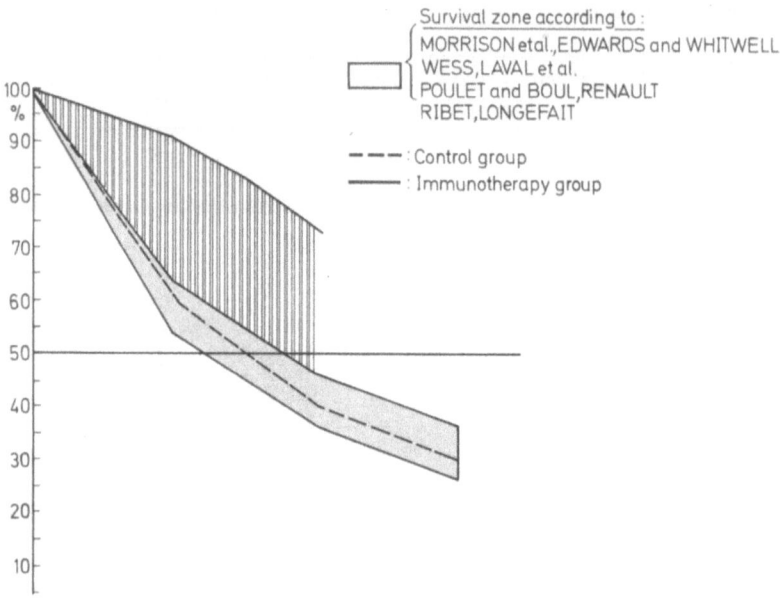

Fig. 2. Survival curves of patients with resected bronchogenic carcinoma according to various authors

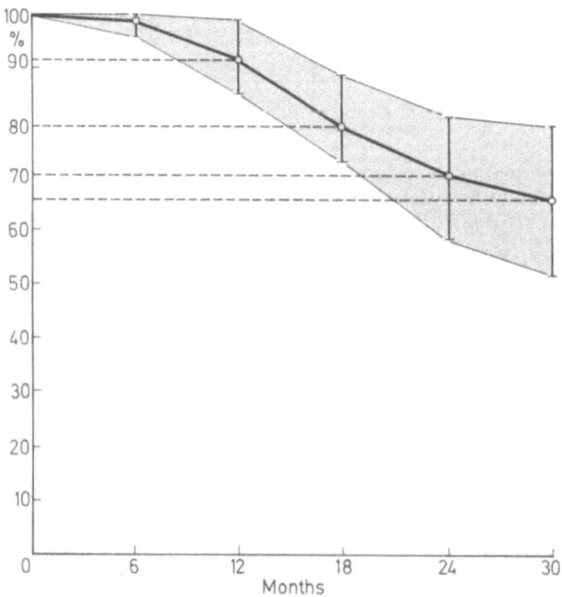

Fig. 3. Survival actuarial curve

The immune status of patients on immunotherapy was monitored essentially by skin testing. The usual tests performed were with protein purified derivative (PPD), candidin, various bacterial extracts, DNCB, and the immunostimulant itself.

These tests were repeated during immunotherapy and served as a guideline for adjusting doses and timing injections.

Only 41% of patients had a positive response before surgery while the number of positive responders 6 months after initiation of immunotherapy rose to 81% (Table 6).

Prolonged postoperative survival is not the only beneficial effect of the immunotherapy used. Patients treated by immunotherapy led a more comfortable existence than those treated by postoperative radiotherapy or chemotherapy (Table 7).

Table 7. Biological data on the 54 patients with an adequately resected primary bronchogenic carcinoma treated postoperatively by immunotherapy (follow-up 12–36 months after surgery)

1. Local reaction to the immunostimulant
   . After 1–4 injections = ±
   . After 4–8 injections = ++

2. Mean sedimentation rate
   . Before surgery = 37
   . 6 months after surgery = 9

3. Mean weight gain 6 months after surgery = 5.4 kg

4. Karnofsky's criteria 6 months after surgery = 80–100

5. Mean age: 61 years

Six months after surgery, the mean sedimentation rate was 9 mn after 1 hour versus 37 mn before surgery. The mean weight gain was 5.4 kg and the mean Karnovsky score was 80–100.

In conclusion, postoperative adjuvant active nonspecific immunotherapy in primary bronchogenic carcinoma has provided some hope in controlling "residual disease" and may, thereby, prevent the development of metastases and prolong postoperative survival.

This form of therapy is economical, well-tolerated, and always procures appreciable improvement in patient comfort.

The immunopotentiator we used has proved to be particularly effective and devoid of any toxic or other untoward effect.

Summary

A postoperative active nonspecific immunotherapy has been conducted in 54 patients operated on for primary bronchogenic carcinoma.

The immunopotentiator used is an original product prepared from a transformed strain of a saprophytic mycobacterium: *M. smegmatis* ATCC 607.

The patients treated show an increase in postoperative survival rates of 60% at 1 year and 50% at 2 years, with regard to the survival rates of a control group and 21 surgical series available totaling over 20,000 patients.

This important increase in the survival rates is accompanied by an appreciable improvement in patient comfort.

References

1. ABBEY SMITH, R.: Long term clinical follow-up after operation for lung carcinoma. Thorax 25, 62 (1970).
2. BAST, R. C., ZBAR, B., BORSOST, T., RAPP, H. J.: BCG and cancer. New Engl. J. Med. 290, 1413 (1974). New Engl. J. Med. 290, 1458 (1974).
3. BROSS, W., ROGALSKI, E. WREZLEWICZ, W.: Our results in the surgical treatment of lung cancer. Bull. Soc. Int. Chir. 31, 614 (1972).
4. CARBONE, P. P., FROST, J. K., FEINSTEINS, A. R.: Lung cancer: perspectives and prospects. Ann. Intern. Med. 73, 1003 (1970).
5. DJUROVIC, V.: Changement de virulence de la souche saprophyte M. Smegnatis ATCC 607 après mélange avec M. Tuberculosis H 37 RV dans la cavité péritonéale de la souris. Rev. Tub. Pneum. 36, 643 (1972).
6. DUBOIS, A., VANDERHOEFT, P.: Exereses pulmonaires pour cancers bronchiques, étude de la survie de 120 malades. Acta Chir. Belg. 5, 337 (1970).
7. EDWARDS, F. R., WHITWELL, F.: Use of BCG as an immunostimulant in the surgical treatment of carcinoma of the lung. Thorax 29, 654 (1974).
8. FRYJORDET, A., KLEVMARK, B.: Bronchial carcinoma—result of treatment in 514 patients. Scand. J. Thor. Cardio-Vasc. Surg. 5, 92 (1971).
9. HIGGINS, G. A.: Use of chemotherapy as adjuvant for surgery for bronchogenic carcinoma. Cancer 94, 539 (1972).
10. HUET, R., BARBE, A., MARTELET, J. P., CHARPIN, P., LONGEFAIT, J.: Le résultat éloigné du traitement chirurgical des cancers bronchiques. Marseilles Med. 112, 565 (1975).
11. ISRAEL, L., CHAHINIAN, P.: De l'impossibilité de guérir les cancers bronchiques par la chirurgie seule. Presse Med. 77, 389 (1969).
12. LAVAL, P., LONGEFAIT, H., KLEISBAUER, J. P., CHARPIN, P., POIRIER, R.: Les cancers épidermoïdes bronchiques opérés. Valeurs pronostique des constatations anatomiques per-opératoires. Rev. Franç. Mal. Resp. 2, (8–9), 702 (1974).
13. MORRISON, R., DEELEY, T. J., CLELAND, W. P.: Treatment of carcinoma of the bronchus: a clinical trial to compare surgery and supervoltage radiation therapy. Lancet 1, 683–684 (1963).
14. NOHL, H. C.: A three year follow-up of classified cases of bronchogenic carcinoma after resection. Thorax 15 (1), 11 (1960).
15. POULET, J., BOUL, M.: Cancer pulmonaire. Pronostic opératoire chez les sujets âgés de plus de 65 ans. Nouv. Presse. Med. 3, 230 (1974).
16. PRIOLLET, D.: La survie à court et à long terme du cancer primitif du poumon opéré. Thèse de Médecine. 1974, Université Paris V. Nouv. Presse. Méd. 37, 2639 (1975).
17. RENAULT, P.: Les cancers épidermoïdes bronchiques opérés. Influence pronostique de divers facteurs histopathologiques. Rev. Franç. Mal. Resp. 2 (8–9), 688 (1974).

18. RIBET, M.: Cancer bronchique et chirurgie. Chirurgie (Mémoires de l'Académie) *96*, (5), 337–344 (1970).
19. SHIELDS, T. W.: Long term survivors after resection of bronchial carcinoma. Surg. Gynec. Obstet. *136*, 759 (1973).
20. SHIELDS, T. W.: Pre-operative radiation therapy in the treatment of bronchial carcinoma. Cancer *30*, 1388 (1972).

The Strategy of Cancer Treatment: Testicular Carcinoma

S. K. CARTER

Testicular tumors are relatively rare tumors accounting for about 1–2% of all malignant neoplasms in man. Estimates of the incidence of all testicular tumors usually lie between two to three per 100,000 men per year [1, 2, 3]. Unlike most malignant tumors, those of the testicle are essentially tumors which attack men in their prime and so the emotional impact is great [4].

Tumors arising from the testis are divided into several histologic types, many of which have several subgroups. The nomenclature of the principle neoplasms has become chaotic as various authors have employed different terminologies and have not always made clear their criteria for defining and naming particular types of tumors. Two of the most important systems in use are those of DIXON and MOORE based on their experience of 900 cases [7], and those of COLLINS and PUGH derived from 995 cases reviewed by the British Testicular Tumor Panel and Registry [3] (see Table 1).

Clinical staging in testicular tumors is useful as a means of planning treatment and evaluating the efficacy of treatment afterward. Of course, a complete case history and physical examination of the patient are an essential beginning to evaluating the extent of disease. This should be followed by more specific diagnostic methods including chest x-rays (including laminograms as indicated to view suspicious nodular densities), excretory urograms, inferior venacavagrams, pedal lymphangiograms, and laboratory measurements of chorionic gonadotropin content. These procedures will permit clinical staging to the best possible extent through the two commonly used systems that are compared in Table 2.

The Walter Reed General Hospital [15] system is based on clinical, roengtenographic, and surgical-pathologic findings. A TNM (tumor, node, metastasis) definition is offered by the Union Internationale Contre le Cancrum [22] but it does not group lesions by stages so that the conflicts between the two systems are minimal. Because of the disagreement surrounding the treatment of testicular neoplasms, it is singularly important to obtain a complete evaluation of the extent of disease at initial diagnosis expressed in one of the staging systems described in Table 2.

One of the major problems encountered in all clinical staging systems is the inability to fully diagnose intra-abdominal lymph node involvement without surgical exploration. Pedal lymphangiography closes this gap to a significant degree. WALLACE and JING [24] have reported that surgical or autopsy findings, or both, correlated well with the results observed in pedal lymphangiograms. Of 18 cases with a positive roetgenographic interpretation, 17 (94%) had a positive finding in the nodes at surgical exploration. In 49 negative lymphangiograms, only eight proved to be false negatives after lymphadenectomy.

Surgery, radiotherapy, and chemotherapy have all been useful in patients with testicular tumors and immunotherapy may ultimately play an important therapeutic role. The problem facing clinicians is how to blend these various modalities into optimum programs of treatment. RUBIN [16] has pointed out the increasing use of combined therapy (i.e., surgery and radiotherapy) that is coupled with the rising cure rate noted in end-result reporting. Twenty years ago, combined therapy was employed in 46% of all patients with testicular tumors. In the period 1960–1964, use of this approach rose to 68% of all cases.

Surgery finds application in the treatment of the primary tumor and regional lymphatic metastases, and in the management of distant metastases. Surgical removal of the primary tumor is always indicated immediately after the clinical diagnosis. This also permits serial section of the testis to determine the proper histopathologic diagnosis. The current practice is to perform an orchiectomy that includes high inguinal ligation of the vas and spermatic

Table 1. Armed Forces Institute of Pathology and British systems for classification of testis neoplasms (partial); Sulak (1970)

Armed Forces Institute of Pathology	Testicular Tumor Panel and Registry of Great Britain and Ireland
Germinal origin	*Germinal origin*

1. Seminoma
   a. Typical (classical)
   b. Anaplastic
   c. Spermatocytic (atypical)
	1. Seminoma(s)

	Uncertain histogenesis
2. Embryonal carcinoma	1. Teratoma differentiated (TD)
3. Teratoma	2. Malignant teratoma intermediate (MTI) a. MTIA—with differentiated or organoid

4. Teratoma with malignant areas
   (teratocarcinoma)
	components
	   b. MTIB—no differentiated or organoid
	      components

5. Choriocarcinoma	3. Malignant teratoma anaplastic (MTA)
6. Compound tumor	4. Malignant teratoma trophoblastic (MTT)
Nongerminal origin	*Combined tumor*—seminoma and teratoma
1. Interstitial cell tumor 2. Gonadal-stromal tumors	*Sertoli cell tumor*
Miscellaneous	*Interstitial cell tumor*
	Orchioblastoma
	Others

vessels, complete removal of the contents of the inguinal canal, and removal of the testis and its adnexa, including the parietal layer of the tunica vaginalis.

There is undoubtedly a curative potential in orchiectomy alone but it is rarely, if ever, used as the sole treatment [26]. Since the prime mechanism of metastasis is by the lymphatics and retroperitoneal lymph nodes are the probable initial site of dissemination, all clinical groups treat these nodes in the same manner. Experience in the last 25 years has shown that surgery to remove the primary lymphatic drainage may be accomplished with a low mortality and acceptable morbidity. In the series of Whitmore [27] and Staubitz et al. [21], combined orchiectomy and retroperitoneal lymph node dissection produced an excellent 5-year survival rate of 87% in patients with "negative" lymph nodes irrespective of tumor type. In the cases of "positive" nodes, the survival rate was 66%.

Radiotherapy is appropriate in the management of both retroperitoneal lymph node metastases and distant metastases and may be either curative or palliative depending upon the precise circumstances. Irradiation may be used to destroy metastatic foci in the lymph nodes without producing clinically important damage to adjacent normal tissues. Radiotherapy has a technical advantage over surgery in that there are no skipped areas at the target end of a properly directed beam.

Seminoma is clearly the most radiosensitive and radiocurable tumor. Friedman [11] has found that the lethal dose for seminoma is in the range of 1000 rad in 10–14 days. By comparison, the dose for "carcinoma" is 4000–5000 rad in 3–6 weeks, although an occasional tumor may be atypically sensitive to a lethal dose of 2500–3000 rad in 2–3 weeks. Chemotherapy agents have been used in the treatment of primary tumor and regional lymphatic metastases and in managing distant metastatic disease. Adjunct chemotherapy is also finding an increasing role in the management of patients with all stages of disease.

Table 2. Comparison of the staging systems of Walter Reed General Hospital and the UICC;
Maier et al. (1968) [15] and UICC (1968) [22]

Walter Reed General Hospital System	UICC System
Stage Ia: Tumor confined to one testis; no clinical or roentgenographic evidence of spread beyond; may include excretory or retrograde urography, lymphangiography, inferior venacavography, and chest roentgenography	T1: Tumor occupying less than one-half of the testis and surrounded by palpably normal gland T2: Tumor occupying one-half or more of the testis, but not producing enlargement or deformity of the testis T3: Tumor confined to the testis but producing enlargement or deformity of the testis NO: No deformity of regional nodes on lymphography
Stage Ib: Same as in Stage Ia, but found to have histologic evidence of metastases to iliac or para-aortic lymph nodes at time of retroperitoneal lymph node dissection	T1–T3: Same as above NX+: When it is impossible to assess the regional nodes, the symbol NX will be used, permitting eventual addition of histologic information, thus NX+ or NX–

Stage II: Clinical or roentgenographic evidence of metastases to femoral, inguinal, iliac, or para-aortic lymph nodes; no demonstrable metastases above the diaphragm or to visceral organs	T1–T3: Same as above
	T4: Tumor extending to the epididymis or beyond the testis
	  a. Tumor extending to epididymis only
	  b. Tumor extending to other structures
	N1: Regional nodes deformed on lymphography
	N2: Fixed, palapable abdominal nodes

Stage III: Clinical or roentgenographic evidence of metastases above the diaphragm or other distant metastases to body organs	TO: No evidence of primary tumor T1–T4: Same as above M1: Distant metastases present including lymph nodes outside the abdomen

The critical questions which cause a great deal of discussion involve how to utilize these various modalities for each histologic type at each stage of presentation.

The therapy of seminoma is relatively uncomplicated with controversy. Orchiectomy is followed by lymphangiography. If the tumor is staged as stage A or I, the management is usually retroperitoneal irradiation with approximately 3000 rad, delivered over a period of 3 weeks to the retroperitoneal lymph node area. From the diaphragm to ipsilateral Poupart's ligament, irradiation to the respective groin, as well as to the contralateral groin and pelvis, can be considered in the event of prior ipsilateral inguinal or scrotal surgery. Extending the radiation therapy to the mediastinum and base of the neck has been advocated by some but the advantage of this has not been proven. If the tumor is shown to be in the retroperitoneal lymph nodes (stage B or II) the extended radiation is recommended. Some investigators utilize adjuvant chemotherapy in this stage, but again conclusive data proving the value of this are not available.

In patients with clinical stage C or III focal irradiation of the metastatic sites with 3000 rad over a 3-week period is potentially curative. In this situation, the logic of adding chemotherapy with alkylating agents is persuasive and is done in most major centers, although still not proven valuable by controlled trials.

For the other cell types which are often lumped as "carcinoma," the controversy is much greater. After orchiectomy and clinical staging the options include: (1) surgery only, (2) radiotherapy only, (3) radiotherapy—surgery—radiotherapy, and (4) chemotherapy or any

Table 3. Cumulative data on the efficacy of single drugs in testicular tumors

Drug	Number of evaluable patients	Number of responses[a] CR	PR	Response rate CR	CR + PR
Phenylalanine mustard	86	0	49	0	57%
Chlorambucil	8	2	2	25%	50%
CPM	2	2	0	100%	100%
MTX	10	0	4	0	40%
FU	10	0	3	0	30%
VCR	7	0	4	0	57%
VBL	25	4	9	16%	52%
Mithramycin	305	33	80	10%	37%
ACT-D	31	5	11	16%	52%
ADR	19	1	12	5%	70%
BLM	38	1	11	3%	31%

[a] CR: complete response; PR: partial response

additional combinations that could be devised. There exist no controlled clinical trial data which prove the value of one approach or another.

At Stanford [8], in the so-called sandwich technique, patients with stage I and II carcinoma (clinical staging) are initially given 3000 rad to the abdominal lymph nodes, as described earlier for seminoma patients. This is followed by a 3-week rest period, at the end of which, each patient is evaluated by an abdominal roentgenogram to study dye-filled lymph nodes and full lung tomography to search for pulmonary metastases. Usually within 2 weeks after bilateral retroperitoneal lymph node dissection, radiation therapy is resumed. Initially, the ports are the same as those used preoperatively. However, oblique fields are employed to deliver over 4000 rads to the periaortic lymph nodes. The total dose is usually 5000 rad when the dissection is negative and 5500 rad when positive. When the abdominal lymph nodes are involved, 4500–5000 rad are given to the mediastinum and supraclavicular regions.

At Stanford, a retrospective comparison with the standard radiotherapy approach has shown no definite value for the sandwich technique except that it allows the separation of patients who do very well from those who will do less well. This should be of value in the designing of adjuvant chemotherapy trial.

It is chemotherapy which is offering the exciting new curative potential in testicular tumors. Testicular tumors are sensitive to a wide range of anticancer drugs (Table 3). In fact, there has been no drug given an adequate evaluation which has not shown some evidence of activity.

It is interesting to note that the concept of combining antitumor drugs, which has proven so valuable in the hematologic malignancies, had one of its first applications more than a decade ago in testicular tumors. Table 4 summarizes the cumulative data on various drug combinations.

In 1960, Li et al. [14] published the first account of treatment with a three drug combination in metastatic testicular cancer. This report and a subsequent one [13] employed a regimen of chlorambucil (10 mg/d p.o. × 16–25 days), methotrexate (MTX) (5 mg/day p.o. × 16–25 days), and actinomycin D (ACT-D) (0.5 mg/day i.v. on days 3–7, 12–16, and 21–25). Among 28 patients treated, there were ten complete (CR) and four partial (PK) remissions; at least one of the complete responses occurred in a patient with choriocarcinoma. Of the 14 responders on triple drug therapy, two were alive and free of disease at the time of Li's second report, seven were alive but in relapse, and five had died following relapse. No data were given on the median duration of remission, but the first report cited a range of 1–18+ months.

Table 4. Cumulative Data on Combination Drug Regimens in Testicular Tumors

Drug combination	Number of evaluable patients	Number of responses[a] CR	PR	Response rate CR	CR + PR
Actinomycin D + chlorambucil + methotrexate	236	29	77	12%	45%
Vinblastine + phenylalanine mustard	11	2	3	18%	45%
Vinblastine + bleomycin	19	3	14	16%	90%
Actinomycin D + chlorambucil	31	5	8	16%	42%
Actinomycin D + mechlorethamine	14	1	3	7%	29%
Mechlorethamine + methotrexate	15	2	3	13%	33%
Vincristine + methotrexate + phenylalanine mustard	12	1	8	8%	75%
Vincristine + methotrexate + cyclophosphamide	22	0	10	0	45%
Vincristine + actinomycin D + cyclophosphamide	10	1	4	10%	50%
Vincristine + actinomycin D + mithramycin + cyclophosphamide	7	3	2	42%	71%
Vincristine + methotrexate + cyclophosphamide + 5-FU	17	5	2	29%	41%

[a] CR: complete response; PR: partial response

In another application of triple therapy, WHITMORE [25] reported objective responses in three patients with seminomas, in 17 of 25 with embryonal cell carcinoma, in 11 of 17 teratocarcinomas, and in seven of ten choriocarcinomas. He stated that "the regression was of no practical value in most instances, either because of its brevity or because of its incompleteness." However, he noted long-term, disease-free survivals of 9+, 33+, and 42+ months in three patients.

For a long time, this combination remained the chemotherapy of choice until the advent of bleomycin's (BLM) activity and its incorporation into combinations with vinblastine (VBL) and other drugs.

BLUM et al. [2] reported 57 evaluable patients with testicular carcinoma treated with BLM. Thirty-seven patients received the drug as a single agent and 20 were treated with BLM and VBL. The overall response was 32% for BLM alone and 90% for the combination. Responses were noted in all cell types, but the duration of response again was short for both the single agent (1.5–2 months) and the combination (2–5 months).

SAMUELS et al. [19] at M.D. Anderson Hospital were the first to combine BLM with VBL for the therapy of testicular tumors. BLM (15 mg i.m.) was administered twice weekly for 5 weeks and VBL was given at 0.4–0.6 mg/kg i.v. in 2 fractions (days 1–2). Fifty patients were treated by this induction scheme and, if response was seen, additional therapy consisted of three or four courses of the same VBL dose and 50% of the dose of BLM. Sixteen patients achieved CR (32%) with this regimen and 15 were free of disease after 2 years. Twenty-two other patients experienced PR (>50% reduction in maximum tumor diameter) with a median survival of 32 weeks. Five patients developed interstitial pneumonitis secondary to BLM therapy.

SAMUELS [17] has modified his approach to a regimen in which VBL is given at 0.4 mg/kg in two fractions (days 1–2) and BLM (30 mg in 1000cc 5% D/W over 24 hours) is started on day 2 for 5 additional days. Courses are repeated every 21–28 days × 3–4. Forty stage III germinal tumors and four extragonadal primary tumors have been studied. In 39 evaluable patients with high tumor volume presentations, there were 19 complete responses (47%) and 10 partial responses. In the extragonadal group, 1 CR and 1 PR were seen. Mean survival of complete responders is 34 weeks with none dead. Toxicity included severe leukopenia in 40, thrombocytopenia in 21, hemolytic anemia in 13, stomatitis in all cases, and BLM pneumonitis in 2 cases. It appears that the complete response rate is superior to intermittent BLM-VBL.

More recently, SAMUELS [18] has compared his experience with velban with biweekly bleomycin in 26 patients with 34 who received velban with continuous BLM. In the biweekly BLM group, seven (20%) achieved CR as against 21 (61%) for the continuous infusion approach. The median survival is also superior in the latter group (78+ weeks) as compared to 48 weeks. These data, SAMUELS feels, show the clear-cut advantage for the infusion approach with BLM.

At the Memorial Sloan-Kettering Cancer Center, daily doses of a three drug combination of BLM (0.4 mg/kg), ACT-D (0.0075–0.015 mg/kg), and VBL (0.025–0.05 mg/kg VAB I) have been tried in testicular cancer [23]. Each drug was given intravenously on days 1, 2, 3 and repeated for two to three doses in 7–14 days as toxicity permitted. Twenty-one patients were treated and 16 were evaluable; of these, eight showed objective responses lasting 1–5 months. Hematologic toxicity was predictable and mucocutaneous toxicity between days 4 and 20 was frequently severe and dose limiting. Pulmonary toxicity was observed in one patient.

In their next study [4] the Memorial Sloan-Kettering Cancer Center group utilized BLM by continuous i.v. infusion (0.5 mg/kg/day × 7) combined with cis-platinum diamine dichloride (1 mg/kg i.v. on day 7) (VAB II). Sixteen previously treated patients with germ cell tumors have been treated with this regimen. All were resistant to conventional weekly i.v. BLM and had been exposed to VBL and ACT-D. Eleven of the patients had partial responses lasting 2–7+ months with one additional patient having a minor response (< 50% > 1 month). The dose-limiting toxicity was mucositis with transient weight loss in most cases. Five patients had transient renal toxicity due to the platinum.

VAB III [5] consists of BLM given by continuous infusion (20 mg/m^2/day) for 7 days, also on day 1 VBL (4 mg/m^2), cyclophosphamide (CPM) (600 mg/m^2), and ACT-D (1 mg/m^2) are given. High dose cis-platinum diamine dichloride (120 mg/m^2) is given on day 8 with prehydration and a sustained mannitol diuresis. Maintenance with velban (4 mg/m^2) every 3 weeks and chlorambucil 4 mg/m^2 p.o. daily is given for 2 of every 3 weeks. ACT-D (1 mg/m^2), adriamycin (ADR) (45 mg/m^2), and platinum (50 mg/m^2) are alternated. The induction phase is repeated at 4–5 month intervals.

In 26 evaluable patients, there are 18 complete responders, six partial responders and still improving, and one minor response. No relapses have been seen as yet with only a 6-month follow-up.

The Eastern Cooperative Oncology Group has reported a study for stage III testicular carcinoma in which patients are randomly assigned to treatment with ACT-D (0.4 mg/m^2 i.v. days 1–5), BLM (15 mg/m^2 i.v. days 1, 8, 15), and vincristine (VCR) (1 mg/m^2 i.v. days 1–8) or to ACT-D at the above disage alone.

So far, 102 patients have been entered on this study and 84 are evaluable. With ACT-D alone 5/42 (12%) have achieved complete remission compared to 8/42 (19%) on the combination. When partial remission status is looked at, the combination is clearly superior with 21/42 (50%) versus 4/42 (10%) for ACT-D alone. The median duration of response is 27 weeks for the single agent and only 12 weeks for the combination, and so there is no meaningful clinical difference between these two regimens.

DANIELS [6] at Stanford has compared two four drug regimens. With a combination of cytoxan, mithramycin, VBL, and BLM, he has achieved complete responses in 4/11. With a second combination of ACT-D, cytoxan, MTX, and VCR, he has 5/12 who achieved CR status. The second schedule was found to be less toxic. Seven of the CR patients remain free of disease in the range of 6–43 months.

EINHORN et al. [9] have utilized just a three drug approach with cis-platinum 20 mg/m^2/day × 5 i.v. q. 3 weeks added to VBL 0.2 mg/kg/day × 2 i.v. q. 3 weeks and BLM 30 u i.v. weekly for 12 consecutive weeks. His results in 20 evaluable patients are a

100% response rate with 15 CR and five PR. Follow-up is still relatively short with a median CR duration of 9+ months and 13/15 CR still in remission.

It is now clear that chemotherapy utilized aggressively can put nearly every patient with stage III testicular carcinoma into some kind of remission. The complete remission potential is high and with that the potential for long-term disease-free control. Patients with this disease should now be referred to major centers where the full therapeutic attack can be mounted since cure is a distinct reality in this tumor even in the advanced stages.

Testicular tumors are potentially controllable by a variety of therapeutic modalities. However, at this time, the only well-defined and uncontroversial therapies are orchiectomy for primary tumor, irradiation in stage I or II seminoma, and chemotherapy for stage III tumors other than seminoma.

The critical need for accurate disease staging has established the role of retroperitoneal lymph node dissection, not only for tumor control but also to identify patients whose prognosis is poor enough to warrant adjunctive x-ray or drug therapy. Controlled clinical trials are needed that will provide vital data required to optimally combine the various modalities.

References

1. BLOM, J., BRODOVSKY, H. S.: Comparison of the treatment of metastatic testicular tumors with actinomycin D or actinomycin D, bleomycin and vincristine. Proc. AACR-ASCO 17, 290 (1976).
2. BLUM, R. H., CARTER, S. K., AGRE, K.: A clinical review of bleomycin—a new actincoplastic agent. Cancer 31, 903–914 (1973).
3. COLLINS, D. H., PUGH, R. C. B.: Classification and frequency of testicular tumors. Brit. J. Urol. 36, (Suppl. 52), (1964).
4. CVITKOVIC, E., CURRIE, V., KRAKOFF, I. H., GOLBEY, R.: Bleomycin infusion with cis-platinum diaminedichloride as secondary chemotherapy for germinal cell tumors. Am. Soc. Clin. Oncol. Abstract #1208, Proc. Amer. Assoc. Cancer Res. 16, 273 (1975).
5. CVITKOVIC, E., HAYES, D., GOLBEY, R.: Primary combination chemotherapy (VAB III) for metastatic or unresectable germ cell tumors. Proc. AACR-ASCO 17, 296 (1976).
6. DANIELS, J.: Testis carcinoma: combination chemotherapy. Proc. AACR-ASCO 17, 282 (1976).
7. DIXON, F. J., MOORE, R. A.: Tumors of the male sex organs. Armed Forces Inst. Path., Washington, D.C. Atlas of Tumor Pathology, Vol. 8, fasc. 31b and 32, 1952.
8. EARLE, J. D., BAGSHAW, M. A., KAPLAN, H. A.: Supervoltage radiation therapy of the testicular tumors. Am. J. Roentgerol. Rad. Therapy & Nuclear Med. 117, 653–661 (1971).
9. EINHORN, L. H., FURNAS, B. E., POWELL, N.: Combination chemotherapy of disseminated testicular carcinoma with cis-platinum diamine dichloride, vinblastine and bleomycin. Proc. of AACR-ASCO 17, 240 (1976).
10. FERBER, B., HANDY, V. H., GERHARDT, P. R., SOLOMON, M.: Cancer in New York State, 1941–1960. Bureau of Cancer Control, N.Y. State Department of Health, 1962.
11. FRIEDMAN, M.: Tumors of the testis and their treatment. In: Clinical Therapeutic Radiology. Portmann, U. V. (ed.). New York: Nelson, Thomas and Sons, 1950.
12. GRISWOLD, M. H., WILDER, C. S., CUTLER, S. J., POLLACK, E. S.: Cancer in Connecticut, 1935–51. Connecticut State Department of Health, 1955.
13. LI, M. C.: Management of choriocarcinoma and related tumors of uterus and testis. Med. Clin. N. Amer. 45, 661 (1966).
14. LI, M. C., WHITMORE, W. F., GOLBEY, R., GRABSTALD, H.: Effects of combined drug therapy of metastatic cancer of the testis. J. Amer. Med. Ass. 174, 1291–1299 (1960).
15. MAIER, J. B., SULAK, M. H., MITTEMEYER, B. T.: Seminoma of the testes: analysis of treatment success and failure. Amer. J. Roentgen. 102, 596–602 (1968).
16. RUBIN, P.: Cancer of the urogenital tract: testicular tumors. J. Amer. Med. Ass. 213, 89–90 (1970).
17. SAMUELS, M. L.: Continuous intravenous bleomycin therapy with vinblastine in testicular and extragonadal germinal tumors. Proc. Amer. Assoc. Cancer Res. 16, (Abstract #448), 112 (1975).
18. SAMUELS, M. L., BOYLE, L. E., HOLOYE, P. V. et al: Intermittent versus continuous infusion bleomycin in testicular cancer. Proc. AACR-ASCO 17, 98 (1976).

19. SAMUELS, M. L., JOHNSON, D. E., HOLOYE, P. V.: The treatment of stage III metastatic germinal cell neoplasia of the testis with bleomycin combination chemotherapy. Proc. Am. Assoc. Cancer Res. *14*, 23 (1973).
20. SILVAY, O., YAGODA, A., WITTES, R., WHITMORE, W., GOLBEY, R.: Treatment of germ cell carcinomas with a combination of actinomycin D, vinblastine, and bleomycin. Proc. Am. Assoc. Cancer Res. *14*, 68 (1973).
21. STAUBITZ, W. J., MAGOSS, I. V., GRACE, J. T., SCHENK, W. G.: Surgical management of testis tumors. J. Urol. *101*, 350– 355 (1969).
22. Union Internationale Contre le Cancrum: TNM Classification of Malignant Tumours. 1968, pp. 68–69.
23. VECHINSKI, T. O., JAESCHKE, W. H., VERMUND, H.: Testicular tumors: an analysis of 112 consecutive cases. Am. J. Roentgen. *95*, 494 (1965).
24. WALLACE, S., JING, B.: Lymphangiography: diagnosis of nodal metastases from testicular malignancies. J. Amer. Med. Ass. *213*, 94–96 (1970).
25. WHITMORE, W.: Some experience with retroperitoneal lymph node dissection and chemotherapy in the management of testis neoplasms. Brit. J. Urol. *34*, 436–447 (1962).
26. WHITMORE, W. F.: Germinal tumors of the testis. In: Proceedings of the Sixth National Cancer Conference. Philadelphia: J. P. Lippencott Company, 1970, pp. 219–245.
27. WHITMORE, W. F.: The treatment of germinal tumors of the testis. In: Cancer Management. Philadelphia: J. P. Lippencott, 1968.

Strategy of Testis Cancer Treatment

G. BRULE

Testicular tumors account for 2% of cancers in males and appear mainly between 20 and 40 years of age.

In a 6-year trial on a series of 232 patients in our institute, observed from 1968 to 1974, 224 (96.5%) had tumors originating in the germ cells, which may undergo three types of malignant change:

1. In 34.8% (78) of the cases, the malignant growth tends to reproduce the same types of cells as those from which it originated. This is the pure seminoma of Chevassu or the gonomia of Masson. These forms are extremely sensitive to radiotherapy and should never, in our opinion, be treated primarily by chemotherapy, even though this technique may well improve the patient's condition. In fact, radiotherapy cures at least 90% of cases.

2. In 35.2% (79) of the cases, malignant transformation of the germ cells results in embryonic carcinomas, which are generally resistant to radiotherapy and drugs.

3. In 5% (11) of the cases, the malignant change is of the trophoblastic type, resulting in a very malignant choriocarcinoma, accompanied by high chorionic gonadotrophic secretion.

This histogenetic theory, which takes into account all the germ cell tumors of the testis, explains why mixtures of cell types may be found in one tumor. Such mixtures are frequent: 25% (56 cases, Table 1).

The first treatment should, therefore, be surgical; castration with section at the upper part of the extra-abdominal spermatic cord for histologic examination of the whole specimen. The treatment of these tumors should have four objectives:

1. To remove the entire primary tumor in all cases
2. To treat the lumboaortic lymph nodes by surgery or irradiation depending on the histologic appearance
3. To prevent disseminated mestastases for the worst histologic forms by chemotherapy
4. To treat distant metastases either by surgery or irradiation if they are isolated or possibly by chemotherapy if they are disseminated

Tumors at Clinical Stages I and II

In our series: stage I   29.7%
              stage II   33.3%

As soon as the histologic evidence of embryonic carcinoma has been established, regardless of the level of chorionic gonadotrophins or α-fetoproteins, we start a 20-day course of chemotherapy with:

MAC protocol

METHOTREXATE (MTX) p.o.	5 mg daily	
ACTINOMYCIN D (ACT-D) i.v.	500 μg, days 1, 2, 3, 4, 5 and 11, 12, 13, 14, 15	
CYCLOPHOSPHAMIDE (CPM) i.m.	200 mg on alternate days	

During this period, lymphography and urography are performed.

Retroperitoneal lymph node dissection is carried out at least 10 days after the cessation of chemotherapy to avoid late toxicity.

Table 1. Germ cell tumors of testis histologic types of testis humors according to WHO classification

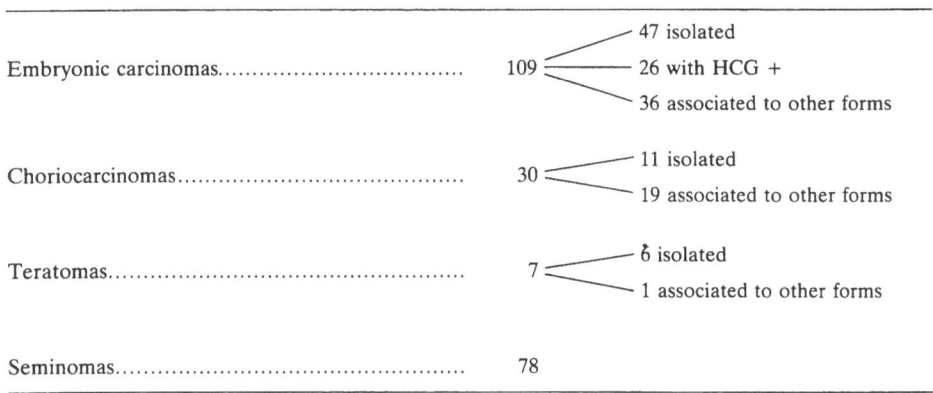

Embryonic carcinomas..................................	109	47 isolated
		26 with HCG +
		36 associated to other forms
Choriocarcinomas..	30	11 isolated
		19 associated to other forms
Teratomas..	7	6 isolated
		1 associated to other forms
Seminomas...	78	

The dissection is:
1. Unilateral if the lymphography is normal
2. With extemporaneous histologic examination of controlateral nodes if palpable or if they present pathologic or uncertain radiologic aspects

In the case of evident malignancy, the malignant lesions (resected or not) are marked with clips.

During the lymphadenectomy, dissection of the spermatic cord should be completed toward the unguinal canal to avoid local relapse.

As soon as possible, after surgery, we start a new course of chemotherapy lasting 20 days.

In all cases, especially if orchidectomy has been done by scrotal incision, inguino scrotal irradiation (4000 rad) is performed.

Chemotherapy is repeated every 2 months for:
1. 1 year only, for patients with negative lymph nodes or normal human chorionic gonadotrophin levels (HCG)
2. 2 years
   a. For patients who had pathologic HCG and/or α-fetoproteins levels
   b. For patients with invaded lymph nodes; in this case radiotherapy at maximal dose is added and focused on the marked zones

The protocol (MAC) is the same for all the courses.

In the case of severe toxicity, each course can be split into two cycles of 10 days, monthly or every 6 weeks.

Tumors at Clinical Stage III

In our series: 36.9%

Most of those cases (27.5%) already have pulmonary metastasis before treatment.

For the treatment of disseminated cases, we reinforce the protocol chemotherapy.

1. A 20-day course of BLEOMYCIN, 15 mg i.m. on alternate days followed by protocol MAC on the same schedule as above is given.

2. The two courses are repeated 6 weeks later: no more than two courses of BLEOMYCIN should be given.

3. In the case of complete remission of multiple pulmonary metastases and after two

supplementary courses of MAC, the possibility of retroperitoneal exploration may be considered.

4. If one solitary pulmonary metastatic node is stabilized, surgical removal by thoracotomy may be considered after six courses of chemotherapy.

5. If satisfactory resection is obtained, secondary retroperitoneal lymphadenectomy may be attempted.

In the case of relapse or failure of the above protocols, other drug combination can be resorted to:

FLUOROURACIL (FU)—PROCARBAZINE (PCB)—VINBLASTINE (VBL) (Table 2)
VINCRISTINE (VCR)—BLEOMYCIN (BLM)—ACT-D (Table 3)
MITHRAMYCIN (MRM) (Table 4)
VELBAN—ACT-D—BLM (Table 5)

Table 2

FU
PCB } Protocol in the treatment of testis tumor according to Institut Gustave-Roussy (1968)
VBL

FU   7.5 mg/kg/day in i.v. infusion at the rate of 250 mg/hour
                                                                              } for 5 days
PCB   200 mg per day in i.v. infusion or orally

VBL   0.1 mg/kg i.v. on the 5th day

      This course may be repeated after 4–6 weeks if bone
      marrow toxicity is not too severe

Table 3

VCR
BLM   } Protocol in the treatment of testis tumor according to Institut Gustave-Roussy,
ACT-D   (protocol LG9)

VCR	1 mg slow infusion	Days 1–2
BLM	15 mg i.v.	Days 1–2
ACT-D	500 μg i.v. infusion	Days 3-4-5-6

Table 4

MRN protocol in the treatment of testis tumor

0.8–1mg/m^2 per day in slow infusion for 10 days

or

2 mg/m^2 in slow infusion on alternate days

This protocol is very toxic

Table 5. VAB protocol in the treatment of testis tumor according to M.D. Anderson Hospital

VAB I	VBL	0.025–0.05 mg/kg	i.v. days 1, 2, 3
	ACT-D	0.0075–0.015 mg/kg	repeated in 2–3
	BLM	0.4 mg/kg	doses in 7–14 days as toxicity permits

| VAB II | Change BLM to 0.5 mg/kg/day × 7 by continuous infusion |
| | Add cis-platinum diamine dichloride 1 mg/kg i.v. on day 7 |

Results

Survival is related:
1. To the initial stage of the disease of the patient at which treatment is started (Fig. 1)
2. To the histologic type of the tumor and the HCG level of the patient (Fig. 2)

Conclusions

With very acute protocols, more patients can be cured and survival has considerably risen in the bad forms (embryonic carcinomas) since systemic chemotherapy is performed before and after surgery.

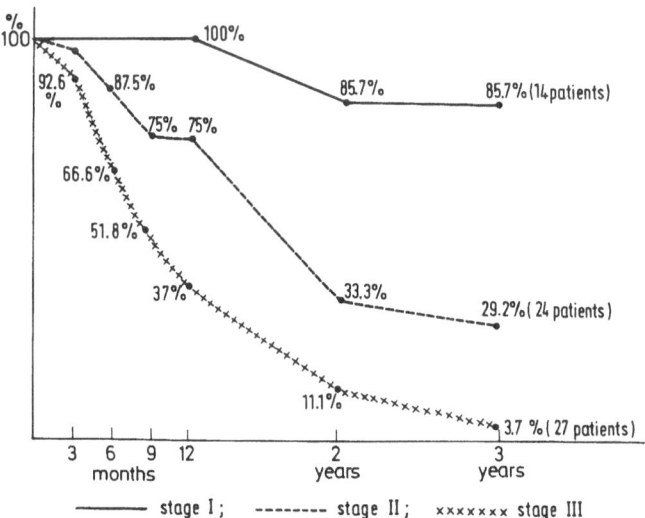

Fig. 1. Survival at 3 years according to the initial stage of disease (patients initially treated at IGR from 1968 to 1972). 65 patients

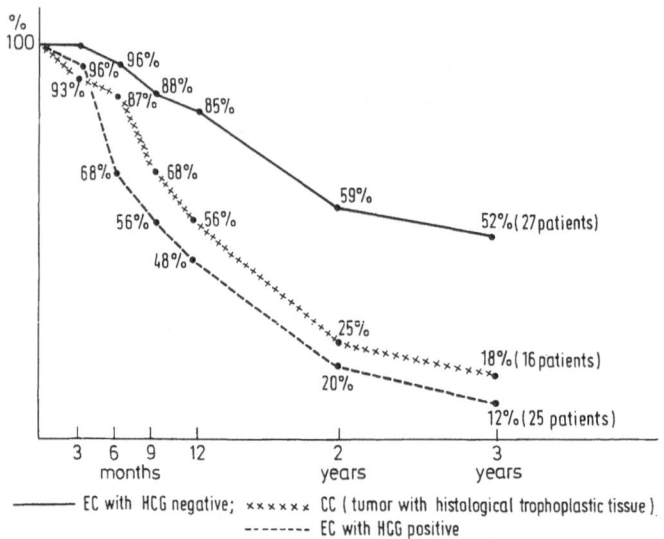

Fig. 2. Survival at 3 years according to histology and hormonology (patients initially treated at IGR from 1968 to 1972). 68 patients

The Combination of Surgery, Radiotherapy, and Chemotherapy in the Treatment of Gastric Cancer

E. Robinson and Y. Cohen

The incidence of gastric cancer in Israel is 28 cases per 100,000 inhabitants per year. Thirteen percent of those dying from cancer die from stomach cancer [16]. Surgical resection is the principal modality, offering the only hope for long-term disease-free survival. However, of the 20–50% of patients who can undergo "curative" resection, four out of five die from recurrent cancer within 5 years [2]. Chemotherapy has been primarily confined to palliative treatment [2, 3]. Since 1969 we have been treating radically operated patients with gastric cancer by adjuvant radio-chemotherapy and inoperable patients by radio- and chemotherapy or chemotherapy alone.

Methods

From 1969 to 1973, 189 patients with gastric cancer were referred to our department. Operable patients were operated on. In Table 1, our policy is shown. The kind of postoperative treatment given varied according to the stage of the disease [7]. Patients with distant metastases received only chemotherapy. Patients with locally advanced disease and regional disease (P3 with any N and N1–2 with any P) were treated with radio- and chemotherapy. When the tumor infiltrated the layers (P2) of the stomach, chemotherapy alone was given. No treatment was given when the tumor was localized to the gastric mucosa.

The radiotherapy technique: the upper abdomen was irradiated by cobalt 60 using two opposing fields the size of which were about 15 × 20 cm. The kidneys were shielded from behind. The daily tumor dose was 200 rad to a total of 3000–4000 rad in 3–4 weeks. The chemotherapy was administered by a daily dose of 500 mg fluorouracil (FU) given in an infusion of 200 ml glucose 5% during 2 hours until a total dose of 150 mg/kg had been given. Afterwards, a maintenance dose of 500–750 mg was given either directly intravenously or as above in infusion once a week. During the last 3 years, the protocol was changed to 5-FU 13.5 mg/kg daily for 5 days once in 5 weeks.

The following patients were excluded from the study:

1. Patients referred 3 months or more after the diagnosis
2. Patients with severe hepatic failure
3. Patients above 70 years of age to whom adjuvant radiotherapy was not administered.

Table 1. Treatment policy for epithelial gastric cancer – the Northern Israel Oncological Center

Treatment policy		
Stage I	P1NOMO	No treatment
	P2NOMO	5-FU − loading dose and maintenance
	P3NOMO	5-FU + radiotherapy and chemo-maintenance
Stage II Stage III	P1-4N1MO P1-4N2MO }	5-FU, radiotherapy, and chemo-maintenance
Stage IV	P1-4NO-2M1	5-FU to escape

Material

Sex: There were 121 male and 68 female patients, a relationship of 1.8:1.
Histology: In Table 2 we see the histology of the tumors. 17.2% of the patients had
anaplastic carcinoma and 51.9% had adenocarcinoma [1].
Stage of disease: In Table 3 the stage of disease of our patients is seen. Of the patients, 29%
had metastases in the lymph nodes and 45% distant metastases. In only 15% was the disease
localized to the wall of the stomach.
The kind of surgical intervention the patient underwent is seen in Table 4. More than 51%
of the patients were inoperable and only 49% underwent a "curative" resection.
Chemo- and radiotherapy treatment: 47% of the patients were treated by the combination
of chemo- and radiotherapy, 34% by 5-FU alone. Thirty patients did not receive any
treatment, *four* of them being in an early stage and *26* in an advanced stage who died before
therapy was started or shortly afterward, as shown in Table 5.

Table 2. Histology (percentage)

	Stomach	Colon	Rectosigmoid	Pancreas
Adenocarcinoma	51.9	82.6	71.4	40
Mucoid carcinoma	18.5	10.1	14.9	—
Anaplastic carcinoma	17.2	4.4	1.1	—
Unspecified, unknown	12.4	2.9	12.8	60
Total	100	100	100	100

Table 3. PNM staging of stomach cancer patients (1968–1973)

			No.	Percent
Stage I	P1NOMO	4		
	P2NOMO	13		
	P3NOMO	11	28	14.8
Stage II	P1-4N1MO		27	14.3
Stage III	P1-4N2MO		28	14.8
Stage IV	P1-4NO-2M1		86	45.5
Unknown			20	10.6
Total			189	100

Table 4. Stomach cancer—surgery

Treatment	No.	%
Total gastrectomy	27	14
Subtotal gastrectomy	65	35
Palliative procedures	17	9
Laparotomy	55	29
Nonoperated	25	13
Total	189	100

Table 5. The Treatment of Stomach Cancer Patients

	No.	%
5-FU	65	34.4
5-FU and radiotherapy	90	47.6
Radiotherapy	4	2.1
No treatment	30	15.9
Total	189	100

Results

Median survival according to therapy: 5-FU combined with radiotherapy gave the longest median survival, 13.5 months. 5-FU alone gave a median survival of 9 months, as shown in Table 6. The results are much better than those published by the Department of Health, U.S.A. which were 5 months [17].

The survival of operable stomach cancer patients treated by adjuvant radiotherapy is seen in Table 7; 82% of the patients survived for 1 year and 40% for 2 years. These results are better than those for surgery alone [8, 9, 14, 17].

Stomach cancer is a fatal disease in most patients. Surgery is, of course, still the best treatment. But half of the patients are inoperable and the median survival time of those operated on is 13 months.

Radiotherapy and chemotherapy have been shown to be of value in patients with advanced disease [10]. Approximately 20% of patients with advanced cancer will show an objective response to 5-FU [4]. In a study of 169 patients 10 years ago [4, 5, 6], it was shown that the response rate of advanced stomach cancer to radiotherapy was zero, 16.6% to 5-FU, and 55% to a combined treatment of 5-FU and radiotherapy.

In 1969, MOERTEL and co-workers [10] confirmed this finding in unresectable gastric cancer and found that the median survival of the placebo plus radiotherapy was 5.9 months while the 5-FU plus radiotherapy was 14 months which is similar to our results.

We have shown that in so-called radically operated patients, adjuvant therapy is also of value. As radiotherapy and chemotherapy are more effective on small tumor volume, treatment should be started immediately after the operation. Our present protocol is to randomize between Methyl CCNU combined with 5-FU and radiotherapy and radio-chemotherapy with MER, which is a methanol extractable residue of BCG [10].

The reason for changing the protocol is that 5-FU with Methyl CCNU has been shown to be more effective than 5-FU alone [11, 13]. MER has been shown to stimulate the immune response and improve the condition of patients with gastrointestinal malignancies and other tumors [12, 15].

Table 6. Median survival time in months according to treatment

Treatment	MST
5-FU	9
5-FU + radiotherapy	13.5
Radiotherapy	7
No treatment	3.2

Table 7. The Survival of Patients with Stomach Cancer

Operation and adjuvant therapy		Operation alone
1 year	82%	40%
2 years	40%	20%
Median survival (months)	23	12.5

References

1. BROOKES, V. S., WATERHOUSE, J. A. H., POWELL, D. J.: Carcinoma of the stomach: a 10 year survey of results and of factors affecting prognosis. Brit. Med. J. *1*, 1577 (1965).
2. COMIS, R. L., CARTER, S. K.: A review of chemotherapy in gastric cancer. Cancer *34*, 1576 (1974).
3. CUTLER, S. J.: Trends in cancers of the digestive tract. Surgery *65*, 740 (1969).
4. FALKSON, G.: Fluorinated pyrimidines as potentiators of ionizing radiations in the treatment of stomach cancer in man. M.D. Thesis, University of Pretoria, 1964.
5. FALKSON, G., SANDISON, A. G., JACOBS, E. L., FICHARDT, T.: Combined telecobalt and 5-fluorouracil therapy in cancer of the stomach. S. African Med. J. *36*, 712–717 (1963).
6. FALKSON, G., VAN EDEN, E. B., FALKSON, H. C.: Fluorouracil, imidazole carboxamide dimethyl triazeno, vincristine and bischloroethyl nitrosourea in colon cancer. Cancer *33*, 1207–1209 (1974).
7. KENNEDY, B. J.: TNM classification for stomach cancer. Cancer *26*, 971 (1970).
8. McMEER, G. T., LAWRENCE, W., ASHLEY, M. P., PACK, G. T.: End results in the treatment of gastric cancer. Surgery *43*, 879 (1958).
9. MODAN, B., KALLNER, H.: Gastrointestinal cancer in Israel. Isr. J. Med. 7, 1475–1478 (1971).
10. MOERTEL, C. G., CHILDS, D. S., REITEMEIER, R. J., COLBY, M. Y., HOLBROK, M. A.: Combined 5FU and supervoltage radiation therapy of locally unresected gastrointestinal carcinoma. Lancet (1969) II, 865.
11. MOERTEL, C. G., MITTELMAN, J. H. et al: Sequential and combination chemotherapy of advanced gastric cancer. Cancer *38*, 678–682 (1976).
12. MOERTEL, C. G., RITTS, R. E., SCHUTT, A. J., Jr., HAHN, R. G.: Clinical studies of methanol extraction residue fraction of bacillus calmette-guerin as an immunostimulant in patients with advanced cancer. Cancer Research *35*, 3075–3083 (1975).
13. MOERTEL, C. G., SCHUTT, A. J., REITEMEIER, R. J., HAHN, R. G.: Therapy for gastrointestinal cancer with nitrosoureas alone and in drug combination. Cancer treatment reports *60*, 729 (1976).
14. RACHMANI, J. et al: Cancer of the stomach. Harefuah *86*, 445–450 (1974).
15. ROBINSON, E., BARTAL, A., COHEN, Y., HAASZ, R.: A preliminary report on the effect of MER on cancer patients. Brit. J. Cancer *32*, 1–4 (1975).
16. STEINITZ, R., COSTIN, C.: Cancer in Israel. Facts and figures 1960–1966. Ministry of Health (1970).
17. U.S.A. Department of Health, Education and Welfare: End results in cancer. NIH, Report No. 4, 47 (1972).

Initial Therapeutic Strategies Applied to Treatment of Common Epithelial Cancers of the Ovary (Stages IIB — III)

"Ovary" Working Party of the E.O.R.T.C

B. ZYLBERBERG, *Secretary* — and M. ABBES, M. BENOIT, D. CREPIN, M. DANA, G. DUTRANOY, R. GENSER, B. JAMAIN, B. KELLER, I. LANSAC, G. LE LORIER, A. LETESSIER, P. MORIN, L. PIANA, J. M. PIQUET, P. POUILLART, H. G. ROBERT, J. SALAT-BAROUX, H. SERMENT, J. H. SOUTOUL, and G. ZOGRAPHOS

Introduction

Ovarian carcinoma now appears as the most common fatal gynecologic malignancy. Surgery and radiotherapy are the most common modalities of therapy used in the treatment of these patients. Surgery provides the initial diagnosis, accurate staging, and initial therapy. Conventionally, radiotherapy has been used as an adjuvant to surgery in localized disease [6, 11]. Unfortunately, because of the poor initial symptomatology, approximately 60% of the patients are initially seen to be in an advanced stage of the disease [13]. In these conditions, the patients may be better helped by chemotherapy [14, 12, 4].

The aim of this communication is to present the first results obtained by the "Ovary" Working Party of the E.O.R.T.C. Three groups of patients were treated respectively, by surgery alone, surgery plus radiotherapy, and surgery plus chemotherapy.

Patients and Method

One hundred and twenty-eight patients with ovarian carcinoma were not selected specifically for three modalities of treatment. It is not a randomized study.

1. 35 patients were treated with extensive surgery alone
   (median age: 53 years, 27–71)
2. 42 patients were treated with extensive surgery and radiotherapy
   (median age: 51 years, 22–70)
3. 51 patients were treated with extensive surgery and chemotherapy
   (median age: 52 years, 23–72 years)

Only the patients with stage IIb and III entered into this therapeutic type II trial. The repartition of patients according to the anatomical stage in these three groups of treatment is presented in Table 1.

Radiotherapy

Two treatment techniques were routinely employed postoperatively in these 42 patients. More often the open field technique was used. It involves radiation through two large fixed

Table 1. Presentation of Patients According to Anatomical Intra-abdominal Extension

	Number of patients	Stage IIb	Stage III
Surgery alone (Group I)	35	4	31[a]
Surgery + radiotherapy (Group II)	42	9	33[b]
Surgery + chemotherapy	51	12	39[c]
	128	25	103

All the patients included in this study are considered as stage IIb and stage III at time of surgery. But seven[a] patients out of 35 (Group 1), six[b] patients out of 42, and 12[c] out of 51 presented an extra-abdominal metastasis in the 3 months after initial surgery.

parts anterior and posterior. Radiation was usually delivered at a rate of 1000 rad per week, and the total dose was of 5500 rad for the lower abdomen and 4000 rad to the para-aortic region. For some other patients [13], the so-called "moving strip" technique was used [6].

Chemotherapy

Fifty-one patients were treated postoperatively with a combination chemotherapy. We used a combination of methotrexate (MTX) (40 mg/m2)—vincaleucoblastine (7 mg/m2)—cyclophosphamide (CPM) (300 mg/m2). Each course of treatment was repeated every 8–15 days according to the hematologic state of the patient.

Tolerance

Four patients out of 42 who were submitted to postoperative radiation therapy presented an intestinal occlusion 2–7 weeks after completion of treatment. Three of them were certainly due to radiotherapy as became clear in the surgical exploration. Two cases of pure necrosis of the small intestine, one case of stenotic sclerosis, and one case of occlusion with both stenotic sclerosis and tumor infiltration were observed. One patient died and another patient required ileostomy and then survived 14 months.

As far as chemotherapy is concerned, the general tolerance was good. The hematologic toxicity was mild and no infection complication of hypoplasia was observed. The psychological tolerance of this long course of chemotherapy was good and no more than 30% of the patients presented a complete, but transitory alopecia.

Results

This report is limited to the study of the actuarial survival curves of each of these patients groups. The actuarial survival curve of the first group of patients treated by surgery alone is

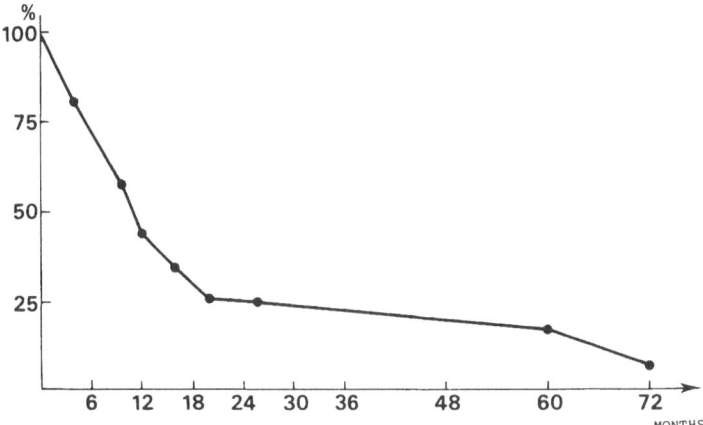

Fig. 1. Ovarian carcinoma. N = 35
Spontaneous course (after surgery alone)
St. IIb–III

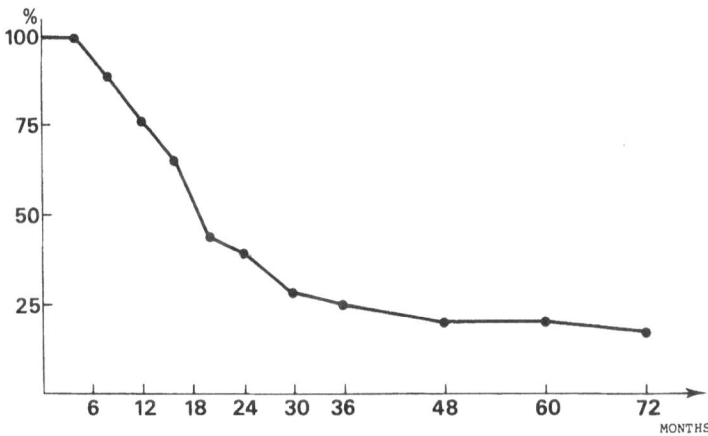

Fig. 2. Ovarian carcinoma. N = 42
Survival curve after surgery + radiotherapy
St. IIb–III

presented in Fig. 1. The median survival time is 11.4 months, and 17% of the patients are still alive and apparently free of disease at the 5th year.

The actuarial survival curve of the second group of patients is presented in Fig. 2. The median survival time is about 19 months, and 20% of the patients are alive after 5 years.

For the patients in the third group of treatment, the actuarial survival curve shows (Fig. 3) that the median survival time was 29 months and that 33% of the patients are still alive after 5 years.

The efficiency of radiotherapy according to complete and incomplete tumor removal is presented in Fig. 4. It shows only a slight difference in survival between these groups. Taking into account only patients with well-documented stage IIb or III disease (eliminating

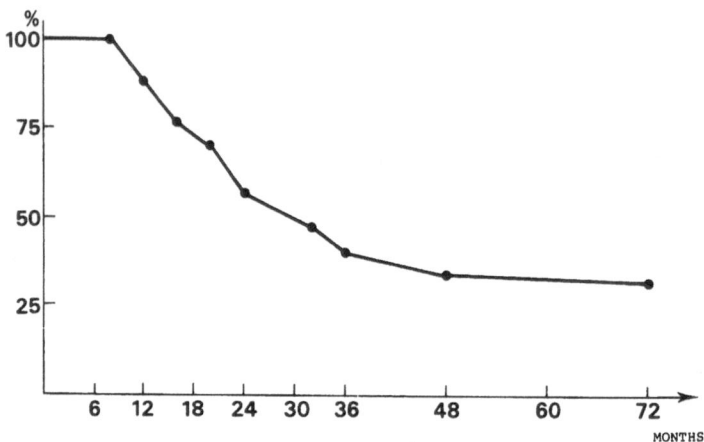

Fig. 3. Ovarian carcinoma. N = 51
Survival curve. Surgery + chemotherapy
St. IIb–III

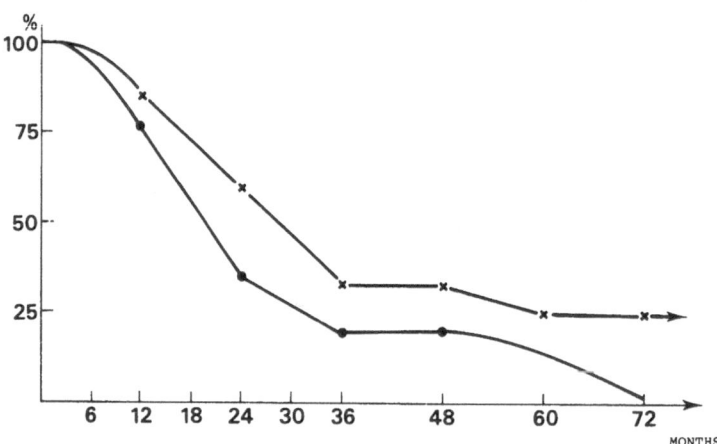

Fig. 4. Ovarian carcinoma.
Survival curves:
after surgery + radiotherapy: N = 14
St. IIb–III ×————×
after incomplete surgery
N = 28
St. IIb–III ●————●

patients with early dissemination), the survival curve according the anatomical stage shows
no difference between both groups identically treated by radiotherapy (Fig. 5). In the same
conditions, the hope of survival of patients submitted to chemotherapy appears to be quite
different in group IIb as compared to group III (Fig. 6).
The role of complete surgery on the evolution of patients secondarily submitted to

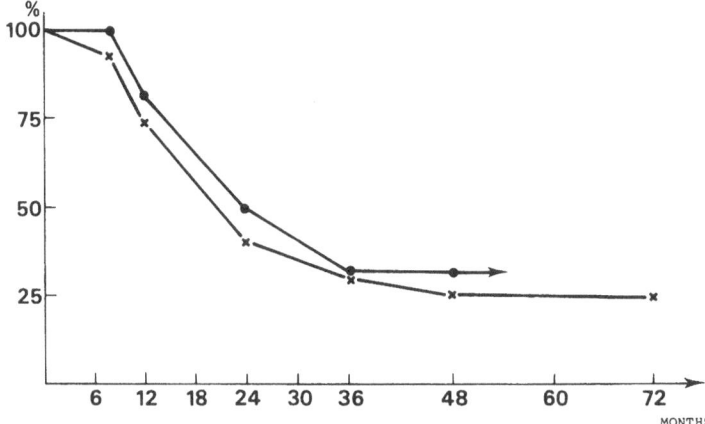

Fig. 5. Ovarian carcinoma. Survival curves
St. IIb ●————●
St. III ×————×

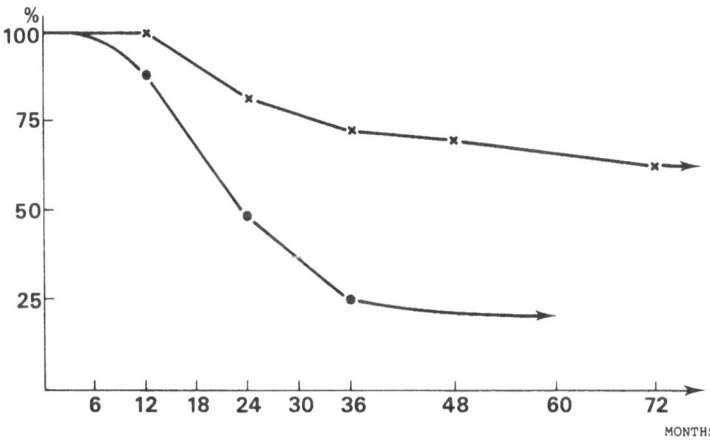

Fig. 6. Ovarian carcinoma. Survival curves after chemotherapy
St. IIb ×————×
St. III ●————●

chemotherapy is presented in Fig. 7. The median survival time of patients, after complete excision of the lesions, is 6 years, and it is only 22 months following incomplete surgical resection.

The administration of chemotherapy in a group of 14 patients initially submitted to radiotherapy, but who relapsed within the first 12 months, gives poor results and seems ineffective in changing the poor prognosis of these patients (Fig. 8).

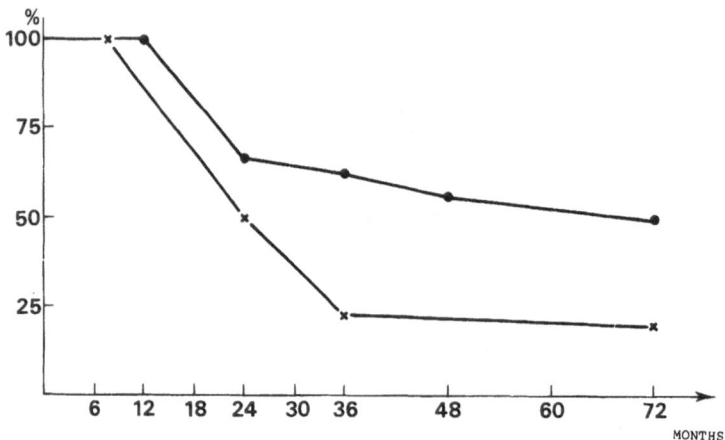

Fig. 7. Ovarian carcinoma. Survival curves
N = 25
after complete surgery ●————●
after incomplete surgery ×————×

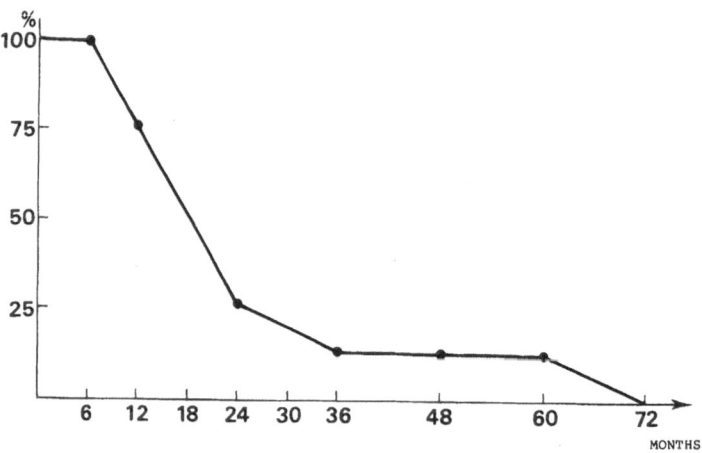

Fig. 8. Ovarian carcinoma. Survival curve of patients in relapse treated with surgery + radiotherapy
and followed with chemotherapy after relapse
N = 21

Discussion

The results presented concern 128 patients with ovarian adenocarcinoma. All the patients of
this trial were initially treated by surgery which provides an accurate staging and initial
therapy. All the patients who entered this nonrandomized study were classified into
stage IIb (25) and stage III (103).

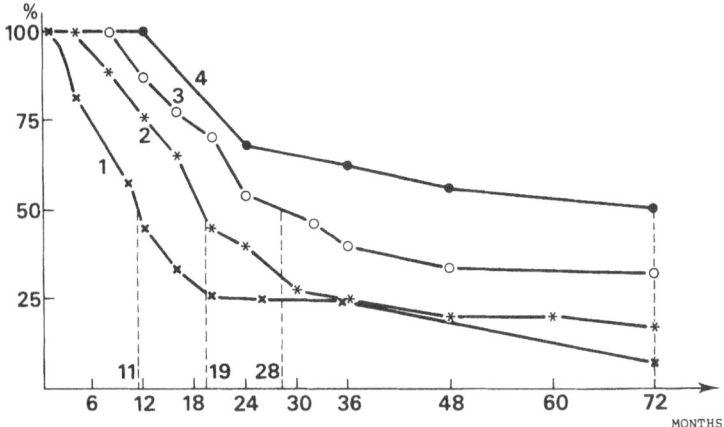

Fig. 9. Ovarian carcinoma: spontaneous course
surgery + radiotherapy   ×————×
surgery + chemotherapy   *————*
complete surgery + chemotherapy   ○————○
                                              ●————●

The comparison of survival rates in the three groups is interesting.

Radiotherapy increases the mean survival time of patients initially treated with surgery from 11 to 19 months; after 5 years, 20% of these patients and only 12% in the group treated by surgery alone survived. Chemotherapy gives better results: the median survival time is 28 months and 30% of the patients are still alive after 5 years. Surprisingly, we found only a slight difference in survival in the radiotherapy group according to the degree of surgical resection. Using the same stratification, the difference appears more evident in the chemotherapy group.

The results we obtained for stage III patients treated with radiation are comparable to those obtained in other studies previously reported [6, 8, 5], and in these cases, chemotherapy for relapse was often poorly tolerated and rarely efficient, probably due to prolonged suppression of bone marrow activity induced by both chemotherapy and previous radiation [6].

In this study with stages IIb and III, cases treated by chemotherapy after surgery seem to have an improved survival rate. In a previous report by SMITH et al. [12], 50% of the stage III patients treated with melphalan after surgery are still alive after 5 years and, in the randomized control group treated by radiation, only 35% of patients are still alive after 5 years. The same difference is found in our study.

It seems to be possible to draw the following conclusions:

1. The preferential use of chemotherapy as complementary treatment of patients with stage III carcinoma of the ovary
2. Radiotherapy and chemotherapy have been frequently combined in the management of patients with advanced disease, but for the moment no advantage in this combination has been clearly demonstrated [13, 1, 10, 2, 9]

The results of this nonrandomized study now suggest to us the possibility of a systematic controlled trial, according to the anatomical stage of the extension of the disease at the time of commencing treatment.

Conclusion

In this nonrandomized study, three groups of patients with stages IIb and III ovarian carcinoma were treated. The results showed that chemotherapy as adjuvant treatment seems able to increase the median survival time of the group of patients and the percentage of patients alive at the 5th year. If no definitive conclusion can be given from these trials, they provide nevertheless, the basis for a new controlled trial with the aim of comparing the respective indications of radiotherapy and chemotherapy according to the anatomical stage of the disease.

References

1. BAGLEY, C. M., YOUNG, R. C., CANELLOS, G. P., DE VITA, V. T.: Treatment of ovarian carcinoma. Possibilities for progress. New Engl. J. Med. *287*, 856–862 (1972).
2. DECKER, D. G., MUSSEY, E., MALKASIAN, G. D.: Adjuvant therapy for advanced ovarian malignancy. Am. J. Obstect. Gynec. *97*, 171–180 (1967).
3. DELCLOS, L., BRAUN, E. J., HERRERA, P.: Whole abdominal irradiation by cobalt-GO moving strip technique. Radiology *81*, 632–641 (1963).
4. DELCLOS, L., SMITH, J. P.: Tumors of the ovary. In: Textbook of Radiotherapy. Philadelphia: Lea and Fibiger, 1973, pp. 690–702.
5. FAZEKAS, J. P., MAIER, J. G.: Irradiation of ovarian carcinoma. A prospective comparison of the open field and moving strip techniques. Am. J. Roengen. Radium Ther. Nucl. Med. *120*, 118–123 (1974).
6. FUKS, Z.: Extremal radiotherapy of ovarian cancer: standard approaches and new frontiers. Seminars in Oncology *2*, 253–266 (1975).
7. GREENSPAN, E. M.: Thiotepa and methotrexate chemotherapy of advanced ovarian carcinoma. J. Mt. Sinai Hosp. New York *35*, 52–67 (1968).
8. HINTZ, B. L., FUKS, Z., RICHARD, L., KEMPSON, R. L., ELTRINGHAM, J. R., ZALOUDEDK, C., WILLIAMSON, T. J., BAGSHAW, M. A.: Results of post operative megavoltage radiotherapy of malignant surface epithelial tumors of the ovary. Radiology *114*, 695–700 (1975).
9. JOHNSON, C. E., DECKER, D. G., VAN HERIK, M.: Advanced ovarian cancer. Therapy with radiation and cyclophosphamide in a random series. Am. J. Roengen. Radium Ther. Nucl. Med. *114*, 136–141 (1972).
10. KOTTMEIER, K. L.: Treatment of ovarian carcinomas with thiotepa. Clin. Obstet. Gynecol. *11*, 428–438 (1968).
11. PEREZ, C. A., BRADFIELD, J. S.: Radiation therapy in the treatment of carcinoma of the ovary. Cancer *29*, 1027–1037 (1972).
12. SMITH, J. P., RUTLEDGE, F. N., DECLOS, L.: Results of chemotherapy as an adjuvant to surgery in patients with localized ovarian cancer. Seminars in Oncology *2*, 277–280 (1975).
13. YOUNG, R. C.: Chemotherapy of ovarian cancer. Post and present. Seminars in Oncology *2*, 267–276 (1975).
14. YOUNG, R. C., HUBBARD, J. P., DE VITA, V. T.: The chemotherapy of ovarian carcinoma. Cancer Treatment Review *1*, 99–110 (1974).

Strategy and Tactics in Prostatic Cancer

P. H. Smith*

Introduction

Strategy is defined as the art of planning and directing larger (military) movements and operations of campaigns or wars; tactics is the art of deploying and manoeuvring such forces as are available.

In considering the necessity for a strategy in prostatic cancer, we need to know whether current treatment is adequate and whether all patients are similar. It is apparent that neither radical surgical excision nor high energy radiation will adequately treat all patients, a situation which is becoming increasingly clear in virtually all forms of cancer. Hormone therapy is known to be hazardous and is not always successful. In addition, patients are dissimilar in that a lesion which may progress remorselessly in a younger patient often has a relatively benign course in an elderly man. It is probable that many elderly patients need no treatment other than relief of their obstruction.

Figures from the Registrar General's Office for England and Wales [1] show that carcinoma of the prostate is the commonest urological cancer in the male forming 6% of all tumours. Almost three-quarters of the patients are over 70 years of age before the condition is diagnosed, whilst the condition is virtually unknown under the age of 50. At the time of presentation, 80% of the patients have disease which has spread beyond the prostatic capsule, the disease being disseminated in 40% [2].

Our knowledge of the natural history of the disease is limited, but it is known that latent carcinoma of the prostate is found at post mortem in 5–10% of males at 50–59 years, 10–20% at 60–69 years and 20–30% over the age of 70 [3] suggesting that the condition may remain clinically silent for many years and that a chance diagnosis at the time of prostatectomy for an apparently benign hypertrophy should not be an indication for active treatment. Further evidence of the long natural history comes from Byar and Mostofi [4] who considered carcinoma of the prostate in patients under 50 years of age and showed a longer survival in patients who were asymptomatic at the time of diagnosis than in those who had symptoms. Also, the Veterans Administration Cooperative Urological Research Group (VACURG) have shown that only 40% of patients with clinical stage III cancer progress to stage IV disease without treatment after 3 years [5]. These facts suggest the desirability, in elderly patients at least, of treatment only if symptoms require it or if the disease is progressing.

In considering treatment, it is important to acknowledge the work carried out by the VACURG during the last 15 years, not only in establishing the hazards of oestrogen therapy and that two-thirds of patients die from intercurrent disease, but also in establishing that radical prostatectomy for stage I prostatic cancer is not superior to conservative or placebo therapy [6]. The place of radiotherapy for tumours clinically confined to the true pelvis remains to be evaluated.

As yet there have been no satisfactory prospective randomised studies between stilboestrol and the agents such as estracyt, anti-androgens and progestogens, whilst many cytotoxic agents await evaluation and immunotherapy has hardly been considered, let alone explored.

---

* Chairman–EORTC Urological Group.

Until such time as more information is available, it will not be possible to progress to trials of the combination of radiotherapy, hormone therapy and chemotherapy which offer the greatest hope. It is, however, quite clear that, as in other forms of cancer, the trend is moving away from radical surgical excision.

Strategy

Having briefly established the current position, it is possible to develop a strategic plan for the next 2–3 years. This must consider not only matters of strictly medical importance but also take account of the differences in language and in medical practice in a community historically as diverse as Western Europe.

The E.O.R.T.C. Urological Group has grown rapidly in the last 3 years. The group includes surgeons, cancer chemotherapists, statisticians, radiotherapists, pathologists, immunologists and scientists keen to develop biochemical markers and to assess the importance of receptors, trace elements and hormonal profiles.

We now have active members in Belgium, Denmark, France, Holland, Italy, Spain, Switzerland and the United Kingdom. All members *must* work as a team, but they can do so effectively only if the group contains enough clinical members to guarantee access to a large number of patients. To overcome this problem we are appointing national coordinators to assist in clinical and scientific recruitment, in translation and the solution of local problems as they arise.

Tactics

At the tactical level, it is important to recognise the different contributions which can be made by the specialist cancer centre in assessing new drugs and encouraging basic research and by the larger cooperative group whose task it must be to carry out prospective trials; each is essential to the other. We have decided to involve ourselves in all urological malignant disease and to promote contact and exchange of information with other groups in all countries.

In prostatic cancer, the urgent clinical tasks are to evaluate the newer hormonal agents by controlled prospective trial, to evaluate cytotoxic agents alone and in combination, and to establish the value of radiotherapy in localised prostatic cancer. On the scientific side, it is necessary to gain further information on the importance of prostatic receptors and trace elements, to develop reliable biochemical markers, and to undertaken immunological studies.

We do not have the resources to attempt to answer all these questions simultaneously but have taken certain tactical decisions which represent our immediate aims. These include:

1. Randomized prospective cooperative trials in new patients with advanced prostatic cancer to evaluate stilboestrol 1 mg t.d.s. against estracyt in one trial and cyproterone acetate in another
2. A pilot study to evaluate procarbazine in patients who have failed to respond or who no longer respond to treatment with stilboestrol
3. The assessment by pilot study of new agents of potential value
4. The development of biochemical markers of predictive value in association with Professor Cooper in Leeds and Dr. Milford-Ward in Sheffield

5. Studies on receptors in prostatic tissue in association with Dr. Hawkins of the Institut Jules Bordet in Brussels and studies of trace metals in association with Professor Stitch of the Department of Steroid Biochemistry in Leeds

We also believe most strongly in the dissemination of information, the encouragement of cooperation and, if possible, the prevention of reduplication. We are hoping to achieve this aim by informal contact with other groups and by meetings such as the International Conference on Prostatic Cancer held in Leeds from 7–9 July 1976.

References

1. Studies on Medical and Population Subject. No. 29. Cancer Mortality, England and Wales, 1911–70. HMSO, 50 (1975).
2. VACURG: Treatment and survival of patients with cancer of the prostate. Surg. Gynae. & Obstet. *124*, 1011–17 (1967)
3. WYNDER, E. L., MABUCHI, K., WHITMORE, W. F., Jr.: Epidemiology of cancer of the prostate. Cancer *28*, 344–360 (1971).
4. BYAR, D. P., MOSTOFI, F. K.: Cancer of the prostate in men less than 50 years old: an analysis of 51 cases. J. Urol. *102*, 726–733 (1969).
5. BYAR, D. P.: Results of clinical trials of estrogen treatment for cancer of the prostate. Proceedings 16th Congress of the International Society of Urology. *2*, 730–739 (1973).
6. BYAR, D. P., VACURG: Survival of patients with incidentally found microscopic cancer of the prostate: results of a clinical trial of conservative treatment. J. Urol. *108*, 908–913 (1972).

Treatment of Trophoblastic Tumours

K. D. Bagshawe

General Historical Background

It is useful to consider the treatment of trophoblastic tumours against the background of the major studies of their pathology by Park and Lees [19], Park [20], and Ober et al. [18]. The therapeutic state before methotrexate (MTX) appeared was indicated in the paper by Brewer et al. [8] which recorded a 20% 5-year survival rate with surgery, radiotherapy and, in some cases, nitrogen mustard.

The dramatic responses to MTX which followed the report of Li et al. [15] took several years to fall into perspective. The fact that advanced disease often showed resistance led to patients being treated earlier and without hysterectomy and, therefore, in many instances, without morphological identification of the type of lesion. Lesions with high potential to kill and lesions with no lethal potential became grouped together as "malignant trophoblastic disease". The criteria for inclusion of cases under this heading were arbitrary and, therefore, different in different parts of the world. To argue that it does not matter whether a lesion is an invasive mole or choriocarcinoma because moles can metastasize or transform to choriocarcinoma misses the point.

What matters is that in order to be able to improve therapy it is necessary to be able to compare results between different centres using different drug regimens. This is an area to be returned to later.

Following recognition that resistance to MTX was frequent [14], a combination of drugs, 6-mercaptopurine (6-MP) with MTX, was used in an attempt to inhibit or defer resistance [1]. The value of 6-MP as a single agent has been studied only on a limited scale in our series, but it was found to be almost as effective as MTX in the report of Sung et al. [25]. Vinblastine (VBL) was reported to have a useful effect on a small series of MTX-resistant cases [13], but there have been few subsequent references to it as a useful agent. In 1962, however, Ross et al. [22] reported that actinomycin D (ACT-D) achieved remissions in 6/13 MTX-resistant cases. Since then, MTX and ACT-D have remained the most effective agents despite the introduction of many new drugs. The addition of an alkylating agent, chlorambucil, to this combination for the treatment of testicular teratomas [16] has been widely transferred to the field of gestational choriocarcinoma and, undergoing a process of fossilization, has become known as 'triple therapy'. With these agents, survival rates in the range 50–90% have been obtained in various centres.

I propose to discuss four of the important problems which have emerged. One is the question of prophylactic therapy for hydatidiform mole. A second is whether drug toxicity can be reduced, coupled with the need for patient stratification. Another is that of comparability of series and the quantification of prognostic factors. A fourth is the question of drug resistance and the associated problem of brain metastases.

Management of the Patient after Hydatidiform Mole

If the risk of malignant sequelae after hydatidiform mole could be eliminated, chorio-carcinoma as a clinical problem would be drastically reduced. Unfortunately, it seems clear that the amount of treatment with MTX or ACT-D which most clinicians feel reasonable to give to all mole patients is inadequate to ensure that none get clinical choriocarcinoma. Histopathological examination of hydatidiform mole provides no reliable guide to malignant sequelae [9]. A reduction in malignancy rate from 8.7 to 4.5% was reported with prophylactic chemotherapy from Singapore [21].

Each year we admit, mostly from abroad, several patients who have failed on prophylactic therapy and who have become more or less resistant to subsequent therapy. In some centres, deaths from prophylactic therapy have occurred but unfortunately these do not get reported. In any case, the policy of giving powerful mutagenic agents to nine or more women for every one who needs them therapeutically is, at best, second best, and those who have used it frequently express reservations [11].

The alternative is close follow-up by human chorionic gouadotrophik (HCG) radio-immunoassay although this is not yet possible in all countries. In the U.K., a national follow-up scheme has been established and works well. The overall rate of admission for chemotherapy is under 10% of registered cases [5]. The general pattern of HCG values following evacuation of hydatidiform mole is quite different from that following normal term delivery or nonmole abortion. Two months postevacuation, almost a half of the patients are still secreting HCG, yet, in all but 10% or less of the total number of patients, the lesion dies out spontaneously. Clearly, if one selects for chemotherapy all those patients who have detectable HCG secretion 2 months postevacuation, one would expect an 80% or better survival rate even if the treatment were totally ineffective. It would seem more rational to select for chemotherapy on the basis of other criteria [5]. Using these criteria, a study of 611 patients followed up at Charing Cross between 1972 and 1974 [24] showed that the risk of requiring treatment was twice as great where the mole was removed by hysterectomy, hysterotomy, oxytocin or prostaglandins compared with those removed by vacuum or dilatation and curettage. This difference may, however, be related to gestational age. The risk of requiring treatment in those taking oral contraceptives whilst HCG was still detectable was almost doubled compared with those not taking oral contraceptives at that time (17.6% compared with 9.3%).

Reduction of Drug Toxicity and Case Stratification

The question of reduction of drug toxicity arose from the fact that even with a cautious follow-up scheme for patients after hydatidiform mole, up to 10% and in some series more than 20% have been given chemotherapy compared with 2–5% known to get chorio-carcinoma. So the question arose whether patients whose tumours posed a relatively small threat to life could be treated successfully without the full rigours of cytotoxic chemotherapy. We found in 1962 that giving MTX by arterial infusion with its antagonist folinic acid by intramuscular route, toxicity could be virtually avoided [2, 17] without detectable loss of effectiveness compared with MTX alone. Further details are given later.

At the other extreme, one saw patients with widespread and massive metastases. This contrast led ultimately to the stratification of cases according to an assessment of risk so that low risk patients receive nontoxic therapy whereas those with a high risk of resistance are treated vigorously [3, 12]. The use of irradiation for CNS metastases reported by Brace [7] was a further step in the direction of attempting to control advanced disease, and the use of plasma/spinal fluid HCG ratios to detect and monitor CNS metastases was also introduced [23].

Prognostic Factors

A broad assessment of risk on the basis of clinical impression only is of limited value. We are left, moreover, with the question of whether the results obtained in centre A are superior to those obtained in centre B because they are treating less advanced disease or because their therapeutic regimen are superior. Within the same centre there is the same problem. Is regimen X better than regimen Y? Clinical trials, other than on a massive scale, are liable to be invalidated by the great variability between different trophoblastic tumours. It is, therefore, necessary to define as precisely as possible those factors which affect prognosis and attach to them the appropriate weight.

Taking our series at Charing Cross up to the end of 1973, there were 317 patients on whom such an analysis could be based [6]. Each definable factor was analysed for its effect on survival. The factors which were defined as influencing prognosis were 1) patient's age, 2) parity, 3) the type of antecedent pregnancy, 4) the interval lapsing between the end of the antecedent pregnancy and the start of chemotherapy, 5) the HCG values in plasma or urine, 6) the ABO group of the patient and her husband [4], 7) the presence and number of metastases, 8) the site of metastases, 9) the size of tumour masses, 10) the extent of mononuclear cell infiltration in the tumour [10], 11) the immunological status of the patient before chemotherapy was given and 12) whether or not the patient had received chemotherapy before referral to us.

On the basis of the outcome of treatment, a provisional scoring system has been devised based on each of these factors as shown on Table 1. The scores obtained for each factor are added together. In broad terms the lower the score the better the prognosis, the higher the score the greater the risk of a fatal outcome. Low risk is associated with scores < 55, medium risk with scores of 55–95 and high risk > 95.

Table 1. Provisional scores given to prognostic factors defined in analysis of 317 cases [6]

	0	10	20	40
Age (years)	< 39	> 39		
Parity	1, 2, > 4	3 or 4		
Antecedent pregnancy	Mole	Abortion	Term	
Interval (AP-chemotherapy) in months	< 4	4–7	7–12	> 12
HCG (plasma mIU/ml or urine IU/day)	10^3–10^4	$< 10^3$	10^4–10^5	$> 10^5$
ABO ♀ × ♂	A × A × B × AB	O × O A × O	B × AB ×	
No. of metastases	Nil	1–4	4–8	> 8
Site of metastases	Not detected Lungs Vagina	Spleen Kidney	GI tract Liver	Brain
Largest tumour mass	< 3 cm	3–5	> 5 cm	
Lymphocytic infiltration	Marked	Moderate, unknown	Slight	
Immune status	Reactive		Unreactive	
Previous chemotherapy	Nil		Yes	

Analaysis of Charing Cross Treatment Series

I now propose to outline the development of treatment in our series in London and to analyse the series.

Between 1958 and the end of 1975, 430 patients were admitted for treatment of trophoblastic tumours. Five patients proved to have no evidence of active disease, 13 were in extremis and died within 4 days before effective treatment could be given. In addition, eight patients had received extensive treatment before referral, or returned abroad before treatment was completed, leaving a total of 404 patients for evaluation.

Of these 404 patients, 64 are known to have died. All the remainder were known to be alive and disease-free for at least 2 years after completing therapy, and only 16 have failed to maintain our minimum annual follow-up routine. A total of 118 patients underwent hysterectomy, 58 before chemotherapy, 38 during chemotherapy and 22 afterwards. On admission, 273 had metastases and 63 of the deaths were in this group. The causes of death are summarized in Table 2.

Table 2

Causes of Death: 64 cases	
Pulmonary embolism	2
Serum hepatitis (both in remission)	2
Infection and drug toxicity	6
Refused retreatment on relapse	4
Initial extent of disease	5
Drug resistance	45

Drug resistance has remained the major cause of failure throughout the period of study. The dangers of severe hepatitis have been somewhat reduced by the detection of Australia antigen. Improved awareness and the mole follow-up scheme has tended to reduce the number of patients being referred with terminal choriocarcinoma. The main thrust of research has, therefore, been towards limiting the risk of drug resistance and at the same time reducing the morbidity and mortality from drug toxicity.

Following the initial report of Li et al. [15], evidence accummulated that drug resistance developed in a high proportion of patients treated with MTX alone. In the London series, only five patients received MTX alone as their initial therapy and three of these died, two from drug resistance. A combination of MTX and 6-MP was used throughout the early years of this study, and a 73% sustained remission rate (Table 3) with this combination was

Table 3

Initial therapy	No. treated	% Surviving
Nonstandard	4	75.0
MTX	5	43.4
MTX + 6-MP ± FA	67	73.2
MTX/FA, ACT-D, CPM/VCR	52	71.2
(6-AZ)MTX + FA	276	90.2

significantly better than the 40–50% rate obtained with MTX alone. Toxic deaths, however, occurred with this combination and alopecia and mucositis were consistent. Moreover, by the early 1960's, patients with nonmetastatic disease and with invasive mole were being referred for chemotherapy so as to preserve reproductive function as well as life. The need for less toxic therapy led first to the addition of folinic acid to the MTX/6-MP regimen [2] and later to the omission of the 6-MP [3].

With this development, MTX was given by continuous arterial infusion for a period of 7 days and folinic acid (FA) given by the intramuscular route every 12 hours with no apparent loss of therapeutic effectiveness but without attendant alopecia and minimal mucositis and myelosuppression.

The only common persisting symptom was pleuritic and sometimes peritoneal pain. This infusion treatment proved effective in cases with pulmonary metastases as well as those without, so that intravenous infusion was substituted and later, the intramuscular regimen was designed to mimic the pharmacokinetic conditions of the intravascular method as closely as possible yet provide for easier administration. The intravascular and intramuscular MTX/FA regimen have proved comparable and effective in a large group of patients. The intramuscular regimen is shown in Table 4.

Table 4

Low Risk	
MTX	1.0 mg/kg q. 48 h × 4 i.m.
FA	6.0 mg i.m. or p.o. 30 h after each MTX

Courses are repeated after 6 days drug-free interval.

Following evidence for the action of 6-azauridine (AZ) on normal murine trophoblast, we found that 6-AZ had a profound though often transient effect on trophoblastic tumours. This was combined with the MTX regimen and apparently increased its effectiveness without significant increase in toxicity in the majority of patients. A few patients, however, went into reversible coma as a result of taking 6-AZ and failing to maintain a high urine output, and for this reason we have now abandoned this regimen. Hydroxyurea also has a similar modest effect on malignant trophoblast and this is now used in combination with MTX/FA for certain patients.

With the (6-AZ)MTX/FA regimen, 188 patients have achieved sustained remissions without any additional drugs. A total of 78 patients failed to go into remission, or relapsed, or it was feared that they would relapse and for these reasons they received treatment with additional agents. Of these, 19 died from resistance to all agents and the remaining 61 achieved remission, i.e. 257 of 276 cases surviving overall.

As the series progressed, so it became possible to analyse it retrospectively and define the prognostic factors relating to the likelihood of developing drug resistance. The question which arose then was whether it was better to start all patients on the 'nontoxic' MTX/FA regimen and introduce additional agents if and when resistance developed, or, alternatively, to define risk categories at the outset and use multiple drug therapy from the outset in those cases where the risk of drug resistance could already be defined as high.

In the early 1970's, the cyclical regimen (Table 5) was introduced for the higher risk patients and in the last 2 years we have further divided this category into 'medium' and 'high' risk according to their prognostic scores.

Table 5. Medium risk: cyclical regimen

Course 1.	ACT-D	10 µg/kg/d	days 5–7 i.v.
Course 2.	VCR	20 µg/kg i.v.	days 1, 3 (5)
	CPM	10 mg/kg i.v.	days 1, 3 (5)
Course 3.	HU	0.5 G 12 hourly × 4	days 1, 2
	MTX	1.0 mg/kg i.m.	days 3, 5, 7, 9
	FA	6 mg i.m.	days 4, 6, 8, 10
	6-MP	1 mg/kg × 3 daily p.o.	days 3–9

A drug-free rest period of 7–9 days intervenes between courses. HU = hydroxyurea.

Table 6. Resistant or high risk cases (CHAMOMA)

HU	500 mg q. 12 h × 4	p.o.	days 1,2
VCR	1.0 mg/m²	i.v.	day 3
MTX	100 mg/m²	i.v.	day 3
+	200 mg/m² 12 h infusion		day 3
FA	12 mg/m² i.m. q. 12 h × 4 starting 12 h post-MTX		
ACT-D	10 µg/kg	i.v.	days 5, 6, 7
CPM	600 mg/m²	i.v.	day 5
ADR	30 mg/m²	i.v. ⎫	
Melphalan	6 mg/m²	i.v. ⎬ day 10	

An interval of 9–14 days is necessary between successive courses

Medium risk patients are treated with the cyclical regimen and high risk patients with a multidrug combination ('CHAMOMA'), as shown in Table 6, which had proved effective in some patients with stage III and IV trophoblastic teratomas. This regimen has proved to be more effective and less toxic in gestational choriocarcinoma than a variety of multidrug regimens used earlier, and some patients with scores > 180 have achieved sustained remission.

Patients in the low risk category who fail to respond to MTX/FA proceed to the cyclical regimen. Patients in the middle risk category who fail to respond to the cyclical regimen proceed to the CHAMOMA regimen.

As indicated earlier cerebral metastases have remained a major hazard. A half of those with cerebral metastases at the start of chemotherapy have responded and achieved sustained remission. In addition to systemic chemotherapy, they received intrathecal MTX 10–15 mg once or twice with each course of systemic chemotherapy. The CHAMOMA regimen incorporates a high dose of MTX to help achieve CNS penetration. Some also received total skull radiation (4000–4500 rad), but the evidence is not adequate to indicate whether this is advantageous. No patient developing intracranial metastases during chemotherapy has survived despite full use of all forms of therapy. In one case, full treatment was directed at the central nervous system following a single abnormal plasma/spinal fluid ratio. The patient went into remission but relapsed with an intracranial recurrence which proved refractory. The use of prophylactic intrathecal therapy or high dose systemic MTX in cases at high risk of developing intracranial metastases is now being investigated.

The duration of chemotherapy is a vitally important issue. To discontinue treatment as soon as pregnancy tests, or even when radioimmunoassays for HCG, become negative, is to invite early relapse. Slow responding tumours need more prolonged treatment after HCG has become undetectable than rapidly responding tumours. From two to eight courses of treatment may be required largely depending on the various prognostic factors outlined above.

Although surgery has only an adjuvant role in trophoblastic tumours, it is an important one. For a demonstrably small uterine lesion in a multiparous woman without evident metastases, hysterectomy at the outset is acceptable and is occasionally curative, but close follow-up by HCG radioimmunassay (RIA) is essential. For large lesions, or in the presence of metastases, it is better deferred until remission has been achieved. Hysterectomy is advisable without delay where resistance to chemotherapy is developing and where residual disease is apparently confined to the uterus. Thoractomy for single resistant metastases is occasionally useful. Craniotomy is best avoided except possibly to remove extensive blood clots and, in contrast to the general results of chemotherapy, is liable to produce residual neurological deficits.

References

1. BAGSHAWE, K. D., MACDONALD, J. M.: Treatment of choriocarcinoma with a combination of cytotoxic drugs. Brit. Med. J. II, 426–431 (1960).
2. BAGSHAWE, K. D., WILDE, C. E.: Infusion therapy for pelvic trophoblastic tumours. J. Obstet. Gynec. Brit. Cwlth. 71, 565–570 (1964).
3. BAGSHAWE, K. D.: Choriocarcinoma. The clinical biology of the trophoblast and its tumours. London: Edward Arnold, 1968.
4. BAGSHAWE, K. D., RAWLINS, G. A., PYKE, M. C., LAWLER, S. D.: ABO blood groups in trophoblastic neoplasia. Lancet (1971) I, 553–555.
5. BAGSHAWE, K. D., WILSON, H., DUBLON, P., SMITH, A., BALDWIN, M., KARDANA, A.: Follow up after hydatidiform mole: studies using radioimmunoassay. J. Obstet. Gynec. Brit. Cwlth. 80, 461–468 (1973).
6. BAGSHAWE, K. D.: Risk and prognostic factors in trophoblastic neoplasia. Cancer 38, 1373–1385 (1976).
7. BRACE, K. E.: The role of irradiation in the treatment of metastatic trophoblastic disease. Radiology 91, 540–544 (1968).
8. BREWER, J. I., SMITH, R. T., PRATT, G. B.: Choriocarcinoma. Absolute 5 year survival rates of 122 patients treated by hysterectomy. Amer. J. Obstet. Gynec. 85, 841–843 (1963).
9. ELSTON, C. W., BAGSHAWE, K. D.: The value of histological grading in the management of hydatidiform mole. J. Obstet. Gynec. Brit. Cwlth. 79, 717–724 (1972).
10. ELSTON, C. W., BAGSHAWE, K. D.: Cellular reaction in trophoblastic tumours. Brit. J. Cancer 28, 245–256 (1973).
11. GOLDSTEIN, D. P.: Prevention of gestational trophoblastic disease by use of actinomycin D in molar pregnancies. Obstet. Gynec. 43, 475–479 (1974).
12. HAMMOND, C. B., BORCHERT, L. G., TYREY, L., CREASMAN, W. T., PARKER, R. T.: Treatment of metastatic trophoblastic disease: good and poor prognosis. Am. J. Obstet. Gynec. 115, 451–457 (1973).
13. HERTZ, R., LIPSETT, M. B., MOY, R. H.: Effect of Vincaleukoblastine on metastatic chorio-carcinoma and related trophoblastic tumours in women. Cancer Res. 20, 1050–1053 (1960).
14. HERTZ, R., LEWIS, J., LIPSETT, M. B.: Five years' experience with the chemotherapy of metastatic choriocarcinoma and related trophoblastic tumours in women. Am. J. Obstet. Gynec. 82, 631–640 (1961).
15. LI, M. C., HERTZ, R., SPENCER, D. B.: Effect of methotrexate therapy upon choriocarcinoma and chorioadenoma. Proc. Soc. exp. Biol. (N.Y.) 93, 361–366 (1956).
16. LI, M. C., WHITMORE, W. F., GOLDBEY, R.: Effect of combined drug therapy on metastatic cancer of testis. J. Am. Med. Ass. 174, 1291–1299 (1960).
17. MARGOULIS, G. B., HAMMOND, C. B., JOHNSRUDE, I. S., WEED, J. C., PARKER, R. T.: Arteriography and infusional chemotherapy in localized trophoblastic disease. Obstet. Gynec. 45, 397–406 (1975).

18. OBER, W. B., EDGECOMB, J. D., PRICE, E. B.: The pathology of choriocarcinoma. Ann. N.Y. Acad. Sci. *172*, 299–426 (1971).
19. PARK, W. W., LEES, J. C.: Choriocarcinoma: a general review with analysis of 516 cases. Arch. Path. *49*, 73–104, 205–241 (1950).
20. PARK, W. W.: Choriocarcinoma. London: Heinemann, 1971.
21. RATNAM, S. S., TEOH, E. S., DAWOOD, M. Y.: Methotrexate for prophylaxis of choriocarcinoma. Am. J. Obst. Gynec. *111*, 1021–1027 (1971).
22. ROSS, G. T., STOLBACH, L. L., HERTZ, R.: Actinomycin D in the treatment of methotrexate-resistant trophoblastic disease in women. Cancer Res. *22*, 1015–1017 (1962).
23. RUSHWORTH, A. G. J., ORR, A. H., BAGSHAWE, K. D.: The concentration of HCG in the plasma and spinal fluid of patients with trophoblastic tumours in the central nervous system. Brit. J. Cancer *22*, 253–5 (1968).
24. STONE, M., DENT, J., KARDANA, A., BAGSHAWE, K. D.: Relationship of oral contraception to development of trophoblastic tumour after evacuation of a hydatidiform mole. Br. J. Obstet. & Gynaec. *83*, 913–916 (1976).
25. SUNG, H. C., WU, P. C., HO, T. H.: Treatment of choriocarcinoma and chorioadenoma destruens with 6-mercaptopurine and surgery. A clinical report of 93 cases. Chin. Med. J. *82*, 24–38 (1963).

The Management of Musculoskeletal Tumours

J. S. MALPAS

Examples of malignant tumours of the musculoskeletal system which commonly occur in children are osteogenic sarcoma and Ewing's sarcoma in bone, and rhabdomyosarcoma in muscle. Osteosarcoma is considered elsewhere, so the principles of management of rhabdomyosarcoma and Ewing's sarcoma only will be discussed.

Rhabdomyosarcoma

This tumour is now thought to be more common. Accurate histology is essential. In the last 22 children proven to have rhabdomyosarcoma at St. Bartholomew's Hospital, only nine were referred with the correct histological diagnosis. The use of the PAS stain and electronmicroscopy may be of help in proving the diagnosis. Careful staging of the children is also important. The staging classification we have adopted has been that shown in Table 1.

Treatment has consisted of radiotherapy to the primary site together with combined chemotherapy using vincristine (VCR), actinomycin D (ACT-D) and cyclophosphamide (CPM). The chemotherapy has started with radiotherapy and has continued at intervals for up to 1 year as shown in Figure 1. Adjustment of dosage has been done in response to signs or symptoms of toxicity (Fig. 1).

This regimen is similar to those described at a number of American centres [1, 2, 4, 6] and is based on the principle of the control of the primary disease by effective radiotherapy and the elimination of micrometastases by long-term adjuvant chemotherapy. Thirteen children who have stage IIa or IIb disease have been treated [5]. Details of care of the seven patients with rhabdomyosarcoma of the head and neck are given in Table 2 and of rhabdomyosarcoma occurring at other sites in Table 3.

These tables show that 'second look surgery', that is the removal of residual disease after completion of radiotherapy or even before, has been successful. Histology of the residual

Table 1. Rhabdomyosarcoma

Staging
Stage I – Localised
All tumour resectable
Stage II – Regional
Adjacent structures involved
Regional lymph nodes involved
IIa – Completely resectable
IIb – Incompletely or nonresectable
Stage III – Generalised
IIIa – Distant metastases with normal bone marrow
IIIb – Distant metastases with marrow infiltration

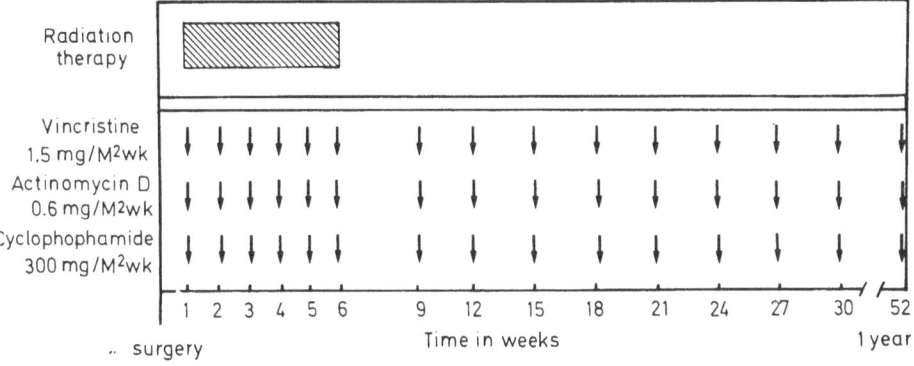

Fig. 1. Schedule for combination therapy of childhood rhabdomyosarcoma

Table 2. Childhood rhabdomyosarcoma of head and neck treatment with combination therapy (March 1976)

Patient	Age	Sex	Stage	Primary site	Response	Duration of survival (months)
G.O.	5	F	IIa	Orbit	Complete[a]	38 N.E.D.
J.S.	3	F	IIb	Orbit	Complete[a]	38 N.E.D.
P.C.	1½	M	IIb	Larynx	Complete	21 N.E.D.
R.B.	2	F	IIb	Mandible	Complete	17 N.E.D.
A.T.	2	M	IIb	Orbit	Complete	16 E.W.D.
S.J.	2	F	IIb	Orbit	Complete	15 E.W.D.
S.B.	2½	F	IIb	P.N.S.	Complete	4 N.E.D.

[a] Second look surgery.   N.E.D. – No evidence of disease   E.W.D. – Expired with disease

Table 3. Childhood rhabdomyosarcoma of chest and pelvis treatment with combination therapy (March 1976)

Patient	Age	Sex	Stage	Primary site	Response	Duration of survival (months)
M.B.	6	M	IIa	Paratesticular	Complete	45 N.E.D.
A.G.	1½	M	IIb	Pelvis	Complete[a]	37 N.E.D.
P.C.	1 month	M	IIb	Paratesticular	Complete[a]	26 E.W.D.
P.M.	8	M	IIb	Intrathoracic	Complete[a]	21 N.E.D.
M.N.	4	M	IIa	Paratesticular	Complete	11 N.E.D.
P.G.	9	F	IIb	Pelvis	Complete	8 N.E.D.

[a] Second look surgery.   N.E.D. – No evidence of disease   E.W.D. – Expired with disease

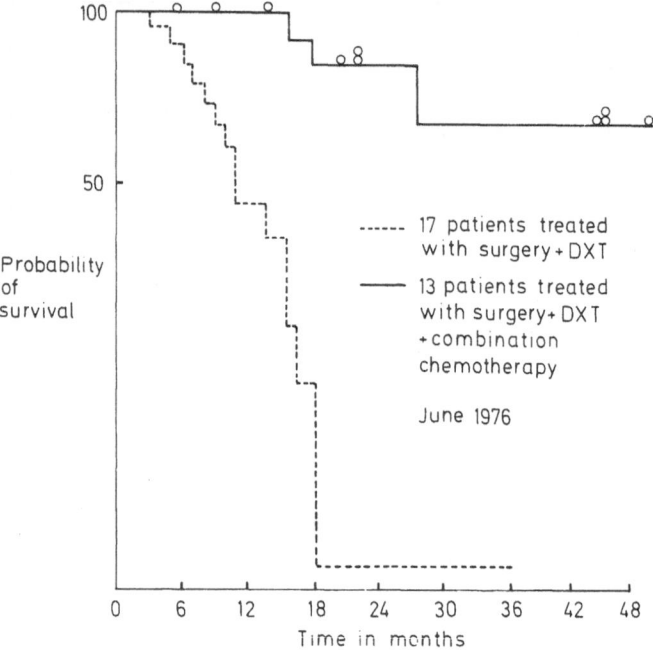

Fig. 2

tumour has shown nonviable tumour in every case. It should be noted that where failure occurred, the relapse was at the primary site. No child died from metastatic disease.

The probability of survival curve for these 13 children calculated in June, 1976 has been compared with the actual survival curve for 17 children of comparable stage treated with surgery or radiotherapy or both. The probability of survival is just under 70% at 4 years, compared with just over 10% in the historical group (Fig. 2).

Ewing's Sarcoma

This is a highly malignant tumour of bone with survival rates of less than 10% in most early series. The considerable improvement in the outlook in other childhood tumours and the reports that Ewing's sarcoma was responding to adjuvant chemotherapy programmes [3, 7] encouraged us to undertake a study of treatment of children having local, regional or disseminated Ewing's arcoma (Bart's-Marsden Children's Solid Tumour Group Protocol for Ewing's Sarcoma). It was thought that adriamycin (ADR) should be given initially instead of ACT-D in the three drug combination with VCR and CPM (Fig. 3).

ADR should be continued to a total dose of 400 mg/M^2 when it is stopped to avoid cardiac toxicity. The adjuvant programme is continued for 2 years. As much chemotherapy as possible is administered early in the programme, but of course adjustment of dose depending on signs and symptoms is carried out (Table 4).

Nine children with local or regional disease are now entered into the study and their details are given in Table 4. Six of these children have remitted completely and are in continuous remission. The other three are approaching complete remission. Their survival is compared

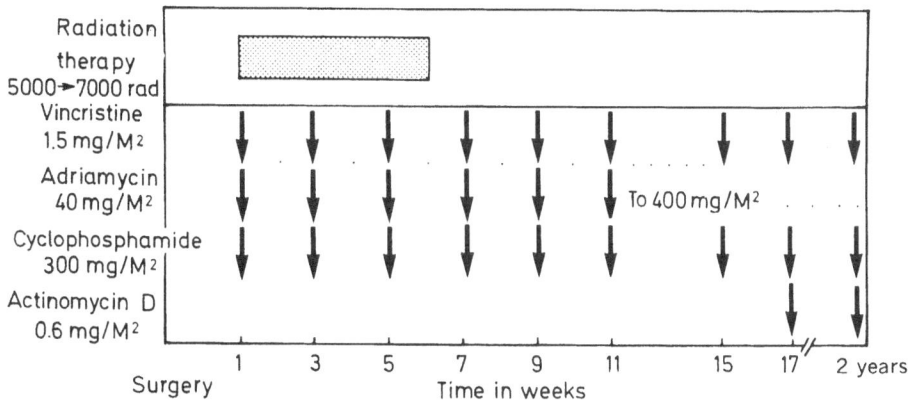

Fig. 3. Combination chemotherapy for Ewing's sarcoma

Table 4. Ewing's sarcoma – local and regional disease in children treated with DXT and chemotherapy

Name	Age	Sex	Site	Response	Disease-free survival months	State
T.M.	13	M	Fibula	CR	40	N.E.D.
A.H.	11	M	Humerus	CR	30	N.E.D.
M.H.	13	M	Cervical spine	CR	29	N.E.D.
P.S.	14	M	Femur	CR	14	N.E.D.
M.Q.	11	M	Humerus	CR	10	N.E.D.
M.R.	12	M	Humerus	CR	4	N.E.D.
S.W.	13	F	Pelvis	—	2	—
J.R.	3/12	M	Skull	—	2	—
R van G	10	M	Pelvis	—	1	—

N.E.D. no evidence of disease.

with an historical group treated with surgery, radiotherapy or occasional single chemotherapeutic agents. There has been an obvious improvement in the natural history of this disease (Fig. 4).

It is more important for the paediatric oncologist to consider the long-term toxic effects of his therapy than anyone else. His patients will have a better chance than any of displaying long-term toxicity of a successful regimen. Considerable damage is inevitably done to developing tissues. In a survey of our children on adjuvant therapy, it was evident that a quarter of them lost weight and did not grow during the year of treatment. It was evident that development was being retarded as 6 months after stopping adjuvant therapy over half had gained weight and started to grow.

All children coming to the end of adjuvant chemotherapy programmes at St. Bartholomew's Hospital are now studied with regard to haematological function, liver function (BSP excretion), renal function (creatinine level), lung function (full studies of volume, ventilation and gas exchange) and cardiac function (echocardiography and measurement of the left ventricular ejection fraction). So far, most children have had normal results, but

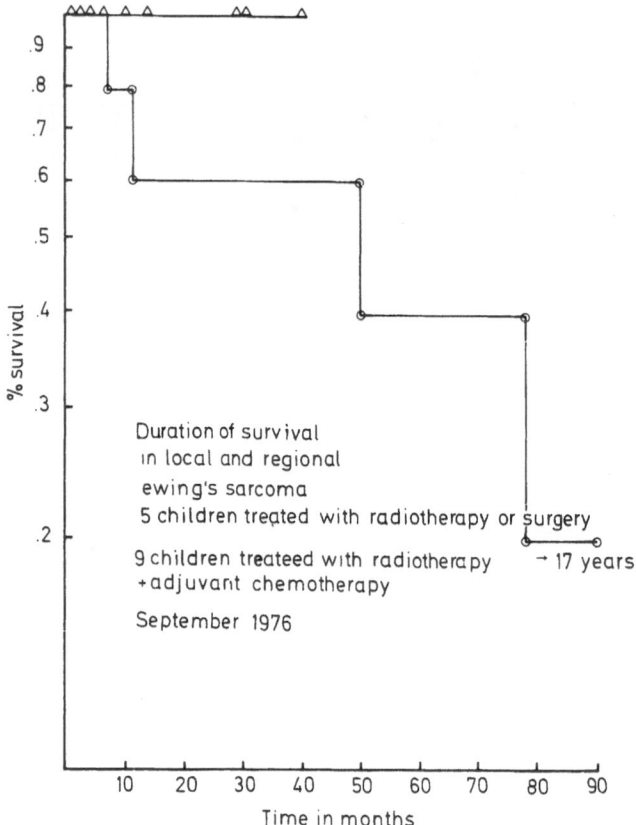

Fig. 4

obviously this study must be repeated for some years to come. The only abnormality that has been found has been the presence of diminished lung volumes or impaired ventilation in some children. A few of the children had had lung irradiation but some had not. These children will be followed carefully and a prospective study of lung function had been started.

Acknowledgement

I am indebted to J. E. Freeman, R. Sandland, A. G. Stansfeld and A. Paxton for their help in the management of the children reported in this presentation.

References

1. Donaldson, S. S., Castro, J. R., Wilbur, J. R., Jesse, R. H.: Rhabdomyosarcoma of head and neck in children: combination treatment by surgery, irradiation and chemotherapy. Cancer 31, 26–35 (1973).

2. HEYN, R. M., HOLLAND, R., NEWTON, W. A., TEFFT, M., BRESLOW, N., HARTMANN, J. R.: The role of combined chemotherapy in the treatment of rhabdomyosarcoma in children. Cancer *34*, 2128–2141 (1974).
3. HUSTU, H. O., PINKEL, D., PRATT, C. B.: Treatment of clinically localised Ewing's sarcoma with radiotherapy and combination chemotherapy. Cancer *30*, 1522–1527 (1972).
4. JAFFE, N., FILLER, R. M., FARBER, S. et al.: Rhabdomyosarcoma in children. Improved outlook with a multidisciplinary approach. Amer. J. Surg. *125*, 482–486 (1973).
5. MALPAS, J. S., FREEMAN, J. E., PAXTON, A., WALKER SMITH, J., STANSFELD, A. G., WOOD, C. B. S.: Radiotherapy and adjuvant combination chemotherapy for childhood rhabdomyosarcoma. Brit. Med. J. *1*, 247–249 (1976).
6. PRATT, C. B.: Response of childhood rhabodmyosarcoma to combination chemotherapy. J. Pediatric. *74*, 791–794 (1969).
7. ROSEN, G., WOLLNER, N., TAN, C., WU, S. J., HAJDU, S. I., CHAM, W., D'ANGIO, G. J. D., MURPHY, M. L.: Disease-free survival in children with Ewing's sarcoma treated with radiation therapy and adjuvant four-drug sequential chemotherapy. Cancer *33*, 384–393 (1974).

The Management of Wilms' Tumor

J. LEMERLE

During the period 1952–1974, 350 initially nonmetastatic cases of Wilms' tumor (stages I, II, III) were treated in our institute. Actuarial survival curves show that, during these 22 years, the cure rate rose from 50% to 80%. However, during the same period, the recurrence-free survival rate did not improve significantly and remained close to 50%. This means that the increase in the survival rate was due to more successful treatment of metastases and local recurrences in recent years rather than to prevention of metastases.

Treatment of the Primary Tumor

Total nephrectomy is the key step in treating the primary tumor. Many authors, mainly in the United States, consider that surgery should be performed immediately on an emergency basis, or at least with the minimum delay. Others, essentially in Europe, consider that in most cases it is better to start the treatment with a course of radiotherapy to shrink the tumor and make surgery easier and safer. The International Society of Pediatric Oncology (S.I.O.P.) conducted a clinical trial to find out which policy was the best [4].

The trial started in September, 1971 and ended in October, 1974; 42 centers in 14 countries took part. One hundred and thirty-seven patients were included in the trial and randomized. Twenty-five patients with very large tumors were excluded because it was considered unsafe to treat them by primary surgery. Patients with preoperative irradiation were given 2000 rad before nephrectomy and postoperative irradiation according to the local extent of the tumor defining the stage, i.e., no additional irradiation in stage I and 1500 rad in stages II and III. Patients randomized for primary surgery were given postoperative radiotherapy in a comparable way. In cases where the tumor was found to be ruptured before or during surgery, with tumor spillage in the abdominal cavity, the whole abdomen was irradiated, with shielding of the opposite kidney above 1200 rad. Taking into account survival rates and recurrence-free survival rates, no significant difference was found between the two groups of patients. However, the most interesting fact revealed by the trial was the high proportion of surgical tumor ruptures which occurred in the group operated on without previous radiotherapy (20/64) compared to the other group (3/73). These accidents were considered a reason to stop entering patients in the trial, since tumor ruptures with contamination of the abdominal cavity lead to more aggressive treatment and castration in girls.

We now recommend the following policy in nonmetastatic cases:

1. Patients under 1 year: surgery first, whenever possible, i.e., in the majority of cases. When the tumor is very large, chemotherapy should precede surgery in order to try to avoid radiotherapy.

2. Patients over 1 year: for average or large tumors, preoperative radiotherapy (2000 rad with a course of actinomycin D). Patients with a small tumor likely to be an easily resectable stage I tumor should undergo surgery first. This is in order to take into account the results of the American National Wilms' Tumor Study (N.W.T.S.) [1] showing that no radiotherapy at all is necessary in actual stage I tumors, and to give the patients a chance to avoid radiation therapy. After nephrectomy, additional radiotherapy (1500 rad) should only be given in stages II and III.

At this point, we consider the following question should be raised: could preoperative radiotherapy be replaced by chemotherapy, as suggested by our experience with metastatic cases? The S.I.O.P. has started a second randomized trial comparing these two modalities of preoperative treatment and aimed at finding out if preoperative chemotherapy with vincristine (VCR) and actinomycin D (ACT-D) is as good as preoperative radiotherapy in avoiding surgical tumor ruptures, and also in terms of recurrence-free survival and survival.

Treatment of Metastases and Local Recurrences

Treatment of undetectable metastases is also wrongly called "prevention" or "prophylaxis" of metastases. It is a very important part of the management of Wilms' tumor as it is clearly better to give a few courses of "maintenance" or "prohylactic" chemotherapy than to have to treat overt metastases with such aggressive procedures as surgery and radiotherapy. One of the most interesting results of the N.W.T.S. [1] has been to establish the usefulness of combined therapy with VCR and ACT-D given during the 8 weeks following nephrectomy, and thereafter at three monthly intervals for 15 months. Patients who were given both drugs (stages II and III) had an 80% 2-year relapse-free survival compared to 63% and 56% respectively for the cases randomized into groups given multiple courses of ACT-D alone or VCR alone. The difference was statistically significant and made obsolete the debate as to which of the two drugs is better. It was also another reason for the S.I.O.P. to stop its Wilms' tumor trial, part of which was aimed at comparing single with multiple courses of ACT-D alone. In this respect, no difference was found between two groups of 80 patients each [4]. The S.I.O.P. recommended the two drug protocol for an interim period of 2 years, and preliminary results of this nonrandomized study seem to confirm the results of the N.W.T.S., showing a marked decrease in the frequency of metastases.

Two questions are now pending with respect to treatment of undetectable metastases:

1. Should adriamycin, a well-known powerful agent against Wilms' tumor, be added systematically despite its cardiac toxicity? This point is being investigated in N.W.T.S. No. 2, in stage II, III, and IV patients.

2. Is it necessary to give maintenance treatment for 15 months as at present, or are shorter periods of treatment as effective? This point is also being investigated on both sides of the Atlantic, in N.W.T.S. No. 2 and in the second S.I.O.P. Wilms' tumor trial and study.

The treatment of clinically detected metastases and local recurrences is difficult, individualized, and can only be given in general outline in a brief report. The location of metastases in radiosensitive tissues such as the lungs coupled with the assumption that occult widely disseminated disease is present in such cases has led us to formulate the following general scheme [3].

In cases of radiologically solitary pulmonary metastases in one or both lungs, the tumor should first be excised and the affected lung carefully palpated. If no other metastasis is found, and if the pathologist's report indicates that the excision has been satisfactory, no radiotherapy is given and the patient undergoes three drug chemotherapy for 1 year. In cases where the tumor proves more disseminated than expected, both lungs are irradiated (2000 rad with air correction). This system has enabled us to cure a few patients without irradiating the lungs at all, which we believe is a great advantage.

When very large, other metastases whether in the lungs or elsewhere, are first treated with a course of chemotherapy. Radiotherapy and surgery are then combined in different ways, depending on each individual situation. Our constant aim is to cure the patient with as little radiotherapy as possible, in view of the late adverse effects of radiation on growing patients, especially babies. With this approach, we have achieved a 50% cure rate in lung metastases.

Complications Arising from Treatment of Wilms' Tumor

Aggressive combined treatment given to children 2–5-years-old may result in many complications, especially in metastatic cases treated with radiotherapy. The chemotherapy given to Wilms' patients cannot be considered very toxic in itself compared to that applied to other pediatric tumors, and adverse complications are mild and foreseeable. However, its combination with radiotherapy can cause several acute conditions such as radiation pneumonitis, radiation hepatitis, and radiation enteritis, which may interfere with the treatment and more particularly with maintenance chemotherapy.

The long-term effects of radiotherapy primarily affect the lung. Serial lung function assessment for patients given 2000 rad to both lungs combined with ACT-D has already shown that, within 2 years, lung complinace diminishes significantly in most cases and so does vital capacity, when it can be measured. We do not yet know to what extent these patients' lung functions will be impaired when they reach adult age, but we consider these first results as good reason to try to avoid lung irradiation in children whenever possible.

Scoliosis is frequent following abdominal irradiation, even when radiotherapy is applied with great care, the fields encompassing the whole vertebral bodies [5]. Scoliosis seems partly due to lack of growth and sclerosis of the soft tissues, and often only becomes apparent during the period of rapid growth preceding puberty. This is one more reason why patients treated for Wilms' tumor should be very carefully watched until they reach adult age.

Prognostic Factors and Individualization of Treatment

The immediate and late adverse effects of treatment raise the question of whether all cases should be given the same treatment. For it now seems clear that although the use of systematic protocols has in recent years improved the results obtained, it has also led to giving some patients more treatment than they actually needed to be cured. On the other hand, we are still unable to cure approximately 20% of Wilms' tumor cases which obviously need more or different treatment. Several prognostic indicators for Wilms' tumor are now well-known [2]: these are age, with better results under 2 years, size of the tumor and its extent at surgery, which establishes the stage. More complicated and difficult to define is the way the histologic pattern of the tumor affects the outcome. All these prognostic indicators and others now being studied such as lymph node involvement should be taken into account when defining the treatment for each individual case. The aim is to improve survival rates of known "bad" cases and avoid complications and sequelae in "good" cases. But the most difficult problem is not to lose the ground recently gained, and we must be very cautious about eliminating treatments of proven efficacy.

References

1. D'ANGIO, G. J., EVANS, A. E., BRESLOW, N. et al.: The treatment of Wilms' tumor. Results of the National Wilms' Tumor Study. Cancer 38, 633 (1976).
2. LEMERLE, J., TOURNADE, M. F., GERARD-MARCHANT, R. et al.: Wilms' tumor, natural history and prognostic factors. Cancer 37, 2557 (1976).

3. LEMERLE, J., TOURNADE, M. F., SARRAZIN, D., VALAYER, J.: Tumours of the kidney. In: Cancer in Children Clinical Management. Berlin-Heidelberg-New York: Springer-Verlag, 1975.
4. LEMERLE, J., VOUTE, P. A., TOURNADE, M. F. et al.: Preoperative versus post operative radiotherapy, single versus multiple courses of actinomycin D in the treatment of Wilms' tumor. Cancer *38*, 647 (1976).
5. RISEBOROUGH, E. J., GRABIAS, S. R., BURTON, R. I. et al.: Skeletal alterations following irradiation for Wilms' tumor, with particular reference to scoliosis and kyphosis. Jour. Bone and Joint Surgery *58a*, 526 (1976).

Present Strategy of Treatment of Neuroblastoma

R. MAURUS

Neuroblastoma is one of the most common tumors of childhood. It ranks fourth in frequency after leukemia, lymphomas, and tumors of the central nervous system.

Given its rather high frequency, one would have expected the therapy of this tumor to have been studied in large randomized trials and to have progressed in the same way as that for some of the other frequent neoplastic diseases of childhood, such as Wilms' tumor or leukemia. In fact, this has not been the case.

Neuroblastoma is treated by multimodal therapy, associating surgery, which may be only partial, radiation therapy in some but not in all cases, and multiple chemotherapy given on a maintenance schedule.

Recently, immunotherapy has been added to this therapeutic arsenal.

However, this pediatric tumor has not shared in the improved survival rates [3] seen in Wilms' tumor [14], rhabdomyosarcoma [6], and Ewing's tumor [13], following the advent of multimodal therapy.

Before analyzing further the reasons for this stagnation and proposing a new strategy, one should first consider some factors which influence the prognosis in individual cases.

Among the most important are age and stage. One year seems to be a critical age. The prognosis is much better in infants. One reason is that they more often have localized, resectable disease.

However, even those babies with extensive disease fare better than older patients [1]. This is especially true for children less than 1 year of age and less so for children from 1–2 years. This is one of the reasons for less aggressive treatments in infants, the other being the fear of higher cost in toxicity of chemotherapy and still more radiation therapy.

Beside the prognostic factors of age and stage, some unique particularities of neuroblastoma also bear on the chances of a therapeutic strategy.

1. Infants may present with a stage IV S, which is characterized by metastases limited to the skin, the liver and the bone marrow, but without x-ray bone lesions.

In this case, the tumor and its metastases may disappear either spontaneously or after a treatment which would classically be considered totally insufficient [2].

2. Even if we consider stages other than IV S, neuroblastoma is among the tumors which have the highest propensity for spontaneous regression, either by complete disappearance or by differentiation in benign ganglioneuroma, although this is a rare occurrence [5].

3. More frequent is the spontaneous regression of metastases once the primary tumor has been removed.

4. Good results have been obtained after partial excision of the tumor.

These facts suggest that host factors may play an important role in the defense against tumor progression and that any strategy for the treatment of these patients should aim at exploiting these factors.

Strong evidence for the existence of immunologic reactions of the patient against his neuroblastoma has been found by HELLSTRÖM and HELLSTRÖM [7]. One can briefly summarize their observations as follows:

1. Patients in remission and some of their relatives have specific cytotoxic antibodies and lymphocytes against autochthonous and allogeneic neuroblastoma cells.

2. Specific cytotoxic lymphocytes are also found in patients with evolutive disease.

3. Blocking antibodies, inhibiting the specific cytotoxicity of lymphocytes, are found during evolutive disease, while unblocking antibodies are found during remission.

The place of the different therapeutic modalities can be summarized as follows:

1. *Surgery* seems to be important even if the tumor tissue is not totally resectable. As already pointed out, metastases may disappear after removal of the primary tumor. Total resection of a single primary tumor evidently gives the best results and is often possible in infants less than 1 year old, but of great interest are the rather satisfactory results afforded by partial resection as compared to a simple biopsy.

KOOP [9] advocates removal of as much tumor tissue as possible, in the hope that endogenous defense mechanisms will take care of the small quantities of tissue left or at least contribute to its eradication with the help of chemotherapy and/or radiation therapy.

2. Although *radiation therapy* has been used for a long time, it is surprising to discover that its effectiveness remains controversial. Some trials on a rather limited number of patients have suggested that radiation therapy is without benefit in stage II on residual disease after surgery, but that it may be efficient on gross residual tumors in stage III. This was shown in a comparative trial of the Children's Cancer Study Group and in a study by KOOP and JOHNSON in Philadelphia [4, 10].

3. *Chemotherapy* is used in stages II and III to complete surgery. In stage IV, combined chemotherapy is used in the hope of inducing complete remissions, or in order to eradicate the metastases and allow a surgical excision of the primary tumor.

The drugs which have been mostly in use are vincristine (VCR), cyclophosphamide (CPM), adriamycine (ADR), DTIC, and peptichemio.

Until now, the addition of chemotherapy to the treatment of neuroblastoma has had disappointing results. Most published data, however, have been obtained by combinations of VCR and CPM given on different schedules. These drugs do induce remission in stage IV patients, but hardly change the survival rate. It should be pointed out that the percentage of complete and partial remissions obtained is at most 40%, which is rather low as compared with the immediate effect of chemotherapy on other childhood neoplastic diseases such as acute lymphoid leukemia or Wilms' tumor, and which is, nevertheless, too low to appreciably change the median survival time [11].

What could be done to improve these results? It is possible that the best drugs have not yet been tried. In recent years, ADR, DTIC, and peptichemio have been added to combination programs, but at present, it is too early to conclude whether or not the survival rate will be changed, although the percentage of complete remissions with a higher median duration does seem to increase.

Probably the efficiency of combined chemotherapy has not yet been tested in large enough controlled studies and one should look for more active combinations or more efficient schedules with the existing drugs.

However, it is possible that the immunosuppressive effects of chemotherapy could be particularly harmful for neuroblastoma patients, whose immunologic defenses seem to play an important role in the control of tumor growth.

This is the rationale for:

1. Use of chemotherapy given as large intermittent pulse doses, considered as less immunosuppressive.

·2. The addition of immunotherapy to the multimodal therapy.

In the United States, a cooperative trial has been elaborated according to these principles [12].

Stage IV patients, over 1 year old, are randomized to receive either intermittent chemotherapy alone or the same chemotherapy plus MER-BCG every month.

Preliminary results suggest that the addition of immunotherapy does increase the number of complete remissions and their duration. This trial will probably be pursued by the CALGB.

Finally, one should also mention that neuroblastoma cells can spontaneously undergo differentiation in vivo and so transform into benign ganglioneuroma cells.

It is most important to know the factors which induce this differentiation process in order to make use of them in the therapy of neuroblastoma.

Cyclic AMP has been shown to inhibit the growth of neuroblastoma cells and to induce their differentiation in vitro.
This led HELSON to include papaverine in the combined therapy of neuroblastoma [8]. Papaverine inhibits phosphodiesterase and thereby is expected to increase in vivo the accumulation of cyclic AMP in tumor cells.
In this regard, it would be interesting to find phosphodiesterase inhibitors or cyclic AMP analogs with a high specificity for neuroblastoma cells.

References

1. BRESLOW, N., McCANN, B.: Statistical estimation of prognosis for children with neuroblastoma. Cancer Res. *31*, 2098–2101 (1971).
2. D'ANGIO, G., EVANS, A., KOOP, C. E.: Special pattern of widespread neuroblastoma with favorable prognosis. Lancet (1971) I, 1046–1049.
3. EVANS, A.: The success and failure of multimodal therapy for cancer in children. Cancer *35*, 48–54 (1975).
4. EVANS, A., D'ANGIO, G. J., KOOP, C. E.: Diagnosis and treatment of neuroblastoma. Pediatric Clin. of N. Am. *23*, 161–170 (1976).
5. EVERSON, T. C., COLE, W. H.: Spontaneous regression of cancer. Philadelphia: W. B. Saunders Co., 1966.
6. GHAVIMI, F., EXELBY, P. R., D'ANGIO, G. J., CHAM, W., LIEBERMAN, P. H., TAN, C., MIKE, V., MURPHY, M. L.: Multidisciplinary treatment of embryonal rhabdomyosarcoma in children. Cancer *35*, 677–686 (1975).
7. HELLSTRÖM, E., HELSTRÖM, L.: Immunity to neuroblastoma and melanomas. Ann. Rev. Med. *23*, 19–38 (1972).
8. HELSON, L.: Chemotherapy of disseminated neuroblastoma. Proc. Am. Soc. Clinic. Oncol. *17*, 263 (1976).
9. KOOP, C. E., SCHNAUFER, L.: The management of abdominal neuroblastoma. Cancer *35*, 905–909 (1975).
10. KOOP, C. E., JOHNSON, D. G.: Neuroblastoma: an assessment of therapy in reference to staging. J. Pediat. Surg. *6*, 595–600 (1971).
11. LEIKIN, S., EVANS, A., HEYN, R., NEWTON, W.: The impact of chemotherapy on advanced neuroblastoma. Survival of patients diagnosed in 1956, 1962 and 1966 in Children's Cancer Study Group A. The Journal of Ped. *84*, 131–134 (1974).
12. NECHELESS, T. F., RAUSEN, A., KUNG, F., POCHEDLY, C.: MER/BCG in the treatment of disseminated neuroblastoma. Proc. Am. Soc. Clin. Oncol. *17*, 258 (1976).
13. ROSEN, G., WOLLNER, N., TAN, C.: Disease-free survival in children with Ewing's sarcoma treated with radiation therapy and adjuvant 4-drug sequential chemotherapy. Cancer *33*, 384–393 (1974).
14. WOLFF, J. A.: Advance in the treatment of Wilms' tumor. Cancer *35*, 901–904 (1975).

Surgery in the Treatment of Pulmonary Metastases

H. Le Brigand, M. Merlier, C. Wapler, P. Levasseur, and A. Rojas-Miranda

Ever since we started treating thoracic tumors surgically, we thought it quite illogical not to operate upon the secondary tumors. Thus, as our surgery was neither severely mutilating nor dangerously threatening to life, we have, earlier than 1950, performed lung resections for metastases. One of our first surgical patients (left inferior lobectomy for a metastasis of colic cancer operated on 3 years earlier) is still alive, and this initial success greatly encouraged us. Our work has evolved into two phases.

1. In the first phase, we operated on essentially single well-delimited metastases of patients in otherwise good health. Somewhat empiricially, according to the original tumor, the precocity of the appearance of the metastasis, and the previous case history of the patient, we have, on a case to case basis, subjected a certain number of our surgical patients to thoracic cobalt therapy or to complementary chemotherapy, without definite and structured planning, with the only aim of reducing the risk of new metastases, but without, however, submitting the patients to overly aggressive treatments, compromising the quality of their further life.

This first experiment gave rise to a publication in l'Academie de Chirurgie in 1974. This paper dealt with the 106 metastases operated on between 1954 and 1972, with only one postoperative death. We were able to perform tumor resections on 83 patients, 18 of whom survived for 3 years and nine for 5 years. These are modest figures, but they are important regarding the very special nature of metastatic surgery. One can, in a way, say that this surgery gave a better and longer life to certain patients, otherwise condemned to die shortly. From this paper one can point out the following facts:

a. The pneumonectomies (15 of the 83 resections) did not lead to a survival of 5 years.

b. Nor did the wedge type resections (peripheral and atypical resections).

c. The group of lobectomies (46 simple or enlarged) included the nine patients who survived for 5 years or more.

d. Four bilateral tumor resections were performed (two in two sessions and two in a single session).

e. The metastases of sarcomas did not lead to patients surviving for 5 years (28 sarcomas out of 106 metastases).

f. The patients who survive for 5 years are found among the metastases of carcinomas (78 out of 106).

g. The metastases arising less than 2 years after the treatment of the original cancer showed poorer results than those which appeared later.

h. Only 19 cases concerned multiple metastases, all the others were apparently single localizations.

i. We did reoperate upon certain patients to treat a recurrence of homo- or controlateral metastases: five patients have thus been the object of repeated resections.

Finally, the results of the series, without being brilliant, are far from being discouraging, and they convinced us that surgery alone could already help in the treatment of pulmonary metastases.

2. Our experiment's second phase, initiated about 4 years ago, rather than being a sum of isolated cases, tends to be integrated into the perspectives of a polyvalent anticancer strategy, the object of the discussion here.

Encouraged by the results of our first series, we continued to operate on similar cases of metastases that could be defined as single and simple. Furthermore, since we have been able to achieve a surgery which is rarely lethal or mutilating, it seemed logical to apply it to cases with apparently less favorable metastases, multiple or very often bilateral; such a surgery could usefully help chemotherapy or immunotherapy since the operation will reduce the tumoral population as far as possible, and this without compromising the respiratory functions.

The techniques of resection limited to small tumoral areas are well-established. They involve enucleation, classical wedge shape resection, or local resection achieved by mechanical staplers, such as the UKL 60, made in the USSR, which we have been using for more than 12 years.

Equally, these well-developed techniques allow us in many cases of bilateral lesions to operate on both sides at the same time; the lungs being approached by the lateral or axillary route, in particular, which are not harmful to chest wall mechanics.

Obviously, this surgery must be integrated into an overall anticancer program; it must be only a therapeutic link in the chain and must precede the treatment of the "residual disease." This is why a large percentage of the patients affected by pulmonary metastases that we receive are sent to us by oncologic teams who are following a therapeutic program, the main characteristics of which are now well-established. We hope that by this collaboration, established in particular with MATHÉ's team, patients suffering from pulmonary metastases will be able to reap appreciable benefits. This paper gives us an opportunity to thank all those of our colleagues and oncologist friends who have shown their confidence in us by sending us their patients.

Thus, although we have operated on 106 metastases in 20 years, more than 70 patients have been operated on in the last 5 years, eight being bilateral cases. Of course, we have not yet done the statistical analyses of this second series, but it does not seem that they should be any more discouraging than those of the first series, and despite an apparently more audacious surgery, there have been no deaths and postoperative morbidity has remained very low.

One of the touchstones of the surgical evolution is that it is only acceptable if it allows the patient, at the end of the series of operations, to lead a normal existence, or, in other words, the treatment of pulmonary metastases is conceivable only if the patient is not turned into a severe invalid. This is, obviously, a general rule of all therapeutics, surgical and others!

Surgical decisions are, therefore, confirmed only at the end of a careful study of the cardiac and respiratory functions, comprising, among others, a global spirometry and a separate lung examination (in which the use of nontraumatic methods, such as the external counting of Xenon 133, allows us to extend the method to all our future surgical patients) and a study, if necessary, of the hemodynmics of the pulmonary circulation. It is thus possible to turn away patients for whom this surgery would risk creating a crippling respiratory insufficiency.

In conclusion, accepting to actively attack pulmonary metastases represents, if one practices a functionally conservative surgery, an "obstinate therapy", which is perfectly justified on two conditions that we consider essential: (1) to integrate the surgical stage into a therapeutic sequence of wider strategy and (2) to repeat that ensuring the comfort of the survivor is finally as important, if not more so, than the length of the patient's life.

Treatment of Cervical Lymph Node Metastases from Carcinomas of the Upper Respiratory and Digestive Tracts

Y. Cachin

The treatment of cervical lymph node metastases consists of surgery, radiotherapy, or a combination of both. The choice of treatment depends upon the site of the primary tumor. Due to the large number of localizations of upper respiratory and digestive tract cancers, it will not be possible to present here in detail the indications for therapeutic intervention site by site; however, the anatomical and physiologic unity of the cervical and facial lymphatic drainage allows us to develop some general principles.

These principles are based on the work of many groups throughout the world, and, in particular, on the experience gathered at the Gustave-Roussy Institute: prospective and retrospective studies dealing with prognostic factors and results as a function of treatment, and statistically controlled therapeutic trials.

First Principle: The Treatment of the Cervical Lymph Nodes is Inseparable from that of the Primary Tumor

One should, therefore, think of treatment in terms of several factors:

1. The Site of the Primary Tumor

All cancers developing in intimate contact with lymphoid structures (Waldeyer's ring, palatine, and nasopharyngeal tonsils) should be treated by radiotherapy of the regional lymph nodes as well as of the primary tumor.

2. The Treatment of the Primary Tumor

A distinction must be made between those cases with and without palpable adenopathy.

a) 1st Category: Palpable Adenopathy Present
If the primary tumor is treated surgically, the lymph nodes are treated by neck dissection, followed by postoperative radiotherapy depending on the results of the histologic examination of the operative specimen.
If the primary tumor is treated by radium implants, the lymph nodes are handled in the same manner. If, however, the primary tumor is treated by external radiation, the lymph nodes are likewise treated by radiotherapy, with surgery reserved for those cases with residual palpable disease following primary therapy.

b) 2nd Category: No Palpable Adenopathy
One must first answer the question of whether it is necessary to treat systematically the cervical lymph nodes, or whether it is possible to await the appearance of palpable adenopathy. Data is currently available to answer some elements of this question:

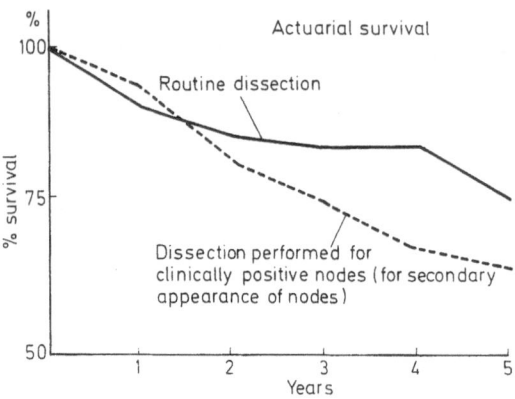

Fig. 1. Therapeutic trial: neck dissection (oral cavity cancers I.G.R. 1967–73)

The results of a *therapeutic trial* carried out at the Gustave-Roussy Institute (1967–1973) comparing systematic performance of neck dissection with therapeutic abstension (with later dissection added in cases of eventual appearance of palpable adenopathy) in cases of oral cavity cancer classified N_0 (Fig. 1).

A study of the results (Table 1) shows the effectiveness of systematically performed neck dissection, although the difference in the 5-year survivals of the two groups (about 10% higher in the treated group) is not quite statistically significant. The difference observed can probably be explained as due to the more frequent evolution of the lymph node invasion to the point of capsular rupture allowed by the delay engendered in waiting for palpable nodes to develop.

The study, undertaken by several groups, of *nodal evolution among patients classified initially* N_0.

FLETCHER [2] studied two groups of patients (with cancers of the nasopharynx and oropharynx) in whom the tumor and adenopathy (eventual) were apparently cured. In one group, radiotherapy had been directed at a portion of the cervical lymph node chains; in the other, at their entirety. Among those patients initially N_0, secondary adenopathy developed in 12% of the first group and in 1.7% of the second (Table 2).

Starting from the same premise, FLETCHER [2] also studied lymph node changes on the contralateral side, initially N_0. Two groups were isolated, depending upon whether or not systematic radiotherapy was delivered to contralateral nodal areas. Secondary contralateral adenopathy developed in 3% of the treated group and in 24% of the untreated group (Table 3).

The results show the effectiveness of systematic radiotherapy in the control of cervical

Table 1. Therapeutic trial of systematic neck dissection for oral cavity cancer initially N_0 Gustave-Roussy Institute 1967–73

	Systematic dissection 39 cases	Dissection for disease only 36 cases
Nodal invasion (N+)	19 cases 49% (NS)	16 cases 44% (NS)
Capsular rupture (N+R+)	5 cases 26% (0,05 < p < 0,10)	9 cases 56% (0,05 < p < 0,10)

Table 2. Appearance of secondary adenopathy in cervical nodes initially N_0 (cancer of Naso and Oropharynx) after FLETCHER 1972

	Number of patients	Appearance of secondary adenopathy
Incomplete therapy	185	12% (22)
Complete therapy	284	1.7% (5)

Table 3. Appearance of secondary adenopathy in contralateral cervical nodes initially N_0 (cancers of the oral cavity, oropharynx, pharyngo-larynx) after FLETCHER 1972

	Number of patients	Secondary adenopathy
No contralateral therapy	187	24% (46)
Contralateral therapy	187	3% (6)

lymph nodes classified N_0. In other words, in the presence of a carcinoma of the upper respiratory or digestive tract, the cervical lymph node chains must be treated in their entirety, in one way or another.

At this point it is necessary to ask a second question: *do surgery or radiotherapy constitute the most valuable form of systematic treatment?* It is impossible to answer this question on the basis of comparative studies. Here also, the decision will depend on the site of the primary tumor and the treatment elected, the lymph nodes being handled either by a functional neck dissection or by moderate dose radiotherapy, of the order of 5000 rad.

Second Principle: The Treatment of Cervical Lymph Nodes depends also on the Volume and Character of the Adenopathy

Preoperative radiotherapy (2000–3000 rad in 3 weeks, or by "flash" technique) must precede excision of very large fixed nodes (N_3) or of rapidly growing ones, but these are relatively rare indications.

Third Principle: The Choice of Surgical Technique must be made in Accordance with Precise Rules

The *classical* (total) radical neck dissection is used for nodes classified N_3, or N_2 and N_1 larger than 2 cm diameter, while a *functional* neck dissection is reserved for nodes classified N_0, or N_1 and N_2 under 2 cm diameter.

The *functional* neck dissection, done according to these indications for therapy, offers the same degree of anatomical excision as the *classical* dissection, in as much as it removes all the lymphatic and adipose tissue of the neck within the aponeurosis. However, the information, currently available, concerning the numbers of lymph nodes removed by the two types of dissection, is not yet sufficient. Moreover, on the oncologic level, data are not yet sufficiently in agreement to allow an appraisal of the effectiveness of the functional dissection in reducing nodal recurrence or in prolonging 5-year survival.

Therefore, two points must be made clear:

1. Functional neck dissection should be performed only by a skilled head and neck surgeon.
2. It should be followed, as is the classical dissection, by postoperative radiotherapy as indicated by the histologic aspect of the operative specimen.

In the case of tumors of the anterior portion of the oral cavity or of the lips, with nodes classified N_0, bilateral suprahyoid neck dissection, with frozen section verification, seems to be a valid procedure and a reasonable alternative to bilateral functional dissection, but final judgment should await analysis of its long-term results.

Fourth Principle: The Choice of Radiotherapy Techniques must also Obey Stringent Rules

One must decide carefully on the nature of the energy source (cobalt or electrons), the use of associated therapy, the fields to be used, and the dose. A dose of 5000 rad permits sterilization of lymph node areas with no palpable adenopathy but with a potential for subclinical involvement. A dose of 5000–7000 rad is necessary when palpable adenopathy is present.

Let us consider as an example a carcinoma of the palatine tonsil with a palpable node just inferior to the angle of the mandible. A dose of 7000 rad should be delivered to the oropharynx and high cervical nodes. A dose of 5000 rad should be used for the lower cervical area, which is without palpable adenopathy and where one can only suspect subclinical invasion.

Fifth Principle: The Choice of Post-operative Radiotherapy

When deciding upon the combined use of surgery and radiotherapy, we have chosen, with only a few exceptions, the use of postoperative radiotherapy. *Preoperative radiotherapy* of cervical lymph nodes is indicated only in a limited number of cases, according to all published data, reviewed by us in a recent article [1].

Postoperative radiotherapy, for a long time disregarded, seems to be very effective despite all theoretical objections. It benefits a great deal from the information provided by the biopsy material, in that it is possible to adjust fields and dosages according to the degree of nodal invasion (capsular rupture, neoplastic emboli in vessels) and to the type of surgery. It seems reasonable to outline the indications for and modes of use of postoperative radiotherapy in the following manner:

1. No lymph node invasion (N−): no postoperative radiotherapy.
2. Lymph node invasion without capsular rupture (N+R−): postoperative radiotherapy should always be used if histologic examination of the operative specimen shows insufficient resection of the primary tumor, and if there has been no contralateral neck dissection. In other cases, where there is no certitude whether or not postoperative radiotherapy is of use, we have chosen to treat patients, in any case, to a dose of 5000 rad.
3. Lymph node invasion with capsular rupture (N+R+): 5000 rad radiotherapy to the entire neck with a 1500 rad boost to the sites of capsular rupture.

The indications for therapeutic intervention used at the Gustave-Roussy Institute are, therefore, determined by theoretical and clinical considerations, and can, in any case, serve as a basis for reasonable discussion between surgeons and radiotherapists. Our aim is to provide the maximum therapy when absolutely necessary, whatever the tissue damage or sequellae, often significant, but also, when possible, to combine a less mutilating surgery with a less damaging radiotherapy.

As for *chemotherapy*, it is known to reduce somewhat the size of cervical nodal metastases, whether administered intra-arterially via the external carotid artery or intravenously. There is very little data available, however, to answer the question of whether complementary chemotherapy is indicated at the end of the surgery/radiotherapy sequence.

It looks as if chemotherapy used in these conditions improves survival in a certain number of cases, but a study of these results shows that the improvement is due to the eventual eradication of distant metastases rather than to an effect on lymph node (or local) recurrence.

Practically then, it would appear necessary to draw a distinction between two categories of patients:

1. First Category

When one is dealing with carcinomas which produce distant metastases in a large proportion of cases, for example poorly differentiated carcinomas of Waldeyer's ring (palatine or nasopharyngeal tonsils) or cervical nodal metastases without detectable primary tumours, one may be justified in utilizing complementary chemotherapy with the expectation of positive results.

2. Second Category

For the other carcinomas of the head and neck, which represent the great majority, one should remember that two-thirds of the therapeutic failures are at the local level (nodal or local recurrence) and that the percentage with distant metastases, as documented by detailed autopsy studies, does not exceed 50%. The decision to use complementary chemotherapy in these cases must be made by weighing the advantages (rather uncertain at this point) against the disadvantages.

References

1. CACHIN, Y., ESCHWEGE, F.: Combination of radiotherapy and surgery in the treatment of head and neck cancers. Cancer Treatment Reviews 2, 177–191 (1975).
2. FLETCHER, G.: Elective irradiation of subclinical disease in cancers of the head and neck. Cancer 29, 1450 (1972).

Recent Results in Cancer Research

Sponsored by the Swiss League against Cancer. Editor in Chief: P. Rentchnick, Genève